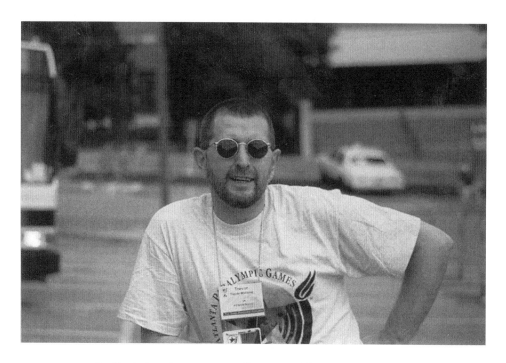

*Dedicated to the memory of Trevor Williams who inspired
the editors in 1997 to write this book.*

Handbook of Sports Medicine and Science
The Paralympic Athlete

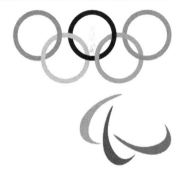

AN IOC MEDICAL COMMISSION PUBLICATION

EDITED BY

Yves C. Vanlandewijck PhD, PT

Full professor at the Katholieke Universiteit Leuven
Faculty of Kinesiology and Rehabilitation Sciences
Department of Rehabilitation Sciences
Leuven, Belgium

Walter R. Thompson PhD

Regents Professor
Kinesiology and Health (College of Education)
Nutrition (College of Health and Human Sciences)
Georgia State University
Atlanta, GA
USA

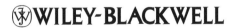

A John Wiley & Sons, Ltd., Publication

Library of Congress Cataloging-in-Publication Data

The Paralympic athlete : handbook of sports medicine and science / edited by Yves C. Vanlandewijck, Walter R. Thompson.
    p. ; cm.
   "An IOC Medical Commission publication."
   Includes bibliographical references.
   ISBN 978-1-4443-3404-3
   1. Athletes with disabilities. 2. Athletes with disabilities—Health and hygiene. 3. Paralympics. 4. Sports for people with disabilities. I. Vanlandewijck, Yves. II. Thompson, Walter R. III. IOC Medical Commission.
[DNLM: 1. Disabled Persons. 2. Sports. 3. Athletes. 4. Sports Medicine. QT 260 P222 2011]
   GV183.5.P37 2011
   796.087—dc22
                                                                                                  2010023430

A catalogue record for this book is available from the British Library.

This book is published in the following electronic formats: ePDF 9781444328363; Wiley Online Library 9781444328356

Set in 8.75/12pt Stone Serif by MPS Limited, a Macmillan Company, Chennai, India

FSC
Mixed Sources
Product group from well-managed forests and other controlled sources
Cert no. SGS-COC-2953
www.fsc.org
© 1996 Forest Stewardship Council

2   2011

Contents

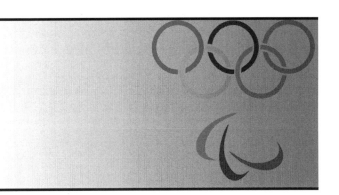

List of Contributors

Marco Bernardi MD
School of Specialization in Sports Medicine,
Department of Physiology and Pharmacology
"V. Erspamer", "Sapienza", Università di Roma, Rome,
Italy and Italian Paralympic Committee

Judith Berzen MSc
Israel Sport Center for the Disabled, Ramat-Gan, Israel

Yagesh Bhambhani PhD
Faculty of Rehabilitation Medicine, University of
Alberta, Edmonton, AB, Canada

Elizabeth Broad PhD
Clinical Services, AIS Sports Nutrition, Australian
Institute of Sport, Canberra, ACT, Australia

Brendan Burkett PhD
School of Health and Sport Sciences, University
of the Sunshine Coast, Maroochydore DC, QLD,
Australia

Marco Cardinale PhD
British Olympic Medical Institute, Institute of Sport,
Exercise and Health, University College London,
London, UK and University of Aberdeen, School of
Medical Sciences, Aberdeen, UK

Emilson Colantonio PhD
Departamento de Biociências, Universidade Federal de
Sao Paulo, Santos, Brazil

Rory A. Cooper PhD
Human Engineering Research Laboratories,
Department of Veterans Affairs, Rehabilitation
Research and Development Service, and the
Department of Rehabilitation Science & Technology,
University of Pittsburgh, Pittsburgh, PA, USA

Varley Teoldo da Costa MS
Department of Physical Education,
University of Belo Horizonte, Belo Horizonte,
Minas Gerais, Brazil

Steven D. Edwards PhD
Department of Philosophy, History and Law in
Healthcare, School of Human and Health Sciences,
Swansea University, Swansea, UK

Sílvio de Araújo Fernandes Jr, PT
Departamento de Psicobiologia, Universidade Federal
de Sao Paulo, São Paulo, Brazil

Marcos Gonçalves de Santana PhD
Campus Jataí, Universidade Federal de Goiás,
Jataí, Brazil

Christine M. Heiner BA
Human Engineering Research Laboratories,
Department of Veterans Affairs, Rehabilitation
Research and Development Service, and
Department of Physical Medicine and Rehabilitation,
University of Pittsburgh, Pittsburgh, PA, USA

Florentina J. Hettinga PhD
Center of Human Movement Sciences, University of Groningen/University Medical Center, Groningen, The Netherlands

P. David Howe PhD
School of Sport, Exercise and Health Sciences, Loughborough University, Loughborough, Leicestershire, UK

Yeshayahu "Shayke" Hutzler PhD
Zinman College of Physical Education and Sport Science, Netanya and Israel Sport Center for the Disabled, Ramat-Gan, Israel

Justin Laferrier MSPT
Human Engineering Research Laboratories, Department of Veterans Affairs, Rehabilitation Research and Development Service, and the Department of Rehabilitation Science & Technology, University of Pittsburgh, Pittsburgh, PA, USA

Laurie A. Malone PhD
Department of Research & Education, Lakeshore Foundation, Birmingham, AL, USA

Jeffrey J. Martin PhD
Department of Kinesiology, Health and Sport Studies, Wayne State University, Detroit, MI, USA

Mike J. McNamee PhD
Department of Philosophy, History and Law in Healthcare, School of Human and Health Sciences, Swansea University, Swansea, UK

Yoav Meckel PhD
Zinman College of Physical Education and Sport Science, Netanya, Israel

Marco Túlio de Mello PhD
Departamento de Psicobiologia, Universidade Federal de Sao Paulo, São Paulo, Brazil

Natalia Morgulec-Adamowicz PhD
Department of Adapted Physical Activity, The Józef Piłsudski University of Physical Education, Warsaw, Poland

Franco Noce PhD
Department of Physical Education, University of Belo Horizonte, Belo Horizonte, Minas Gerais, Brazil

Kevin Orr BS
Canadian Wheelchair Sports Association, Ottawa, ON, Canada

Ian Rice MS, OTR
Human Engineering Research Laboratories, Department of Veterans Affairs, Rehabilitation Research and Development Service, and the Department of Rehabilitation Science & Technology, University of Pittsburgh, Pittsburgh, PA, USA

Luiz Oswaldo Carneiro Rodrigues PhD
Departamento de Educação Física, Universidade Federal de Minas Gerais, Belo Horizonte, Brazil

Lee Romer PhD
Centre for Sports Medicine and Human Performance, Brunel University, London, UK

Dietmar Martin Samulski PhD
Department of Physical Education, Federal University of Minas Gerais, Belo Horizonte, Minas Gerais, Brazil

Federico Schena MD, PhD
Department of Neuroscience & Faculty of Exercise and Sport Science, University of Verona, and Center of Bioengineering and Sport Science, Verona, Italy

Andressa da Silva Msc
Departamento de Psicobiologia, Universidade Federal de Sao Paulo, São Paulo, Brazil

Michelle L. Sporner MS
Department of Rehabilitation Science & Technology, University of Pittsburgh, Pittsburgh, PA, USA

Matthias Strupler MD
Institute of Sports Medicine, Swiss Paraplegic Center, Nottwil, Switzerland

Sergio Tufik PhD
Departamento de Psicobiologia, Universidade Federal de Sao Paulo, São Paulo, Brazil

Sean Tweedy PhD
The University of Queensland, School of Human
Movement Studies, Brisbane, QLD, Australia

Peter Van de Vliet PhD
International Paralympic Committee, Bonn,
Germany and Health, Leisure and Human Performance
Research Institute, Faculty of Kinesiology and Recreation
Management, University of Manitoba, MB, Canada

Nick Webborn MBBS
Chelsea School Research Centre, University
of Brighton, East Sussex, UK

Stuart Willick MD
Division of Physical Medicine and Rehabilitation
University of Utah Orthopaedic Center,
Salt Lake City, UT, USA

Garry Wheeler PhD
Vice President Edmonton Chapter and Alberta
Division, MS Society of Canada, Psychologist,
Glenrose Rehabilitation Hospital, and Faculty
of Physical Education and Recreation,
University of Alberta, Edmonton, AB,
Canada

Foreword

By Dr Jacques Rogge

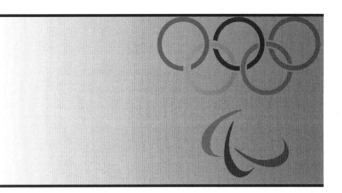

The physiology, biomechanics, and medical care of athletes must be studied and interpreted with special relationships to age, gender, and genetic potential. Each athlete must base programs of nutrition, physiological and psychological conditioning, and skill development on a base of what has been inherited from the parents. The special features brought to the competitive venues by athletes with a wide variety of disabilities must be carefully reviewed and understood in order to better serve their health, safety, and performance needs.

As levels of both interest and participation in sports by disabled athletes have grown markedly in recent years, so has the amount and sophistication of related research by sports medical personnel and sport scientists. Profs. Vanlandewijck and Thompson and their contributing authors have produced a handbook in which the research has not only been synthesized and summarized but also presented with practical applications of great use to sports medicine doctors, sports scientists, coaches and trainers, and the athletes themselves.

A major section of the handbook is devoted to all aspects of the science of disability sport: biomechanics, physiology, medicine, and the social sciences of philosophy, sociology, and psychology. A second major emphasis of the handbook is allocated to exercise testing and exercise prescription for Paralympic Sports. This includes aerobic and anaerobic power, strength, nutrition, mental preparation, and preparation for different meteorological environments.

The collaborative efforts of the International Olympic Committee and the International Paralympic Committee to produce this handbook have resulted in a major contribution to the health and welfare of many thousands of athletes.

Dr Jacques Rogge
IOC President

Foreword

By Sir Philip Craven

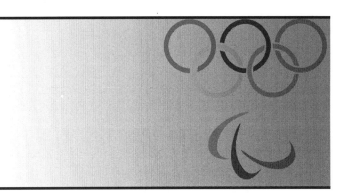

Since its founding in 1989, the International Paralympic Committee (IPC) has experienced exponential growth in the number of sports but more importantly, the number of athletes competing against each other with the Paralympic Gold Medal as the ultimate prize. While much has been learned about the Paralympic athlete in these past two decades, there is still much more to be discovered. Scientists all over the world are now actively engaged in the study of Paralympic athletes. Much of the credit for the increased interest has to be attributed to the IPC Sports Science Committee.

This book, *The Paralympic Athlete*, introduces for the first time a comprehensive evaluation of the athlete from several different perspectives: basic science, applied science, social science, nutrition, and performance enhancement in both cold and hot environments. This book will be used to stimulate more research but can also be utilized by the coach and the athlete as a guide to improving athletic performance. The book can be a source of valuable information for coaches and athletes and will also be important in the classroom where now entire college and university courses are dedicated to the understanding of the Paralympic athlete.

Prof. Dr. Yves Vanlandewijck of Katholieke Universiteit (Leuven, Belgium) and Prof. Dr. Walt Thompson of Georgia State University (Atlanta, GA, USA), both members of the IPC Sports Science Committee, have successfully recruited the world's best and most respected scientists to write exemplary chapters and then amalgamated this handbook into the most comprehensive book on the subject of the Paralympic athlete. The IPC Governing Board, Paralympic Sports, coaches and athletes, member nations, and the Paralympic Movement are indebted to all who contributed to this book.

Philip Craven

Sir Philip Craven, MBE
President
International Paralympic Committee

Preface

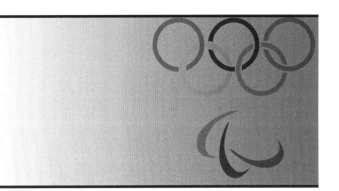

The idea for this book was raised for the first time in a hotel room in Chateau Frontenac in Quebec, Canada in 1997 by Dr. Trevor Williams, a true pioneer in research on the Paralympic Movement. Trevor's aim was two fold: he wanted to review the knowledge available within the main sport scientific disciplines addressing questions relevant to the Movement; and he wanted to apply this available knowledge to the current training and coaching strategies of Paralympic athletes. The first outline of the book conceived by us respected this double aim, reviewing – after a historical review of the Paralympic Movement and a comprehensive explanation of the role of classification in Paralympic Sports in chapter 1 – Biomechanics, Physiology, Medicine, Philosophy, Sociology, and Psychology of Sport research in chapters 2 to 7, and providing coaching information on how to train and prepare the Paralympic athlete for competition in chapters 8 to 15. When all the pieces started to take form in this book, the line between science and its application to the Paralympic athlete became very thin, mainly because of the high involvement of all the contributing authors in the Movement. We first thought that researchers would be interested in the first part of the book while coaches and athletes would be more interested in the second half. However, we now believe that all who are interested in the Paralympic Movement will read this book cover-to-cover.

This book was initiated through the International Paralympic Committee Sport Science Committee (IPC SSC), originated in 1994 under the leadership of Prof. Dr. Gudrun Doll-Tepper as the IPC Sport Science, Research and Education Committee. Trevor was a member of the committee from its inception until his untimely death in 1998. The mission of the IPC SSC is to seek interaction with the scientific community, formulating actual research questions relevant to the Movement, hand the questions over to the academic community, and activate strategies to come to solutions. In its efforts, the Committee collaborates with the leading associations in sport science such as the International Council of Sport Science and Physical Education (ICSSPE), the Medical and Scientific Working Group of the International Olympic Committee (IOC), the American College of Sports Medicine (ACSM) and the International Federation of Sports Medicine (FIMS). It is the hope of the Editors that this book will also find its way to the shelf of the members of these associations, amalgamating the strength of researchers from both sport for the able-bodied and athletes with a disability.

The Paralympic Movement is very young but evolving extremely fast. At the time that Trevor initiated this idea, one book could perhaps have encompassed all of the research questions and answers of the time. Today, however, to address in detail all the issues important for the Paralympic athlete to perform at the most optimal level in the most health protective conditions, each Paralympic sport and each academic discipline addressing the Paralympic athlete has enough substance for a separate book. The IPC SSC will therefore initiate a series of Sport-specific and Discipline-specific monographs in the future to address research relevant to the Paralympic Movement and all its stakeholders.

The editors would like to thank all of the authors who spent countless hours writing manuscripts for this book and who put up with the seemingly endless questions and comments from the editors. We would also like to thank the International Olympic Committee, and especially Prof. Dr. Howard Knuttgen and Dr. Jacques Rogge, for this extraordinary opportunity to once again partner for the betterment of all athletes. The editors would like to thank the International Paralympic Committee, and especially Dr. Peter Van de Vliet, Mr. Xavier Gonzales and Sir Philip Craven who always were encouraging us to complete this project so that others could see the work of research within the Paralympic Movement. We would like to thank Lieven Coudenys for greatly enhancing the book by including his incredible photographs. He has always been a good friend to the Movement, and for that we especially thank him for lending us his talent. We also thank our publisher, Wiley-Blackwell and especially Cathryn Gates and Geetha Williams for their guidance and for their patience. Finally, we thank all of the athletes who have demonstrated to us that no physical impairment can keep anyone from excelling in sport and for allowing us to be fans as well as scientists.

Yves C. Vanlandewijck
Walter R. Thompson

PART 1
INTRODUCTION

Chapter 1
Introduction to the Paralympic Movement

Sean Tweedy[1] and P. David Howe[2]

[1]The University of Queensland, School of Human Movement Studies, Brisbane, QLD, Australia
[2]School of Sport, Exercise and Health Sciences, Loughborough University, Loughborough, Leicestershire, UK

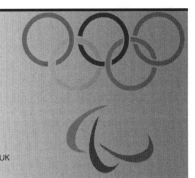

Part 1 of this book provides the reader with a comprehensive overview of the Paralympic Movement, describing the principle events and ideas that have shaped the movement to date, and considering the key issues for the future. It comprises two sections—*History of the Paralympic Movement* and *Classification in Paralympic sport.* This structure provides the reader with an historical account which flows logically and is not broken up by detailed consideration of the evolution of Paralympic classification, an area that is so important and complex that it warrants stand-alone treatment. The first section, History of the Paralympic Movement, was co-authored by Drs. Sean Tweedy and David Howe and the second section, Classification in Paralympic Sport, was authored by Dr. Tweedy.

the development of the movement is divided into six key periods: 1944–1952; 1952–1959; 1960–1964; 1964–1987; 1987–present; and the future. For each period an overview is provided and in some instances key events are identified and expanded upon.

Throughout the history of the movement it is clear that Paralympic sport has grown and developed for three main reasons:

1. Sport is an effective means of augmenting rehabilitation outcomes for people with disabilities.
2. People with disabilities have a right to participate in sport and should have the same opportunities as others.
3. Paralympic sport is elite, exciting, and inspiring (Figure 1.1).

These factors have rarely operated in isolation, and at most points in the history of the movement, a

History of the Paralympic Movement

Introduction

History of the Paralympic Movement commences with background information for the reader— antecedents of the Paralympic Movement, the life and achievements of Sir Ludwig Guttman, and etymology of the term "Paralympic". Following that,

The Paralympic Athlete, 1st edition. Edited by Yves C. Vanlandewijck and Walter R. Thompson. Published 2011 by Blackwell Publishing Ltd.

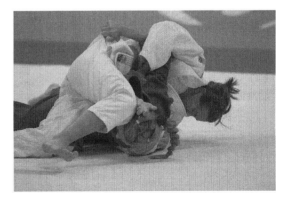

Figure 1.1 Paralympic sport is elite, exciting, and inspiring.

combination of these factors has driven development. Equally, however, each of these factors has pre-
dominated at certain periods and each of the five key
periods includes consideration of the principal factors
that drove development at that time. The reader is
also referred to Table 1.1 which presents a chronological summary of the key events in the history of the
movement.

Table 1.1 Chronological summary of key events in the history of Paralympic sport.

Year	Event [*Significance of the event in square brackets and italicized*]
1922	• Establishment of Comité International des Sports des Sourds/International Committee for Deaf Sports (CISS) [*Significance—first international sports organization for people with disabilities*]
	• Establishment of the Disabled Drivers Motor Club (UK) [*Significance—one of the earliest sports organization for people with physical disabilities (Brittain, 2010)*]
1924	• First International Games for the Deaf [*Significance—first international sports event for people with disabilities*]
1932	• Establishment of British Society of One-armed Golfers [*Significance—one of the earliest organizations to emphasize sports of physical prowess for people with physical disabilities*]
1939	• Start of World War II [*Significance—theatres of war lead to a large increase in the number of fit, young soldiers and civilians sustaining permanent physical impairments, including SCI*]
1944	• Dr. Ludwig Guttmann begins tenure as inaugural Director of the National Spinal Injuries Unit in Stoke Mandeville, UK [*Significance—Guttmann had free reign to develop and implement his quite radical approach to management of SCI. The inclusion of competitive sports activity was a key component of this approach and it became increasingly important over the years*]
1945	• Finish of World War II
1948	• First Stoke Mandeville Games, an archery competition between patients from Stoke Mandeville and those from the Star and Garter Home in Richmond, Surrey (Bailey, 2009; Brittain, 2010) [*Significance—occurred the same day as the opening ceremony of the London Olympic Games being held just 35 miles away, an important, though possibly coincidental initial link with the Olympic Movement (Bailey, 2009; Brittain, 2010)*]
1949	• Second Stoke Mandeville Games, known at the time as the *Grand Festival of Paraplegic Sport*—Brittain, 2010 [*Significance—the Games became an established annual event and grew substantially, from 16 competitors and two hospitals in the previous year, to 37 competitors from six hospitals—(Brittain, 2010); Guttmann gives a speech in which he declares his hope that the Games would become international and achieve "world fame as the disabled men and women's equivalent of the Olympic Games (Bailey, 2007; Goodman, 1986).*]
	• First Winter Games for the Deaf
1950	• Ski School for amputees established in Salzberg, Austria [*Significance—first winter sports organization for persons with a disability (Jahnke, 2006).*]
1952	• First International Stoke Mandeville Games, known at the time as the *First International Inter-Spinal Unit Sports Festival* (Bailey, 2009) with an official team from the Netherlands competing in a program of five sports (Gold 2007; Brittain 2010; Bailey, 2009) [*Significance—Recognized as the first ISMGs; First International Games for Athletes with a Physical Disability; second Stoke Mandeville Games to be held in the same year as the Olympic Games.*]
1953	First media record of the term "Paralympic", in the *Bucks Advertiser and Aylesbury News* (Brittain, 2010)
1956	• Fifth International Stoke Mandeville Games [*Significance—third Stoke Mandeville Games to be held in the same year as the Olympic Games.*]
	• Guttmann awarded the Fearnley cup by the IOC for "outstanding achievement in the service of Olympic ideals" [*Significance—first official engagement with the Olympic Movement.*]

Year	Event [*Significance of the event in square brackets and italicized*]
1957	The term "Paralympic" in common colloquial use to describe the Stoke Mandeville Games (Gold, 2007)
1959	Establishment of International Stoke Mandeville Games Committee (ISMGC) (Bailey, 2009)
1960	• First Paralympic Games held in Rome (also officially known as the Ninth International Stoke Mandeville Games); Competitors were SCI athletes only [*Significance—first ISMGs held outside Stoke Mandeville; first time the Olympic Games and Stoke Mandeville Games were held in the same city, venue, and year, strengthening links between the movements; recognized by IPC as first Paralympic Games.*]
	• Formal decision by International Stoke Mandeville Games Committee to align the International Stoke Mandeville Games with the Olympic cycle, so that in the year of an Olympic Games the Committee would endeavor to hold the annual Games in the same city (or country) as the Olympic Games
1964	• Second Paralympic Games held in Tokyo, also officially known as the Thirteenth International Stoke Mandeville Games; competitors were SCI athletes only [*Significance—ISMGC achieves goal of linking the Games with the Olympics, which they set in 1960; Paralympic athletes share accommodation and sporting facilities used by Olympic athletes.*]
	• Establishment of International Sports Organization for the Disabled (ISOD), a multi-disability sports organization that aimed to provide sports opportunities for people with disabilities other than SCI
1966	• Ludwig Guttmann knighted for services to the disabled and becomes President of ISOD
	• World Games for the Deaf replace International Games for the Deaf (est'd 1924)
	• First International Sports Competition for Amputees, held at Stoke Mandeville and hosted by the British Limbless Ex-Serviceman's Association (Brittain, 2010)
1967	• ISOD transfers headquarters to Stoke Mandeville
	• ISOD begins development of rules of sports and classification for amputee athletes
1968	• Third Paralympic Games held in Tel Aviv, Israel, also officially known as Seventeenth International Stoke Mandeville Games; competitors were SCI athletes only [*Significance—despite promising early negotiations with Instituto Mexicano de Rehabilitación, ISMGC failed for the first time to secure a host for the Games in Mexico, the 1968 Olympic City; credible alternative bids from Israel and United States indicated the growing international stature of the Games.*]
	• Establishment of Sports and Leisure Group by International Cerebral Palsy Society
1972	• Fourth Paralympic Games held in Heidleburg, Germany, also officially known as the Twenty-first International Stoke Mandeville Games; competitors were SCI athletes only
	• ISMGC changes name to International Stoke Mandeville Games Federation (ISMGF) (Bailey, 2007)
1975	• United Nations (UN) General Assembly adopts *The Declaration on the rights of Disabled Persons* (Resolution 3447), article 9 of which states that "Disabled persons have the right to . . . participate in all social, creative or recreational activities."
1976	• Fifth Paralympic Games held in Toronto, Canada (also officially known at the time as the Toronto Olympiad for the Physically Disabled, or Torontolympiad); competitors were SCI athletes and, for the first time, amputee and vision impaired (VI) athletes [*Significance—first Paralympic Games not auspiced by the ISMGC alone, but in cooperation with ISOD; first games which included athletes other than those with SCI—viz. amputee and les autres.*]
	• First Winter Paralympic Games held in Örnsköldvik, Sweden (also officially known at the time as the *Winter Olympic Games for the Disabled* (Jahnke, 2006)); competitors were amputee and VI athletes
	• United Nations adopted resolution 31/123, declaring 1981 the International Year of Disabled Persons
1977	• ISOD creates Les Autres Classification system, a single classification system for athletes not eligible to compete in competitions for people with SCI, CP, amputation, VI, or hearing impairment (Bailey, 2009)
1978	Establishment of Cerebral Palsy-International Sports and Recreation Association (CP-ISRA), replacing Sports and Leisure Group of the International Cerebral Palsy Society (est'd 1968) (Brittain, 2010)

(continued)

Table 1.1 (*Continued*)

Year	Event [*Significance of the event in square brackets and italicized*]
1980	• Sixth Paralympic Games in Arnhem, the Netherlands (also officially known at the time as Olympics for the Disabled); competitors were SCI, amputee, VI athletes and, for the first time, athletes with CP. • Establishment of International Blind Sports Association (IBSA) [*Significance—first international sports organization for people with VI.*] • Second Winter Paralympic Games held in Geilo, Norway (also officially known at the time as the Second Winter Olympic Games for the Disabled (Jahnke, 2006)); competitors were amputee and VI athletes and, for the first time, athletes with SCI. • World Health Organization publishes International Classification of Impairment Disability and Handicap (ICIDH). [*Significance—this document defined and used a standardised language for describing the consequences of disease and injury. It also provided a framework to code information relating to the consequences of disease and injury*]
1981	United Nations declares International Year of the Disabled
1982	• Establishment International Coordinating Committee of World Sports Organizations for the Disabled (ICC), comprising representatives from CP-ISRA, IBSA, ISMGF, ISOD (Bailey, 2007; Brittain, 2010) • First Cerebral Palsy World Games, held in Denmark and hosted by CP-ISRA • United Nations adopts Resolution 37/53, proclaiming 1983–1992 the *United Nations Decade of Disabled Persons*
1983	United Nations declares Decade of Disabled Persons (GA resolution 37/52)

1984	• Seventh Paralympic Games held in two locations:
	  • New York, USA (also officially known at the time as the New York International Games for the Disabled); competitors were SCI, amputee, VI, CP, and, for the first time, LA athletes
	  • Aylesbury, UK (also officially known at the time as International Stoke Mandeville Games); competitors were SCI athletes only
	• Third Winter Paralympic Games, held in Innsbruck, Austria (also officially known at the time as the III World Winter Games for the Disabled (Jahnke, 2006)); competitors were SCI, amputee, VI, CP, and, for the first time, LA athletes

1985	Establishment of International Association for Sport for Persons with Mental Handicap (INAS-FMH)
1986	CISS and INAS-FMH join ICC
1988	• Eighth Paralympic Games, held in Seoul Korea [*Significance—first Games since 1964 held in the same city as the Olympic Games, sharing venues and facilities*]; competitors were SCI, amputee, VI, CP, LA athletes, and, for the first time dwarves were included under the banner of LA • Fourth Winter Paralympic Games, held in Innsbruck, Austria (also officially known at the time by two names—the *IV World Winter Games for the Disabled—Winter Paralympics 1988* and *IV World Winter Games for Physically Disabled Innsbruck 1988* (Jahnke, 2006)); competitors were SCI, amputee, VI, CP, and LA athletes
1989	• Establishment of International Paralympic Committee (IPC)
1990	ISMGF changes name to International Stoke Mandeville Wheelchair Sports Federation (ISMWSF)
1992	• Ninth Paralympic Games, held in Barcelona, Spain; competitors were SCI, amputee, VI, CP, and LA athletes • First Paralympic Games for athletes with ID, held in Madrid, Spain • Fifth Winter Paralympic Games held in Tignes-Albertville, France • Conclusion of United Nations Decade of Disabled Persons • United Nations declares December 3 the annual International Day of Disabled Persons (GA resolution 47/3)
1993	• First World Dwarf Games, Chicago, USA • Establishment of the International Dwarf Athletic Federation (IDAF)
1994	• Sixth Winter Paralympic Games held in Lillehammer, Norway; competitors were SCI, amputee, VI, CP, and LA athletes.
1995	• CISS withdraws from Paralympic Family, having joined in 1986
1996	• Tenth Paralympic Games, held in Atlanta, USA; competitors were SCI, amputee, VI, CP and LA athletes, and, for the first time at the same venue, ID athletes

Year	Event [*Significance of the event in square brackets and italicized*]
1998	• Seventh Winter Paralympic Games held in Nagano, Japan; competitors were SCI, amputee, VI, CP and LA athletes, and, for the first time, ID athletes
1999	INAS-FMH changes name to International Association for Sport for Persons with Intellectual Disability (INAS-FID)
2000	• Eleventh Paralympic Games held in Sydney, Australia; competitors were SCI, amputee, VI, CP, LA, and ID athletes
2001	• INAS-FID suspended from the Paralympic Movement by the IPC at the 2001 General Assembly following revelations that 69% of athletes who had won medals in the intellectually disabled events at the Sydney Paralympic Games did not have a necessary verification of an ID • Deaflympics replace World Games for the Deaf (est'd 1966)
2002	• Eighth Winter Paralympic Games held in Salt Lake, USA; competitors were SCI, amputee, VI, CP, and LA athletes
2004	• Twelfth Paralympic Games held in Athens, Greece • ISMWSF and ISOD merge to form the International Wheelchair and Amputee Sports Federation (IWAS)
2006	• Ninth Winter Paralympic Games, held in Torino, Italy
2007	• IPC endorses the IPC Classification Code [*Significance—details policies and procedures that should be common to classification in all sports; sets principles to be applied by all sports within the Paralympic Movement, including mandating development of evidence-based systems of classification.*]
2008	• Thirteenth Paralympic Games, held in Beijing, China
2009	• INAS-FID reinstated to the Paralympic Movement at the IPC General Assembly • Publication of International Paralympic Committee Position Stand – Background and scientific principles of Classification in Paralympic Sport [*Significance—provides a scientific background for classification in Paralympic sport; defines evidence-based classification; and provides guidelines for how evidence-based classification may be achieved*]
2010	Tenth Winter Paralympic Games, held in Vancouver, Canada
2012	• Thirteenth Paralympic Games, to be held in London, UK; competitors will be SCI, amputee, VI, CP, LA, and ID athletes
2014	• Eleventh Winter Paralympic Games, to be held in Sochi, Russia; competitors will be SCI, amputee, VI, CP, LA, and ID athletes
2016	• Fourteenth Paralympic Games, to be held in Rio, Brazil

Background to the Paralympic Movement

Antecedents of the Paralympic Movement

It is commonly accepted that the Paralympic Movement began in England in the 1940s. However the concept of providing sports opportunities specifically for people with disabilities was pioneered much earlier. The first Sports Club for the Deaf was founded in Berlin in 1888 (Gold & Gold, 2007). An international sports federation for the deaf—Comité International des Sports des Sourds (CISS)—was founded in 1922 (Bailey, 2007; Gold & Gold, 2007). The first two International Silent

Games were held in the year of the Olympic Games and in the same city: the 1924 Paris Games and the 1928 Amsterdam Games (http://www.deaflympics.com/games/). However, since 1935 the International Games for the Deaf have been held in the year immediately following the staging of the Olympic Games. In 1966, the Games were renamed the World Games for the Deaf and the current official name—Deaflympics—was adopted in 2000. Winter Games for the Deaf have been held since 1949 and are held in the year following the Winter Olympics (http://www.deaflympics.com/games/).

Among the earliest sports organizations for people with physical disabilities were the Disabled Drivers Motor Club (1922) and the British Society of One-Armed Golfers (1932) (Brittain, 2010).

Sir Ludwig Guttmann—Founding Father of the Paralympic Games
"Dr Guttmann, you are the de Coubertin of the paralysed!"

(His Holiness Pope John XXIII, 1960)

Sir Ludwig Guttmann (1899–1980) was born into a Jewish family in Germany on July 3, 1899. He qualified as a medical doctor in 1924 (MD, Frieburg) and, as a new graduate, began his lifelong specialization in neurology and neurosurgery under the tutelage of Prof. Otfrid Foerster (Whitteridge, 2004). In 1933, the National Socialists came to power and, because he was Jewish, Guttmann was forced to leave his post and become a neurologist and neurosurgeon in the Jewish hospital in Breslau. In 1937, Guttmann became medical director of that hospital. In 1939, Guttmann and his family were granted visas to visit England. On that visit he made contact with the Society for the Protection of Science and Learning and, through this connection, was invited to interview at Oxford University where he secured a research position (Whitteridge, 2004). He worked at Oxford until 1943 when, frustrated by the lack of clinical work in the University environment, he accepted an offer to become inaugural Director of the National Spinal Injuries Unit at the Ministry of Pensions Hospital, Stoke Mandeville, Aylesbury. He became a naturalized Briton in 1945 (Whitteridge, 2004).

It was at Stoke Mandeville that Guttmann began a number of highly innovative methods of rehabilitation for people with spinal cord injury (SCI). Chief among these was the inclusion of sport as an integral part of physical rehabilitation, an initiative which ultimately led to the establishment of the Paralympic Games. Guttmann's considerable contribution in this area is covered in more detail in the remainder of this section. As instrumental as Guttmann was in the establishment of the Games, he made other contributions that were similarly impressive—he founded the scientific journal *Paraplegia* (currently published as *Spinal Cord*) as well as the *International Medical Society for Paraplegia* (now the *International Spinal Cord Society*) and wrote a Textbook of Sport for the Disabled (1976). He also trained medical staff from many countries at Stoke Mandeville and, in recognition of the outstanding education he provided, medical training centers in Spain, West Germany, and Israel have been

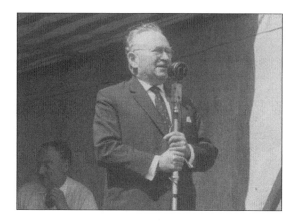

Figure 1.2 Sir Ludwig Guttmann, the founding father of the Paralympic Movement (photographer unknown).

named in his honor (Whitteridge, 2004). Guttmann became Sir Ludwig Guttmann in 1966 when he was knighted by Queen Elizabeth II for services to the disabled. He died on March 18, 1980, prior to the Olympics for the Disabled in the Netherlands later that year.

There is little doubt that, just as Baron Pierre de Coubertin is considered the founder of the modern Olympic Games, Sir Ludwig Guttmann deserves to be considered founding father of the Paralympic Movement (Figure 1.2).

The term "Paralympic"

Originally, the term "Paralympic" was considered a pun combining "paraplegic" and "Olympic" although its origins are unclear. The term was first used in the media in 1953 in the *Bucks Advertiser and Aylesbury News* and until 1960 the term was used as an alternative or colloquial means of referring to the annual International Stoke Mandeville Games (ISMGs) (Brittain, 2010). Although Guttmann was a determined promoter of the link between the Olympic and Paralympic Movements, the record shows that he preferred the "International Stoke Mandeville Games" to be used officially and did not promote use of the term Paralympic. The term remained colloquial following the 1960 Rome Games although, from that time, Paralympic tended to be used in the press only when referring to the ISMGs that occurred in the same year as the Olympics (Brittain, 2010; Gold & Gold, 2007).

The first attempt to use the term officially was by the self-titled "1984 Paralympics Steering Committee", which was preparing to host games for the spinal cord injured in Chicago. The United States Olympic Committee (USOC) registered its disapproval of the term at that time, indicating that it felt that the term was too closely aligned with "Olympic", but the Games in Chicago did not eventuate and so use of the term at that point was not tested (Brittain, 2010). Subsequently, the International Olympic Committee (IOC) approved the use of the term Paralympic in connection with the 1988 Seoul Games and following these Games the term was incorporated into the name of the new governing body for the Games, the International Paralympic Committee (IPC). The term Paralympic has been the correct term of reference for the Games and the movement ever since (Figure 1.3) (http://www.paralympic.org/Media_Centre/).

Officially the IPC has retrospectively recognized the 1960 Rome Games as the first Summer Paralympics and the 1976 Örnsköldvik Games as the first Winter Paralympics. The meaning of the term has also been defined to indicate its meaning in the current context—the English prefix "para" (i.e., a bound morpheme derived from the Greek) meaning alongside and the stem "Olympic" referring to the Games, with the term Paralympic indicating that the Olympic and Paralympic movements exist side by side (http://www.paralympic.org/Media_Centre/).

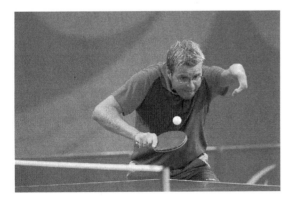

Figure 1.3 Modern Paralympic athlete competing in a recent Paralympic Games. Reproduced courtesy of Lieven Coudenys.

1944–1952: sport as rehabilitation

Dr. Ludwig Guttmann's tenure as inaugural Director of the National Spinal Injuries Unit in Stoke Mandeville began on March 1, 1944. His patients were principally ex-servicemen who had sustained war-related SCIs, although there were an appreciable number of civilian injuries admitted as well (Howe, 2008). It was believed that a unit specializing in management of spinal injuries would ensure that patients would receive better treatment than could be given in general medical, surgical, orthopedic, or neurosurgical wards (Scrutton, 1998).

Guttmann's early work was influenced by Dr. D. Munro, a neurosurgeon from Boston, USA, who had developed methods of management that reduced the incidence and recovery time from decubitus ulcers, and who also achieved some success in the treatment of urinary tract infections. Guttmann began by implementing Munro's measures, but soon made important advances himself. For example, he showed that antiseptics retarded the healing of bedsores, which were best managed by excision of necrotic tissues, skin grafting, and the training of patients to self-monitor on a regular basis (Whitteridge, 2004). A hallmark of rehabilitation at Stoke Mandeville was that patients were always encouraged to extend themselves physically—whether sitting up in bed during early rehabilitation or using calipers in the later stages. Upon discharge from the Unit, patients were expected to have high levels of physical independence (Scrutton, 1998).

Inspiration for incorporating sport into the Stoke Mandeville rehabilitation methods came from the patients themselves. While doing his rounds, Guttmann saw a group of patients frantically moving in their wheelchairs outside the dormitory blocks using a puck and an upside down walking stick, a game subsequently dubbed wheelchair polo. Attractive as this game was for the patients, the use of the stick at the same time as propelling the wheelchair made the game unacceptably dangerous, and it was soon replaced by a variety of other sports, including archery, netball, javelin, and snooker.

In the context of postwar spinal rehabilitation, the notion that sport could be used to enhance outcomes was entirely novel. It is arguable that, unless Guttmann had helped establish sport as a legitimate feature of comprehensive rehabilitation, the growth of the Paralympic Movement could have been delayed by 40 years. Guttmann promoted sport as "the most natural form of remedial exercise, restoring physical fitness, strength, coordination, speed, endurance and overcoming fatigue" (Guttmann, 1976). He also held that sport ". . . had a psychological impact of restoring pleasure in life and contributing to social reintegration". In essence, Guttmann believed that sport was a vital means of achieving what he regarded as the ultimate aims of rehabilitation—to make the spinally injured person ". . . as independent as possible and to restore him to his rightful place in social life" (Guttmann, 1976).

On July 29, 1948, Guttmann officially extended the reach of his sports program beyond the patient population at Stoke Mandeville, inviting a team of patients from the Star and Garter Home in Richmond, Surry, to compete against his own patients in an archery competition at the Hospital. This was the first Stoke Mandeville Games and it occurred on the same day as the opening ceremony of the 1948 London Olympic Games. With the benefit of hindsight, this co-occurrence appears highly symbolic, although Guttmann himself did not claim that he had selected the date for that reason (Brittain, 2010).

The second Stoke Mandeville Games were held exactly one year later and grew substantially in that short space of time—at the 1948 Games, 16 patients from two hospitals had competed; in the 1949 Games, 37 patients from six hospitals competed. It was at these Games that Guttmann made his Paralympic pretensions explicit. In a remarkably prescient speech, Guttmann foreshadowed the possibility that the movement would eventually mature into one which would fully embrace the ethos of elite sport, speaking of the day when the Games would become truly international and when it would be "the disabled men and women's equivalent of the Olympic Games" (Bailey, 2007; Goodman, 1986). In the ensuing years, the growth of the Games continued apace and at the 1951 Games, 126 patients from 11 hospitals throughout the United Kingdom competed in four sports—archery, netball, javelin, and snooker.

The year of the Helsinki Olympic Games (1952), was the first year that the Stoke Mandeville Games became international. Known at the time as the *First International Inter-Spinal Unit Sports Festival*, a team from a spinal unit for war veterans at Aardenburg in the Netherlands traveled to Stoke Mandeville to compete in the Games (Bailey, 2007; Gold & Gold, 2007). Over the next 7 years, the Games became officially known as the ISMGs and were held annually at the Hospital. The number of international teams grew markedly, and at the 1959 Games, 360 competitors from 20 countries (principally from the industrialized nations) took part (Brittain, 2010).

1952–1959: leaving the hospital

During this period of internationalization (1952–1959), rehabilitation remained an important driver for development of Paralympic sport. Specifically, medical specialists and staff from rehabilitation units were a crucial engine for growth of the Games. Staff who visited the hospital to train, and Stoke Mandeville staff who moved on to positions in other countries, spread knowledge of and enthusiasm for the Hospital's approach to paraplegic care and the role of sport in rehabilitation (Gold & Gold, 2007). Guttmann himself also spread the word though *The Cord*—a newsletter published from Stoke Mandeville which Guttmann contributed to regularly and which often devoted space to sports reports from the Hospital—and through international conference presentations, at which he frequently challenged key delegates to bring teams to the Games (Brittain, 2010; Gold & Gold, 2007).

During the same period, however, Paralympic sport grew beyond rehabilitation. This occurred principally through continued participation in the Games by patients who had completed their rehabilitation and been discharged into the community. This increasingly large group of people was no longer comprised of patients completing an externally imposed rehabilitation regime in order to achieve augmented rehabilitation outcomes—rehabilitation was over. These people—community-dwelling people with SCI who continued to compete at ISMGs following discharge—can therefore rightly be identified as the first Paralympic athletes who were NOT doing sport as rehabilitation. Instead, people in this group competed in sport for the same reasons as other people in the community are known to, including enjoyment, social interaction, recreation, competition, and enhanced health and well being (Vallerand & Rousseau, 2001). In 1952, athletes were selected to represent their countries, rather than their rehabilitation hospital, another change that aligned Paralympic sport with nondisabled sport, and which served to de-emphasize sport as rehabilitation.

An important antecedent of elite Paralympic sport also appeared during this period, with the first official link between the Paralympic and Olympic movements. The Olympic Movement is synonymous with elite sport; and in 1956, one of the guests invited to the ISMGs was Sir Artur Porritt, a surgeon and a British member of the IOC. Porritt was apparently so impressed by the Games that he nominated the Games for the Fearnley Cup, an IOC award for "outstanding achievement in the service of the Olympic ideals" (Guttmann, 1976). At this point the symbol of the International Stoke Mandeville Games Federation (ISMGF) was three entwining wheels that represented friendship, unity, and sportsmanship, a clear echo of the symbolism of the five Olympic rings.

1960–1964: a material link to the Olympic Games

The 1960 ISMGs were tremendously significant in the development of the Paralympic Movement and are officially recognized by the IPC as the first Paralympic Games (http://www.paralympic.org/Media_Centre/). They were the first ISMGs ever held outside the Hospital grounds, and they were conducted in the same city as the Olympic Games had been. The association with the Olympic Games was strengthened by the fact that competitors at the ISMG competed at Olympic venues. The capacity to conduct the Games was due largely to strong working links between Guttmann and the unit at Stoke Mandeville on one hand, and key rehabilitation institutions in Italy on the other (namely Instituto Nazionale per l'Assicurazione contro Infortuni

sul Lavoro—INAIL—and the Ostia Spinal Unit, Rome).

The Rome Games were the first to be conducted under the auspices of the ISMG Committee (ISMGC), which was formed in 1959. Inspired by the great success of the Rome Games, the ISMGC made a formal decision to align the ISMGs with the Olympic cycle, so that in the year of an Olympic Games the Committee would endeavor to hold the annual Games in the same city (or country) as the Olympic Games (Bailey, 2007; Brittain, 2010). This highly ambitious aim was achieved in 1964, when the ISMG were held in Tokyo. The 1964 Tokyo Games were similar to the Rome Games in a number of ways—they were held in the same city and year as the Olympic Games, Olympic facilities were used by ISMG competitors and these arrangements were facilitated by very strong links between Stoke Mandeville and the medical rehabilitation community in the host country—in this case with Dr. Nakamura a doctor of rehabilitation from Beppu (Brittain, 2010). At this point in time, the factors helping to drive the development of Paralympic sport were derived from each of the three themes identified in the introduction to this section: sport for rehabilitation, promoting participation, and elite sport.

Unfortunately, despite the best efforts of people within the movement, it was not until 24 years later, at the 1988 Games in Seoul, that the Olympic and Paralympic Games were once again held in the same city re-establishing the close alignment that characterized the Rome and Tokyo Games.

1964–1987: defining the scope of the movement and the beginnings of a unified voice for Paralympic sport

In 1964, only athletes with SCI participated in Paralympic sport and only Summer Games were held. By 1987, the scope of the movement had expanded dramatically to include all the groups that are currently eligible to compete in Paralympic sport; the Winter Paralympic Games had been established; and the first international umbrella organization for Paralympic sport—the International Coordinating Committee of World Sports Organizations for the Disabled (ICC)—had been formed.

Expansion of the disability groups comprising the movement

Initially it was intended that a single organization—the International Sports Organization for the Disabled (ISOD), established in 1964—would develop opportunities for people who were not eligible to compete under ISMGC rules (i.e., the spinal cord injured). In 1966, Guttmann became President of ISOD and the Headquarters shifted from Paris to Stoke Mandeville. ISOD commissioned writing of sports rules and a classification system for amputees and other forms of limb deficiency in 1967 (Bailey, 2007). By 1976, ISOD had also developed sport rules and classification systems for people with vision impairment (VI) and cerebral palsy (CP), however, establishment of independent sports organizations for athletes with CP in 1976 (the Cerebral Palsy-International Sport and Recreation Association—CP-ISRA) and those with VI in 1980 (the International Blind Sports Association—IBSA) meant that the systems developed by ISOD were never widely implemented (Brittain, 2010). Amputee and VI athletes first competed at the Summer Paralympic Games in Toronto in 1976 and CP athletes competed at the Arnhem Games 4 years later.

ISOD also developed sports rules and a classification system for Les Autres (LA), a French term which literally means "the others". As the name suggests, the system served as a catch-all, catering for people with movement-related impairments who were not eligible to compete under the rules of other sports organizations for the disabled at that time (i.e., ISMGF, CP-ISRA, ISOD [rules for Amputees], or IBSA). More specifically LA athletes were those with "locomotor disabilities[1] regardless of diagnosis", but specifically excluding those with "severely reduced mental capacity . . . heart, chest, abdominal, skin, ear and eye diseases without locomotor disability" (ISOD, 1993). It included athletes affected by conditions such as multiple sclerosis, arthrogryposis, muscular dystrophy, as well as those with injuries that permanently affected muscles, nerves, or bones and caused permanent weakness and/or loss of range of movement. LA athletes first competed at the Summer Paralympic Games in 1984 in New York. Dwarves were included under the LA banner after 1984 and first competed at the Seoul Paralympics in 1988 (http://www.paralympic.org/Media_Centre/).

In 1986, toward the end of this period of expansion, the International Association for Sports for Persons with a Mental Handicap (INAS-FMH) was established and was later renamed the International Association for Sports for Persons-Federation for the Intellectually Disabled (INAS-FID). Athletes with an intellectual disability (ID) competed in their first Paralympic Games in 1992, although a decision by the local organizing committee meant that they were not permitted to compete in Barcelona. Instead INAS-FID organized separate games in Madrid, after the Barcelona Games which, although separate, were officially recognized as part of the Paralympic Games (Brittain, 2010).

The Winter Games

Winter sports for persons with a disability began in Europe in the late 1940s and, in contrast to the summer sports which began with sports for people with SCI, the first sports organization for people with a disability was a ski school for amputees (Jahnke, 2006). The school was established in Salzburg, Austria in 1950 and during the 1960s organizations for people with VI also began. The concept of an International Winter Games for persons with a disability was proposed by Sweden at an ISOD meeting in 1974, and in 1976 the first Winter Paralympic Games—also officially known at the time as the *Winter Olympic Games for the Disabled*—were hosted by ISOD in Örnsköldvik, Sweden (Jahnke, 2006). Competitors at the games were amputees and athletes with VI. The second Games were held in Geilo, Norway in 1980 and athletes with SCI competed for the first time. LA athletes and those with CP first competed at the third Winter Paralympic Games in 1984 at Innsbruck, Austria.

Examination of historical accounts of this phase of Paralympic sports development does not indicate that provision of sport as rehabilitation drove growth in the variety of groups participating and provision of opportunities in winter sports. More specifically the strong involvement of the medical fraternity that was evident in the early development and expansion of the ISMGs were not as evident in these new sports organizations.

Rather, it appears that this significant period of broadening was related to growing international acceptance of the view that people with disabilities had a right to participate in the full spectrum of activities that comprised community life, and that sport and recreation were an integral part of this spectrum. For example, in 1975 the United Nations (UN) General Assembly adopted *The Declaration on the rights of Disabled Persons* (Resolution 3447), article 9 of which states that "Disabled persons have the right to . . . participate in all social, creative or recreational activities." In 1976, the United Nations adopted resolution 31/123, declaring 1981 the International Year of Disabled Persons and in 1982 (Resolution 37/53) proclaimed the period 1983–1992 the United Nations Decade of Disabled Persons. While these UN initiatives are not explicitly linked to the broadening of the Paralympic Movement, they certainly indicate that the international conditions were right for an expansion of the types of sporting opportunities available to people with disabilities, as well as an extension of the number of people with disabilities served by Paralympic sport. The official philosophy of INAS-FID, one of several international sports organizations for people with disabilities that was established during this period, supports this view, stating that " . . . persons with intellectual disability are members of society entitled to the same rights, opportunities, and duties as everyone else. They are not special, but have specific needs, just as the old, the young, the blind, and physically impaired have specific needs."

Development of a unified voice

By 1981, four international organizations of sport for the disabled existed—ISMWSF (representing athletes with SCI), ISOD (representing amputee and LA athletes), CP-ISRA (representing CP athletes), and IBSA (representing VI athletes)—and no single organization existed that had the authority to speak or act on behalf of this collective. This made dealings with the Paralympic Movement very complicated and fractious, concerns that had been expressed on a number of occasions by the IOC (Bailey, 2007). In March 1982, the four international organizations held the founding meeting of what was later named the ICC. In 1986, CISS and INAS-FMH were admitted as members of the ICC (Brittain, 2010).

The explicit aim of the ICC was to become the organizing body for the Paralympic Games and it gave the Paralympic Movement its first united voice, permitting improved lines of communication with the IOC and relevant Olympic Games organizing committees. The advantages conferred by a unified voice undoubtedly facilitated arrangements that permitted the 1988 Summer Olympic and Paralympic Games to be held in the same city and in close cooperation for the first time since 1964. Following on from this, the 1992 Winter Olympic and Winter Paralympic Games also engaged in a similar shared organization for the first time ever.

During the period 1964–1987, recognition that Paralympic sport was elite and inspiring did not make a major contribution to the growth of Paralympic sport. This was due principally to the fact that for the majority of this period the movement had been too fractured and disparate to develop effective working relations with the IOC, relations that later proved pivotal in developing the image of Paralympic sport as elite. However, there were two developments that helped develop the image of Paralympic sport as elite.

The first was the inclusion of wheelchair racing (men's 1500 m and women's 800 m) as demonstration events for the first time at the 1984 Olympic Games (Brittain, 2010). This raised the profile of Paralympic sport enormously and, because of the status of the Olympic Games as an elite sports event, made a clear statement that Paralympic sport is elite sport. The other notable trend toward elitism from within the movement was the tailoring of the Paralympic events program so that it became more closely aligned with the Olympic sports program. Table 1.2 presents sports and events that were culled from the Paralympic program during this period, clearly demonstrating a tendency to remove events that might be perceived as novelty events, rehabilitation events or recreational events. Whether culling such events was necessary in order to project an image of elite Paralympic sport is debatable, however, there is little doubt that elitism motivated the trend.

Table 1.2 Sports and events culled from the Paralympic program 1960–1987.

Sport/event	Year in	Last year on program
Dartchery*	1960	1980
Snooker	1960	1976
Precision javelin	1960	1976
Wheelchair slalom	1964	1988
Kick ball	1988	1988
Lawn bowls	1968	1996

*Dartchery: a sport in which competitors score points by shooting arrows onto a target that is configured in the same way as a dart board.

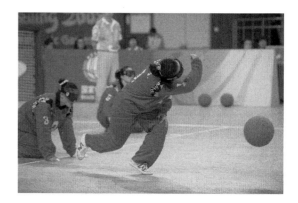

Figure 1.4 Athletes competing in the 2008 Beijing Paralympic Games. Reproduced courtesy of Lieven Coudenys.

1988–present: Paralympic sport comes of age

This period began with the 1988 Seoul Paralympic Games, the Games that heralded the arrival of Paralympic sport as an elite international sporting event. At the conclusion of the games, the first President of the IPC, Dr. Bob Steadward commented: "the 1988 Seoul Paralympics dramatically demonstrated the effects of proper organisation and the shift from sport as rehabilitation to sport as recreation to elite sport . . . The winning athlete was the elite athlete, one at the peak of training and conditioning. Thus these Games are considered the first Games of the modern Paralympic era" (Bailey, 2007). Indeed, with 3951 athletes competing at the Beijing Games in 2008 (Figure 1.4), the Paralympics are now the second largest international sports gathering of *any* type after the Summer Olympics (Gold & Gold, 2007).

During this period, the predominant factor that has driven development of the movement has been recognition that Paralympic sport is elite, exciting, and inspiring. Specifically, factors that have contributed to this recognition have included an evolution from the ICC to the IPC and closer, more functional ties between the IPC and the IOC.

Evolution from the ICC to the IPC

The ICC was established in 1982 and achieved its intended purpose, coordinating the staging of both the Summer and Winter Paralympic Games

of 1988 and 1992. On the whole these four Games were considered outstanding successes, bearing testimony to the effectiveness of the organization and the advantage of having a single representative organization for Paralympic sport (Brittain, 2010).

The IPC was formed in 1989 and replaced the ICC as the lead agency for organization of the Summer and Winter Games in 1992. Organizationally the principal difference between the ICC and the IPC was that while the ICC membership comprised only the six International Sports Organizations for the Disabled (IOSDs[2])—ISMWGF, CP-ISRA, IBSA, ISOD, INAS-FMH, and CISS—IPC membership also included 41 member nations, each of whom had voting rights. This structure was more democratic and ensured that a greater diversity of voices could be heard. CISS withdrew from the IPC in 1995, resuming the independent position that had been characteristic of the organization since its inception in 1922 (Bailey, 2007).

Currently, the IPC is the global governing body of the Paralympic Movement, as well as the organizer of the Summer and Winter Paralympic Games. There are 20 Summer Paralympic sports, and four Winter Paralympic sports and these are presented in Table 1.3, together with Wheelchair Dance Sport which is not contested at the Paralympic Games but which is governed by the IPC.

As indicated in Table 1.3, the IPC acts as international federation for eight sports (seven Paralympic and one non-Paralympic), whereas the remaining

Table 1.3 Sports governed by the IPC and its member federations as of January 2009.

Sports governed by IPC	Sports governed by IPC Member Federations			
	IOSDs		International Federation Sports	
	Sport	Organization	Sport	Organization
Alpine Skiing (W)	Boccia	CP-ISRA	Archery	Fédération International de Tir à l'Arc
Athletics	Football 5-a-Side	IBSA	Cycling	Union Cycliste International
Ice Sledge Hockey (W)	Football 7-a-Side	CP-ISRA	Equestrian	International Equestrian Federation
Nordic Skiing (Biathlon & Cross Country Skiing) (W)	Goalball	IBSA	Rowing	International Rowing Federation
Powerlifting	Judo	IBSA	Sailing	International Foundation for Disabled Sailing
Shooting	Wheelchair Fencing	IWAS	Table Tennis	International Table Tennis Federation
Swimming			Volleyball (Sitting)	World Organization for Volleyball for Disabled
Wheelchair Dance Sport			Wheelchair Basketball	International Wheelchair Basketball Federation
			Wheelchair Tennis	International Tennis Federation
			Wheelchair Curling (W)	World Curling Federation
			Wheelchair Rugby	International Wheelchair Rugby Federation

Acronym key: IOSD, International Organizations of Sport for the Disabled; CP-ISRA, Cerebral Palsy-International Sport and Recreation Association; IBSA, International Blind Sport Association; IWAS, International Wheelchair and Amputee Sports Federation; W, Winter sport.

17 Paralympic sports are governed by international federations that are structurally independent, but which have been admitted to the membership of the IPC. These international federations comprise International Organizations of Sport for the Disabled (IOSDs) which provide sports opportunities for people with specific disabilities (e.g., CP or VI); and International Sport-Specific Federations (e.g., Union Cycliste Internationale or International Wheelchair Basketball Federation).

The IPC celebrated its 30th anniversary in 2009 and in this time it has had only two Presidents—Dr. Robert Steadward (1989–2001) and Sir Philip Craven (2001–present). It has unprecedented resources that, in a relatively stable organizational environment, have permitted development of a corporate culture and systems that have aided the advancement of the movement, including cultivation and projection of Paralympic sport as elite and entertaining. Figure 1.5 presents the current IPC organizational structure.

Closer and more functional ties between IPC and IOC

Between the 1964 Tokyo Games and the 1988 Seoul Games relations between the IOC and the Paralympic Movement were not strong. This was due in part to the absence of a functioning umbrella organization that could legitimately speak on behalf of the Paralympic Movement. However, during this period the IOSDs did demonstrate an ability to resolve differences and work together for mutual benefit. The first meeting between the newly established ICC and then IOC President Juan Antonio Samaranch took place in 1983 and was called to resolve a dispute over naming of the third Winter Paralympic Games. Outcomes from the meeting were: the originally

IPC GENERAL STRUCTURE

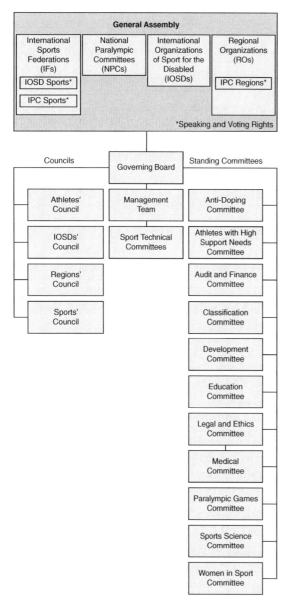

Figure 1.5 IPC organizational structure.

Sarajevo Winter Olympics and the Los Angeles Olympics (Brittain, 2010).

In the lead-up to the 1988 Games the IOC agreed to the term "Paralympic" being used for the Seoul Games and all games from then onward. With the naming issue finally settled, tensions arose over the logo selected for the Korean Paralympic Games—5 Tae geuks—which the IOC considered was too similar to the Olympic rings (Figure 1.6). Sanctions were threatened and the IPC agreed to change the logo to 3 Tae-geuks in 1992 (Figure 1.7), though the original logo remained in limited use until the 1994 Winter Games (Bailey, 2007; Brittain, 2010). In 2003, the

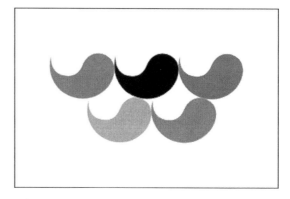

Figure 1.6 Five Tae-geuks, the logo developed for the 1988 Summer Games (Seoul) and used at the 1992 Summer Games (Barcelona) and the 1994 Winter Games (Lillihammer). It was also the original logo for the IPC but, at the urging of the IOC, was changed in 1992—see Figure 1.7 (http://www.paralympic.org/IPC/Paralympic_Symbol_Motto.html).

Figure 1.7 Three Tae-geuks, symbolizing "Mind, Body Spirit". This logo was adopted by the IPC in 1992 and was used until 2003, when it was replaced by the current logo (see Figure 1.8). From 2003 it remained in limited used until the 2004 Athens Paralympic games (http://www.paralympic.org/IPC/Paralympic_Symbol_Motto.html).

named "Third Winter Olympic Games for the Disabled" would remove the word "Olympic" from the name, becoming the "World Winter Games for the Disabled"; IOC would provide patronage and financial support to the ICC; and demonstration of Paralympic events would be included at the 1984 current logo—3 agitos symbolizing spirit in motion was adopted (Figure 1.8).

In 2001, relations between the IPC and IOC reached an unprecedented level of formality with the signing of a detailed cooperative agreement which stipulated, *inter alia*, bids for the Olympic

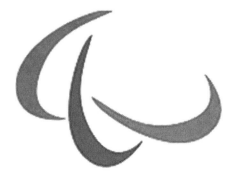

Figure 1.8 Current official logo for the IPC, adopted in 2003. It comprises three Agitos, symbolizing "Spirit in motion".

and Paralympic Games would be contractually linked and new levels of financial support for the IPC. In 2003, this agreement was amended to transfer "broadcasting and marketing responsibilities of the 2008, 2010, and 2012 Paralympic Games to the Organizing Committee of these Olympic and Paralympic Games".

Currently the Olympic and Paralympic Movements have become so closely aligned that it is reasonable to posit that Guttmann's 1948 vision—that the Paralympic Games would become the "disabled men and women's equivalent of the Olympic Games"—has been realized. Closer ties between the IPC and IOC have been the hallmark of the IPC stewardship to date, and this relationship has been instrumental in transforming Paralympic sport into the high performance spectacle that it currently is, as well as facilitating unprecedented growth in terms of athlete numbers (Figure 1.9a and b) and number of countries competing (Figure 1.10a and b).

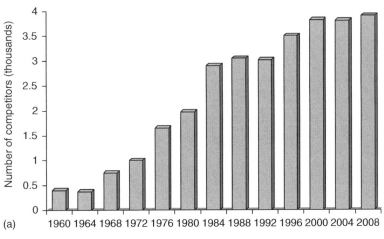

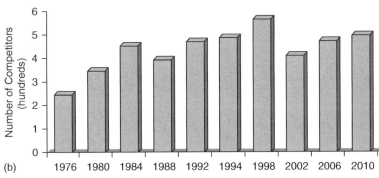

Figure 1.9 Number of competitors at (a) the Summer Paralympic Games 1960–2008 and (b) the Winter Paralympic Games 1976–2010.

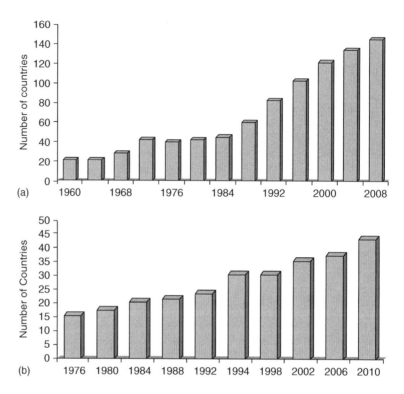

Figure 1.10 Number of countries competing at (a) the Summer Paralympic Games 1960–2008 and (b) the Winter Paralympic Games 1976–2010.

The Sydney 2000 classification fiasco

At the 2000 Paralympic Games in Sydney, the Spanish team defeated Russia in the gold medal play-off in the basketball competition for athletes with an ID. Following the Games, Carlos Ribagorda, a member of the winning team and a journalist with the magazine *Capital* published an article in which he revealed that, *inter alia*, 10 of the 12 members of the Spanish gold-medal-winning team in Sydney were not intellectually disabled (Brittain, 2010). Subsequent investigation by the IPC revealed that, "Of the possible medals awarded for ID events at the Sydney 2000 Paralympic Games, 69% were awarded to athletes from various countries whose INAS-FID registration forms did not meet the proper requirements of the eligibility verification process" (International Paralympic Committee, 2006). As a result, INAS-FID was suspended from the Paralympic Movement by the IPC General Assembly in 2001.

Athletes with an ID were re-admitted to the Paralympic Movement in November 2009. The timing and extent of readmission depends on the progress of international research being conducted in order to determine the relative strength of association between different measures of intellectual impairment and performance in four sports—athletics, swimming, table tennis, and rowing.

The future

This historical account posits that the Paralympic Movement has grown for three main reasons:
1. Sport is an effective means of augmenting rehabilitation outcomes for people with disabilities.
2. People with disabilities have a right to participate in sport and should have the same opportunities as others.
3. Paralympic sport is elite, exciting, and inspiring.

Each of these reasons has been predominant at different periods during the growth of the Paralympic Movement. The future health of the Paralympic Movement depends on recognition and cultivation of all three of these historically important areas of growth.

Sport as rehabilitation

The long-term prospects of the movement will be improved by active engagement with the rehabilitation sector. Just as Stoke Mandeville served as a hot-house for Paralympic sport in the 1940s, rehabilitation centers that include sport as a component of comprehensive management methods provide a vital avenue for recruiting participants. Rehabilitation units that provide modern exemplars of practice in this area include the Swiss Paraplegic Center and Association at Nottwil, the Beitostølen Healthsports Center in Norway and the Zahal Disabled Veteran's Organization in Israel. Innovative programs in developing countries are also important (Carvalho & Farkas, 2005), as is publication of the results of sports and lifestyle interventions in scientific journals and conference proceedings (Carvalho & Farkas, 2005; Røe, 2008).

Sport as a right for people with disabilities

Away from rehabilitation centers in community settings, effective methods for promoting sports participation must be studied and implemented. Within the IPC's current structure the IOSDs— IWAS, CP-ISRA, IBSA, and INAS-FID—have a central role in developing and growing opportunities for participation among the populations within their remit. Although evidence regarding participation rates among people with disabilities in sport is limited, available evidence indicates that rates are particularly low—in Australia, in 2003, 24.0% of adults with disabilities participated in organized sport, compared with 62.4% of nondisabled adults (Australian Bureau of Statistics, 2006). The IPC has an obligation to provide opportunities, pathways, and incentives for sports participation.

Paralympic sport which is elite, exciting, and inspiring

This is an area in which the IPC has excelled recently—a dedicated media department, the advent of ParalympicSport.tv and an increasingly professional website provide outstanding access to a product that is highly attractive. However, efforts to promote Paralympic sport as *elite* must be clear about what elite performance is in the Paralympic context. Specifically, elite should not be a descriptor reserved for performances that are comparable with nondisabled performances—an athlete in a severely disabled class that breaks a world record should receive similar attention and kudos within the Paralympic family as Oscar Pistorius, another Paralympic record holder who performs in a class in which records are, quite understandably, reasonably close to those of nondisabled athletes. Failure to discharge this duty toward the more severely disabled in the movement threatens the authenticity of the IPC, including its role as legitimate representative of all Paralympic athletes.

Finally, the single issue that is likely to have the greatest bearing on the future of the Paralympic Movement is that of classification which is addressed in the second section of this Introduction.

Classification in Paralympic sport

Classification is a critical aspect of Paralympic sport for two key reasons.

1. Classification determines who is and who is not eligible to compete in Paralympic sport. As the stature of Paralympic sport increases—increased public awareness, increased media attention—there is a proportional increase in the importance of decisions which determine eligibility for Paralympic sport.

2. Classification is the sole means by which success in Paralympic sport is legitimized. If stakeholders in Paralympic sport—athletes, coaches, administrators, the media, or the public—suspect that the athletes who succeed in Paralympic sport are simply those who have disabilities that are less severe than their

competitors, then the value of success in Paralympic sport becomes questionable.

What is classification?

Classification is a process in which a single group of entities (or units) are ordered into a number of smaller groups (or classes) on the basis of observable properties that they have in common (Bailey, 1994; Fleishman & Quaintance, 1984).

Taxonomy is the science of how to classify, its principles, procedures, and rules (Fleishman & Quaintance, 1984). It is applied in most scientific fields to develop systems of naming and ordering that facilitate communication, understanding, and identification of interrelationships.

Classification in sport

As a science in its own right, taxonomy is made meaningful through its application in other fields of science, such as pathology, botany, and zoology for classification of diseases, plants, and animals, respectively. Classification is also a feature of most modern sports. The units of classification most commonly used in sport are age, sex, and body mass. The effect of these forms of classification is to minimize the impact of the unit/s of classification on the outcome of competition.

To illustrate, if all the boys at a school athletics carnival competed together, the age of each child would have a huge impact on where each child finished in the field—the top-placed children would likely be older, and the youngest would be among the last-placed children. This is because age is closely related to physical maturation and, for a range of reasons, the more physically mature children are, the faster they are able to run. However, if the children at the carnival were classified according to how old they were, then the impact of maturation on the order of finishing would be minimized. As a consequence, the relative importance of other attributes—amount of training, psychology, physiology, and anthropometry—would be increased.

From a sociological perspective, classification in sport encourages and fosters participation. This is because, as the previous example illustrates, classification increases the prospects of close competition and empirical evidence indicates that close competition is one of the key factors that motivate people to participate in sport (Vallerand & Rousseau, 2001). If children were not classified according to age and 6-year-old boys competed against 13-year-old boys at the school carnival, the prospects of close competition would be low and the 6-year-olds would have little motivation to participate. Classification according to age minimizes the impact of age on competition outcome, and this encourages younger children to participate.

Classification in Paralympic sport

The first sports competitions for the hearing impaired were held in the late 19th century. From a sports classification perspective these competitions were significant because it was the first time that impairment had been used as a unit of classification in a sporting context. Later, in the 1940s, Dr. Ludwig Guttmann's decision to incorporate sport as an element of comprehensive spinal injury rehabilitation lead to the development of the impairment-based systems of classification that are now the basis of Paralympic sport.

Originally, probably because Paralympic sport originated as an extension of the rehabilitation process, early systems of classification were medically based. The organizational structure of medically based classification systems reflected the structure of a rehabilitation hospital, with separate classes for people with SCIs, amputations, brain impairments, and those with other neurological or orthopedic conditions. Athletes received a single class based on their medical diagnosis, and competed in that class for all sports—athletics, swimming, archery, and any other sports offered. An athlete with a complete L2 SCI—resulting in lower limb paresis but normal arm and trunk power—would compete in a separate wheelchair race from a double above-knee amputee because their medical diagnosis was different. The fact that the impairments resulting from their medical condition caused roughly the same activity limitation in wheelchair propulsion was not considered in the classification process because classification was based on medical diagnosis.

As the Paralympic Movement matured, sport ceased to be a mere extension of rehabilitation and became important in its own right. The focus on sport, rather than rehabilitation, drove the development of functional classification systems. In functional systems, the main factors that determine class are not diagnosis and medical evaluation, but how much the impairment of a person impacts upon sports performance. For example, in Paralympic Athletics, an athlete with a complete L2 SCI now competes in the same wheelchair racing class as a double above-knee amputee (class T54). This is because these impairments have an impact on wheelchair propulsion that is approximately the same.

In contrast to the medical classification approach, in which athletes competed in the same class for all sport, functional systems of classification are necessarily sports-specific. This is because any given impairment may have a significant impact in one sport and a relatively minor impact in another. For example, the impact that bilateral below elbow amputation has on swimming is relatively large compared with the impact on distance running. Consequently, in sport-specific functional classification systems, an athlete with such impairment would compete in a class that had relatively severe activity limitation in swimming and a class that had relatively minor activity limitation in track athletics. Currently, most Paralympic sports use systems of classification that are described as functional, a notable exception being the classification system used by the IBSA which remains medically based.

The IPC Classification Code and Position Stand on scientific principles of classification

In general terms, the preceding account of the historical evolution of classification in Paralympic sport is accurate. However, there are currently 25 Paralympic systems of classification and while the majority share some key features—for example, class should reflect how much an impairment impacts performance in a specific sport—there is considerable variability on a range of fundamental issues, including definition of key terms, the stated purpose of each of the systems, and the basis for determining minimum impairment criteria. These differences have arisen partly for historical reasons—most Paralympic sports predate unification under the IPC by many years and therefore, naturally, developed quite independently—but also because, until recently, the domain of Paralympic classification was almost entirely atheoretical (Sherrill, 1999; Tweedy, 2002). However, classification is of such fundamental importance to Paralympic sport that in order for the movement to advance requires greater unity in this domain. The issue of minimum impairment criteria illustrates why unity is required.

In order for Paralympic sport to exist requires methods for classifying prospective athletes as eligible or not eligible, commonly known as minimum impairment criteria. But what should be the principle that determines what the minimum impairment criteria should be? Is the presence of a clinically verifiable impairment sufficient? Or should the impairment not only be clinically detectable, but also have an impact on sport (i.e., have different criteria from sport to sport)? What if the impairment does not impact on a particular sport, but impacts on a person's ability to train for the sport—should these people be eligible? Or should the criteria be that the impairment causes a disadvantage compared to nondisabled athletes? This is not an exhaustive list of the possibilities, yet each of these approaches leads to eligibility criteria that differ vastly from each other. Each approach also makes a fundamental statement about what Paralympic sport stands for and the values of the movement. Moreover, in order for science to make a contribution to the development of criteria, the principle should remain consistent. Therefore, in order for Paralympic sport to advance, a unified, coherent position on such issues is required across Paralympic sports.

Recently, the IPC has endorsed two documents that have aimed to bring cohesion to a range of classification issues—the IPC Classification Code and

International Standards (International Paralympic Committee, 2007), approved by the IPC General Assembly in November 2007; and the IPC Position Stand—Background and Scientific Principles of Classification in Paralympic Sport (Tweedy & Vanlandewijck, 2009), passed by the IPC Sports Science Committee, Classification Committee and Governing Board in June 2009. At the time of writing, the IPC were overseeing a self-audit process in which each of the sports was determining where their respective systems were in accord with the code and where they were not. Until all systems align with the code it will remain very difficult to make accurate, general statements about Paralympic classification. Therefore, the remainder of this part of the Introduction summarizes the main resolutions to come from these two documents, highlighting areas where major discrepancies still exist, and challenges for the future. The five areas of resolution are that all Paralympic systems of classification must:

- be consistent with the International Classification of Functioning Disability and Health (ICF);
- be based on scientific evidence;
- define eligible types of impairments;
- define minimum impairment criteria;
- classify impairments according to the extent of activity limitation caused.

Consistency with ICF

The ICF (World Health Organization, 2001) is currently the most widely accepted classification of health and functioning. It is a broad, multipurpose classification that provides a standardized language and structure that may be applied to describing and understanding health-related functioning in a wide variety of contexts and sectors. Further information, including copies of the ICF, is available at: *http:// www.who.int/classifications/icf/en/*. The Position Stand on Classification indicates that Paralympic systems of classification should be consistent with the ICF language and structure in order to reduce the considerable barriers to international communication that currently exist, and to help to promote research by ensuring the language used to describe classification is unambiguous and uniform across sports. This introduction uses terms as defined by the ICF, the most important of which are presented in the Glossary.

Evidence-based

In Paralympic sport, an evidence-based system of classification is one that has the following two features.

1. The system has a clearly stated purpose: To date, one of the most significant barriers to the development of evidence-based systems of classification is that many systems of classification either do not have a stated purpose or have a statement of purpose that is ambiguous. For example, many classification systems simply state that the purpose is to provide "fair and equitable competition". This statement is ambiguous because fair and equitable sports competition can be achieved in ways that are not consistent with the aims of Paralympic classification. For example, grouping athletes who have similar levels of performance—such as the handicap system used in golf or the belt system used in martial arts—is recognized as fair and equitable within those sports. However, this form of fair and equitable is not an acceptable basis for Paralympic classification.

To facilitate development of evidence-based systems of classification, all Paralympic systems of classification should indicate that the purpose of the system is to promote participation in sport by people with disabilities by *minimizing the impact of eligible types of impairment on the outcome of competition*. From a taxonomic perspective the proposed statement of purpose is critical because "impairment" is explicitly identified as the unit of classification. When impairment is the unit of classification then the relative impact of other performance determinants—for example, volume and quality of training and psychological profile—is increased and the athletes who succeed will do so because they are stronger in these areas, rather than because they have an impairment that causes less activity limitation.

2. Empirical evidence indicates that the methods used for assigning class will achieve the stated purpose: Most current systems of classification have little scientific evidence to support them. In some instances, this is not problematic because decisions make innate sense—for example, as previously described, an athlete with L2 SCI competes in the same class as a double above-knee amputee because the impairments have a comparable impact on wheelchair propulsion. However, there are many instances when decisions become more difficult. For example, in the sport of athletics a wheelchair racing athlete with a SCI, who has paralyzed legs, but unimpaired arms and trunk muscles, will compete in the T54 class. However, if the athlete also has a permanently injured elbow which he/she cannot straighten, the classification decision is more difficult. If the elbow restriction is small and is deemed to have little impact on wheelchair propulsion, the athlete would stay in the T54 class. But if the restriction is severe enough to significantly hinder the athlete's ability to push a wheelchair they would compete in the T53 class, which is for athletes who have normal arm muscle power but no muscle power in their trunk muscles or in their legs. Classifiers assessing such an athlete must ask themselves an important question: *"How much elbow restriction will cause the same amount of difficulty as the complete loss of trunk muscle function?"* Unfortunately there is no research or evidence which can help to answer this question. This sort of decision-making is the basis of all functional Paralympic classification systems. Because there is no research, currently these decisions are necessarily based on the experience and judgment of the classifiers who write and administer the classification systems. However, the IPC is committed to scientific studies that will develop evidence to support decision-making in classification. An overview of the methods required for developing such an evidence base is provided in the Position Stand.

In the absence of research evidence, the current best practice for estimating the extent of activity limitation resulting from impairment requires assessment of four key areas:

1. Impairment(s)—tests of impairment include, but are not limited to:
   - manual muscle test scores for individual movements (e.g., elbow flexion, elbow extension), assessment of hypertonia at different joints, residual limb length, and range of movement for athletes with physical impairment;
   - assessment of static and dynamic visual acuity, visual field, motion detection, contrast sensitivity,

and color vision in athletes with visual impairment; or
   - testing of general and sport intelligence (generic name for component of intellectual functioning or cognition that relate to performance, such as response process, manner and content; executive functioning; and attention/concentration) for athletes with intellectual impairment.

2. Novel activities—these are activities or movements that are new to the athlete and which are unlikely to have been practiced by them in the usual course of training for their sport. Performance on these tests is likely to be quite consistent with findings from the impairment tests. Examples of novel tests include:
   - foot tapping tasks, hand rubbing, isolated finger flexion/extension, static balance exercises in athletes with physical impairment;
   - general orientation and object-discrimination tasks in athletes with visual impairment; or
   - memory, visualization, choice reaction time, spatial orientation tasks in athletes with intellectual impairment.

3. Practiced activities—these are activities which incorporate elements of strength, range of movement, coordination, intellectual functioning, and/or any other sport-specific demands which are highly likely to have been practiced by the athlete in the course of training for their sport. Performance on these tests is likely to be quite different from the novel tests for well-trained athletes, while for untrained athletes performance is not likely to differ markedly. Examples of practiced activities include:
   - assessment of wheelchair rugby players would include dynamic warm-up routines, ball catch and throw drills, wheelchair maneuverability, and exercises;
   - assessment of goalball players would include audio-spatial orientation;
   - assessment of intellectual impaired table tennis players would include items such as service return, return to target skills, player positioning with respect to the table.

4. Training history and other personal and environmental factors affecting how well the athlete will do the activity—this will include questions about frequency, intensity and duration

of training, periodization of training, coaching standard (e.g., coach qualifications), use of sports medicine/sports science services. Other factors such as athlete age and gender may also be relevant. Intelligent, cogent questioning of athletes regarding training habits will provide insight into how well the athletes are trained—even athletes of low intellect who are well trained will be likely to answer questions about their training that indicates the frequency, duration, and intensity of training they do.

These four sources of information need to be evaluated by the classification team and considered on balance in order to determine how much of the activity limitation experienced by an athlete is attributable to impairment.

Defining eligible *types* of impairment

Sports should clearly identify which impairment types are eligible and define them according to the ICF codes. To date only 10 types of impairment have been eligible for Paralympic sport, these being VI, impaired strength, impaired range of movement, limb deficiency, leg length difference, hypertonia, ataxia, athetosis, short stature, and intellectual impairment. Table 1.4 presents eligible impairment types. Impairments are not to be confused with health conditions—SCI, CP, spina bifida, retinitis pigmentosa—which are useful for identifying the disease processes which lead to eligible impairment types, but which should not be the basis for determining eligibility.

Section 5 of the Code states that the type of impairment must be permanent (IPC, 2007; Tweedy & Vanlandewijck, 2009) indicating that it should not resolve in the foreseeable future regardless of physical training rehabilitation or other therapeutic interventions. The motivation for requiring permanence is clear—a person should not be eligible for Paralympic sport if they, for example, rupture a cruciate ligament and, as a result of casting or disuse during the acute phase, muscle strength, and/or joint range become temporarily impaired. To account for instances when a classified athlete receives an intervention that will materially alter measures

of impairment (e.g., botox to reduce hypertonia; tendon releases; Harrington rods; corrective eye surgery), classification systems should have a Notifiable Interventions policy which requires the athlete to notify the Head of Classification or Chief Classifier and make them aware of the intervention and to make arrangements for reclassification. A sound Notifiable Interventions policy also positions Paralympic sports to manage future scientific advances, for example, in the fields of neural regeneration, neural plasticity, and gene therapy.

The requirement that impairments should be permanent is based, at least in part, on the premise that eligible impairment types do not alter significantly in response to physical training—that athletes cannot "train away" spastic hypertonia, athetosis, or neurological paresis. However, in the recent past there have been instances of athletes claiming that, through sheer hard work and training intensity, impairments such as hypertonia which had previously been clearly clinically evident—to the extent that they had been deemed eligible by classification panels—had become clinically undetectable. The current state of research does not permit such claims to be dismissed out of hand nor accepted at face value. Decision-making in this area would benefit greatly from research investigating the responsiveness of impairments to sustained high level training, particularly the responsiveness of minimal impairments.

It is important to note that many health conditions that cause eligible impairment types affect multiple body structures and functions. For example, in addition to impaired strength, SCI may also result in impaired sensation (tactile sensation, proprioception, or pain), impaired thermoregulatory function and impaired cardiac function. While some of these associated impairment types—notably impaired cardiac function—may have a significant impact on sports performance, they are currently not eligible impairment types and therefore should not impact classification. Whether the types of eligible impairments should be expanded is a matter for debate. However, a decision to expand should not be taken lightly—expansion of the types of impairment that are classified

Table 1.4 The 10 impairment types that are eligible for various Paralympic sports: In order to compete in Paralympic sports, a person must be affected by at least one of the impairments listed in first column of this table. Note that the impairments presented must result directly from a health condition (e.g., trauma, disease, or dysgenesis), examples of which are presented in column 2. Impaired muscle power resulting from disuse (e.g., due to pain, hysterical conversion) is not eligible.

Working descriptor	Examples of health conditions likely to cause such impairments	Impairment as described in the ICF*	Relevant ICF Impairment Codes
Hypertonia (e.g., hemiplegia, diplegia/ quadriplegia, monoplegia)	CP, stroke, acquired brain injury, multiple sclerosis	High muscle tone *Inclusions*: hypertonia/high muscle tone *Exclusions*: low muscle tone	b735
Ataxia	Ataxia resulting from CP, brain injury, Friedreich's ataxia, multiple sclerosis, spinocerebellar ataxia	Control of voluntary movement *Inclusions*: ataxia only *Exclusions*: problems of control of voluntary movement that do not fit description of ataxia	b760
Athetosis	Chorea, athetosis (e.g., from CP)	Involuntary contractions of muscles *Inclusions*: athetosis, chorea *Exclusions*: sleep-related movement disorders	b7650
Limb deficiency	Amputation resulting from trauma or congenital limb deficiency (dysmelia)	Total or partial absence of the bones or joints of the shoulder region, upper extremities, pelvic region or lower extremities	s720, s730, s740, s750 *Note*: These Codes would have the extension 0.81 or 0.82 to indicate total or partial absence of the structure, respectively
Impaired Passive Range of Movement (PROM)	Arthrogryposis, ankylosis, scoliosis	Joint mobility *Exclusions*: hypermobility of joints	b7100–b7102
Impaired muscle power	SCI, muscular dystrophy, brachial plexus injury, Erb palsy, polio, spina bifida, Guillain-Barré syndrome	Muscle power	b730
Leg length difference	Congenital or traumatic causes of bone shortening in one leg	Aberrant dimensions of bones of right lower limb OR left lower limb *Inclusions*: shortening of bones of one lower limb *Exclusions*: shortening of bones of both lower limbs; any increase in dimensions	s75000, s75010, s75020 *Note*: For coding purposes aberrant dimensions of bones of right lower limb is indicated by addition of the qualifying code 0.841 and in the left lower limb, 0.842
Short stature	Achondroplasia or other	Aberrant dimensions of bones of upper and lower limbs or trunk which will reduce standing height	s730.343, s750.343, s760.349
Vision impairment	Trauma, retinitis pigmentosa, glaucoma	Vision acuity functions Visual field functions	b2100 b2101
Intellectual impairment	Down syndrome	Psychomotor control (quality) Higher-level cognitive functions (abstraction, cognitive flexibility, judgment problem solving)	b1471 b1640, b1643, b1645, 1646

*For further information on ICF codes, including how to obtain a copy of the ICF, visit the website at http://www.who.int/classifications/icf/site/ icftemplate.cfm.

in Paralympic sport has the potential to have a significant impact on the culture and fabric of Paralympic sport.

Finally, it should be noted that while it is theoretically possible to develop systems of classification in which people with all 10 types of impairment compete together, this approach is not favored by the IPC. Sports are encouraged to group impairments in a way that promotes face validity—when a spectator looks at an event, it should make sense. As Tweedy has previously proposed (2003), there are sound taxonomic reasons for treating the ten eligible impairment types as *at least* three distinct groups: (a) neuromusculoskeletal (or biomechanical impairments), comprising the eight neuromusculoskeletal impairments—impaired strength, impaired range of movement, limb deficiency, leg length difference, hypertonia, ataxia, athetosis, and short stature; (b) visual impairments; and (c) intellectual impairments. In fact there are cogent arguments in favor of breaking down neuromusculoskeletal impairments into smaller "fundamental competitive units": can a spectator be expected to understand how the effects of dwarfism and SCI can be readily equated in the sporting context? Those responsible for developments in classification should give this matter appropriate consideration.

Define minimum impairment criteria

Section 5 of the Code indicates that in order to be eligible, an impairment must impact on sports performance (IPC, 2007). The origin of the notion that impairments should impact on sports performance in order to be eligible can be traced back to the establishment of the IPC. Prior to that time, international sport for people with disabilities was organized along diagnostic lines—CP-ISRA for people with CP, ISMGF for people with SCI, etc. The mission of such organizations was based around provision of sports opportunities for people with those conditions and consequently the most logical inclusion criteria was diagnostic—a person with a SCI should be catered for within ISMGF. The purpose of minimum impairment criteria was to ensure impairment was not trivial—finger or toe amputees were not eligible for amputee sport. Under this organizational structure, through wrist amputation

makes sense as a minimum impairment criterion for amputees for any sport they wanted to compete in—running, throwing, swimming, etc. Legitimacy of the criteria derives from the fact that the aim of the sports organization was to provide sports opportunities for amputees. Moreover, when an organization only provides sports opportunities for a single disability group, then the organization is not challenged to develop criteria for different impairment groups that are equitable.

However, when IPC took charge of the governance of the movement in 1989, the focus of Paralympic sport became considerably more elite and, because the IPC mandate covered a range of impairment groups, it became more important to develop minimum impairment criteria which were equitable across impairment groups. In these circumstances, equity is required and the most logical standard is that all eligible impairments should impact on sports performance. In the elite sporting milieu, the legitimacy of minimum impairment criteria is not derived from a charitable standpoint in which the objective is to provide sports opportunities to everyone with a particular impairment type—rather, legitimacy is derived from the fact that the sports people that deserve a "parallel Olympic Games" are those who have an impairment which materially and directly impacts sports performance.

To ensure that only impairments which impact on the sport are eligible, each Paralympic sport should develop minimum impairment criteria (IPC, 2007; Tweedy & Vanlandewijck, 2009). More specifically, each Paralympic sport should identify those activities that are fundamental to performance in that sport, and then operationally describe criteria for each eligible impairment type that will impact on the execution of those fundamental activities. For example, determination of minimum impairment criteria for VI in alpine skiing should be set by analyzing the vision requirements for optimum downhill performance—visual acuity, visual field, contrast sensitivity, etc.—and then, once they have been identified, developing an operational description of the minimum VIs that will sufficiently compromise those requirements to be considered eligible.

There are two important consequences arising from accurately described minimum impairment criteria.

1. It will be possible for an athlete to have an eligible *type* of impairment but to be ruled ineligible because the impairment does not meet the relevant minimum impairment criterion. For example, while a person who has had a single toe amputated is technically an amputee (an eligible type of impairment), the impairment does not cause sufficient activity limitation in running and therefore does not meet the minimum impairment criteria for IPC Athletics (Tweedy & Bourke, 2009).

2. Minimum impairment criteria will be specific to each sport. Consequently, it will be possible for a person to have an impairment that is eligible in one sport, but not in another.

Note that minimum impairment criteria should describe impairments that directly cause activity limitation in the sport and should exclude impairments that may cause activity limitation in training but do not directly impact on activities that are fundamental to a sport (Tweedy & Vanlandewijck, 2009). For example, although the loss of the fingers on one hand will cause activity limitation in certain resistance training exercises considered important in sprinting (e.g., the snatch and the power clean), the impairment will cause negligible activity limitation in the sprint events themselves and therefore such an impairment is not eligible in IPC sprint events (Tweedy & Bourke, 2009).

To some extent determining how much activity limitation will be sufficient is affected by sports culture and more than one view may sometimes be considered valid. Consequently, determination of minimum impairment criteria should draw on empirical evidence when it is available, but also ensure that it reflects the views of key stakeholders in the sport—athletes, coaches, sports scientists, and classifiers.

Classifying impairments according to extent of activity limitation caused

Impairments which meet the eligibility criteria should be divided into classes according to how much activity limitation they cause. To date a number of other phrases have been used to describe the conceptual basis of classification in Paralympic sports. Table 1.5 identifies two of the main ones and illustrates why each is not suitable. Note

Table 1.5 Previously proposed statements regarding the conceptual basis of Paralympic classification and why they are unsuitable.

Conceptual basis	Problem with this conceptual basis
Place athletes into classes according to their *degree of function*	Although function is affected by impairment, a range of other factors also affect how well a person functions. These factors include age, fitness, and motivation. A person who is old, unfit, and unmotivated will not function as well as when they were young, fit, and motivated. Moreover, we know that training affects function—if it did not, then athletes would not train. If athletes was placed into classes according to function, then an athlete who was young, motivated, and well trained would be placed in a more functional class than someone who was older, unmotivated, and poorly trained. Paralympic systems of classification should ensure that young, well-trained athletes should gain a competitive advantage, and therefore classifying athletes according to their degree of function is not a suitable conceptual basis for classification in Paralympic sport.
Place athletes into classes according to their *degree of performance potential or innate potential*	The performance potential or innate potential of an athlete is determined by an array of natural attributes including, but not limited to, impairment. For example, in discus, performance potential or innate potential is obviously negatively influenced by impaired strength. However, performance potential is enhanced by increased standing height, arm span and increased proportion of type II (fast twitch) muscle fibers. If athletes were classified according to such constructs, then tall athletes with long arms and an ideal muscle fiber composition would compete in higher classes than short, endurance-type athletes. Paralympic classification systems should ensure that athletes with the best combination of natural attributes have a competitive advantage over others, therefore classifying athletes according to their performance potential is not a suitable conceptual basis for classification in Paralympic sport.

that while it is common to refer to "classifying athletes", the IPC has recently reinforced that the unit of classification in Paralympic systems should be impairments, not athletes. This distinction is important because it emphasizes the fact that each athlete is a unique, sentient human being whose diversity and individuality cannot be captured by assigning a label or a class (Tweedy, 2002; Tweedy & Vanlandewijck, 2009).

To conclude this section on classification, an outline of the administrative and scientific challenges facing the movement is provided.

- Administrative challenges include:
  - Capacity building: The research questions that must be addressed in order to develop evidence-based classification methods are both conceptually and methodologically challenging. While the IPC maintains strong links in the medical fraternity, it does not have a strong scientific culture—particularly in classification—or broad engagement with the scientific community. Efforts to build scientific capacity are therefore required.
  - Realistic time frames: As important as changes are in this area, the IPC must be realistic about the time frames for developing and funding research projects, conducting them and implementing results. Years, not months, is the most appropriate metric.
  - Informed media management: Until evidence-based systems are in place, the information provided by the IPC to the media regarding classification, particularly the information provided when classification controversies inevitably arise, must be accurate and consistent. Moreover, the message must strike a balance between explaining that classification is a "work in progress", and causing the media to call into question the legitimacy of the Paralympic Movement.
  - Stakeholder involvement: The Paralympic Movement has been doing many things well for a long time, and the pressing need for reform in this area may not be immediately obvious to all. The movement must be careful to ensure that accurate, lay-language materials, and open forums explaining the urgency of the reforms are readily available.

- Scientific challenges include:
  - Developing research designs which evaluate the relative strength of association between eligible types of impairment—intellectual, strength, range of movement, coordination, etc.—and sports performance.
  - Recruiting samples of sufficient size to ensure credible results.

Acknowledgments

Sean Tweedy's work was supported by the Motor Accident Insurance Commission, Australia. This research was supported by the Australian Research Council (grant LP0882187), the International Paralympic Committee, the Australian Sports Commission, and the Australian Paralympic Committee.

Glossary

Activity An activity is the execution of a task or action by an individual. The term activity encompasses all sports-specific movement, including running, jumping, throwing, wheelchair pushing, shooting, and kicking.

Activity limitations Activity limitations are difficulties an individual may have in executing an activity. In Paralympic sport, activity limitations refer to difficulty executing the sports-specific movements required for a particular sport. Running is a core activity in the sport of athletics and a person who has difficulty running is said to have an *activity limitation* in running.

Body functions The body functions are the physiological functions of body systems (e.g., cardiovascular functions and sensory functions). The body functions of central concern in Paralympic sport are neuromusculoskeletal function, visual function, and intellectual function.

Body structures The body structures are anatomical parts of the body such as organs and limbs and their components. The body structures of central concern in Paralympic sport are those related to movement and include the motor centers of the brain and spinal cord, as well as the upper and lower limbs.

Function and disability In the ICF the terms "function" and "disability" are nonspecific umbrella terms that refer to several components of the ICF. For example, function can refer to neurological function (e.g., nerve conduction velocity), the ability to perform an activity (e.g., ability to run or jump) or functioning of a person in the community (e.g., to conduct financial affairs or access health services). To minimize ambiguity, the terms functioning and disability should be avoided when describing the purpose and conceptual bases of Paralympic classification.

Handicap The term "handicap" is not used in the ICF because of its pejorative connotations in English.

Health conditions Health conditions are diseases, disorders and injuries and are classified in the ICD-10: International Statistical Classification of Diseases and Related Health Problems (World Health Organization, 1992–1994), not the ICF. CP, spina bifida, and multiple sclerosis are examples of health conditions.

Impairments Impairments are problems with body functions or body structures. A person with a contracture at the right elbow would be described as having *impaired* range of movement. Paralympic classification systems should specify eligibility in terms of ICF impairment types (e.g., in the sport Judo, the classification system should specify that only VIs are classified).

The ICF The ICF is the acronym for the International Classification of Functioning, Disability and Health (ICF), published in 2001 by the World Health Organization. The ICF is an international standard for describing the functioning and disability associated with health.

Notes

1. The term locomotor here is inaccurate—it included people with upper limb weakness or loss of range of movement, impairments with minimal impact on locomotion.

2. Note: IOSD is not the name of an organization, but the collective acronym used to refer to international sports organizations that provide sports opportunities for people from different disability groups (e.g., CP-ISRA). The term should not be confused with ISOD, the umbrella organization founded in 1964 and which, in 2004 merged with ISMWSF to form the International Wheelchair and Amputee Sports Federation (IWAS).

References

Australian Bureau of Statistics. (2006). Sport and Recreation: a statistical overview, Australia, Canberra: Author.

Bailey, K.D. (1994). *Typologies and Taxonomies: An Introduction to Classification Techniques*. Sage Publications, Inc., Thousand Oaks, CA.

Bailey, S. (2007). *Athlete First: A History of the Paralympic Movement*. John Wiley and Sons Inc., Hoboken.

Brittain, I. (2010). *The Paralympic Games Explained*. Routledge, Abingdon.

Carvalho, J. & Farkas, A. (2005). Essay: Rehabilitation through sport—pilot project with amputees in Angola. *Lancet*, **366**, S5–S6.

Fleishman, E.A. & Quaintance, M.K. (1984). *Taxonomies of Human Performance*. Harcourt Brace Jovanovich, Orlando.

Gold, J.R. & Gold, M.M. (2007). Access for all: the rise of the Paralympic Games. *The Journal of the Royal Society for the Promotion of Health*, **127**, 133–141.

Goodman, S. (1986). *Spirit of Stoke Mandeville: the story of Ludwig Guttmann*. London: Collins.

Guttmann, L. (1976). *Textbook of Sport for the Disabled*. St. Lucia, Australia: University of Queensland Press.

Howe, P.D. (2008). *The Cultural Politics of the Paralympic Movement*. Abingdon: Routledge.

International Sports Organisation for the Disabled. (1993). *Handbook*. International Sports Organisation for the Disabled, Newmarket, ON.

International Paralympic Committee. (2007). *IPC Classification Code and International Standards*. Bonn, Germany.

International Paralympic Committee. (2006). *Position Statement Regarding the Participation of Athletes with an Intellectual Disability at IPC Sanctioned events*. Bonn, Germany.

Jahnke, B.S. (2006). *30th Anniversary Paralympic Winter Games 1976–2006*. RLC, Paris, France.

Røe, C., Dalen, H., Lein, M. & Bautz-Holter, E. (2008). Comprehensive rehabilitation at Beitostølen Healthsports Centre: influence on mental and physical functioning. *Journal of Rehabilitation Medicine*, **40(6)**, 410–417.

Scruton, J. (1998). *Stoke Mandeville: Road to the Paralympics*. Aylesbury: The Peterhouse Press.

Sherrill, C. (1999). "Disability sport and classification theory: a new era." *Adapted Physical Education Quarterly* **16(3)**, 206–215.

Tweedy, S.M. (2002). Taxonomic theory and the ICF: foundations for a unified disability athletics classification. *Adapted Physical Activity Quarterly*, **19(2)**, 220–237.

Tweedy, S.M. (2003). Biomechanical consequences of impairment: a taxonomically valid basis for classification in a unified disability athletics system. *Research Quarterly for Exercise and Sport*, **74(1)**, 9–16.

Tweedy, S.M. & Bourke, J. (2009). *IPC Athletics Classification Project for Physical Impairments: Final Report—Stage 1*. IPC Athletics, Bonn, 104.

Tweedy, S.M. & Vanlandewijck, Y.C. (2009). International Paralympic Committee Position Stand—background and scientific rationale for classification in Paralympic sport. *British Journal of Sports Medicine*. Published online 22 Oct 2009.

Vallerand, R.J. & Rousseau, F.L. (2001). Intrinsic and extrinsic motivation in sport and exercise. In: R.N. Singer, H.A. Hausenblaus, C.M. Janelle (eds.) *Handbook of Sport Psychology*, 2nd ed. John Wiley & Sons, Inc., New York.

Whitteridge, D. (2004). Guttmann, Sir Ludwig (1899–1980). In: *Oxford Dictionary of National Biography*, online ed. Oxford University Press, Oxford.

World Health Organization. (2001). *International Classification of Functioning, Disability, and Health*. Geneva, Switzerland.

Recommended readings

History of the Paralympic Movement

Bailey, S. (2007). *Athlete First: A History of the Paralympic Movement*. John Wiley and Sons Inc., Hoboken.

Guttmann, L. (1976). *Textbook of Sport for the Disabled*. University of Queensland Press, St. Lucia, Australia.

Howe, P.D. (2008). *The Cultural Politics of the Paralympic Movement*. Routledge, Abingdon.

Jahnke, B.S. (2006). *30th Anniversary Paralympic Winter Games 1976–2006*. RLC, Paris, France.

Paralympic Classification

International Paralympic Committee. (2007). *IPC Classification Code and International Standards*. Bonn, Germany.

Tweedy, S.M. & Vanlandewijck, Y.C. (2009). International Paralympic Committee Position Stand—background and scientific rationale for classification in Paralympic sport. *British Journal of Sports Medicine*, published online 22 Oct 2009.

PART 2
PARALYMPIC SPORT SCIENCE

Chapter 2
Biomechanics

*Ian Rice[1,2], Florentina J. Hettinga[3], Justin Laferrier[1,2],
Michelle L. Sporner[2], Christine M. Heiner[1,4], Brendan Burkett[5]
and Rory A. Cooper[1,2]*

[1]Human Engineering Research Laboratories, Department of Veterans Affairs,
 Rehabilitation Research and Development Service, Pittsburgh, PA, USA
[2]Department of Rehabilitation Science & Technology, University of Pittsburgh, Pittsburgh, PA, USA
[3]Center of Human Movement Sciences, University of Groningen/University Medical Center, Groningen,
 The Netherlands
[4]Department of Physical Medicine and Rehabilitation, University of Pittsburgh, Pittsburgh, PA, USA
[5]School of Health and Sport Sciences, University of the Sunshine Coast, Maroochydore DC, QLD, Australia

Introduction: sports for athletes with lower-limb disabilities

The wheelchair athlete and his/her wheelchair are inseparable and must seamlessly interface as a complete unit. After injury or trauma resulting in some degree of lower body paralysis, work once done by the legs is taken over by the arms. Arm work is less efficient and more strenuous compared to leg work, and can lead to lower physical capacity. Risks of mechanical overuse are higher and because of overuse injuries, mobility can decrease. Nevertheless, high-level sports performance is possible with subsequent increases in physical fitness, health, and mobility. Not only wheelchair athletes, but also individuals with lower-limb loss compete at high levels in Paralympic running events with prosthetic devices. At the elite level, runners with artificial limbs/lower-limb prostheses have even been suggested to have the potential to outperform able-bodied runners, which is an ongoing topic of debate.

The Paralympic Athlete, 1st edition. Edited by Yves C. Vanlandewijck and Walter R. Thompson. Published 2011 by Blackwell Publishing Ltd.

Knowledge of user interfaces and the study of wheelchair propulsion biomechanics have shaped equipment design and improved athletic performance. Impact on wheelchair racing, basketball, rugby, and handcycling will be discussed in the first part of the chapter. Then, athletes with major limb loss will be discussed separately in the final section, as their equipment needs are distinct from the wheelchair athletes.

Wheelchair–user interface

The question of how to minimize injury and maximize performance is vital to the long-term success of any wheelchair athlete. Numerous performance-determining factors relate to one's potential for achievement in everyday propulsion as well as in sports. It has been suggested that the wheelchair–user interface may be the most critical, yet least understood performance-determining factor. An optimized user interface should maximize the user's functional abilities without restricting them in any way. The user's goals and abilities must be considered while aligning critical chair dimensions to the athlete's anthropometrics. Subsequently, the equipment and user should be thought of as one unit and the chair as an extension of the body. Many of the principles for fitting a sports wheelchair are similar to those for fitting a prosthetic limb. For instance, wheelchair technology has led to task-specific devices individually adjusted to the user, further leading to enhanced mobility and efficiency. For example, handcycling has become increasingly popular for long-distance everyday travel, recreation, and elite sport. Handcycling was added as an official event to the Paralympics in 2004. Particularly for elite sports performance, high-tech wheelchairs and handcycling (Figure 2.1) options are available and are commonly customized and tuned to individual characteristics (Figures 2.2–2.4).

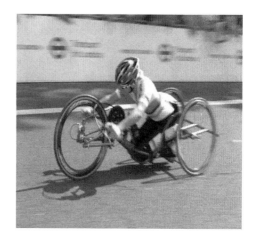

Figure 2.1 Female handcycling (kneeling position).

Classification Handbikes

AP	AP1	AP2	AP3	1	ATP	ATP1	ATP2	ATP3
Arm-Power				2	Arm-Trunk-Power			
wheelchair-sit	recumbent 60°	recumbent 30°	recumbent 0°	3	wheelchair-sit	car-seat	long-seat	knee-seat
upright	reclined	reclined	reclined	4	forward	forward	forward	forward
attach-unit	rigid frame	rigid frame	rigid frame	5	attach-unit	rigid frame	rigid frame	rigid frame
				6				
100%	62.6%	39.6%	33.3%	7	96.8%	82.8%	60.9%	60.3%
tour	tour	competition	competition	8	tour	tour	competition	competition
		H1,H2,H3	H1,H2,H3	9			H3	H4

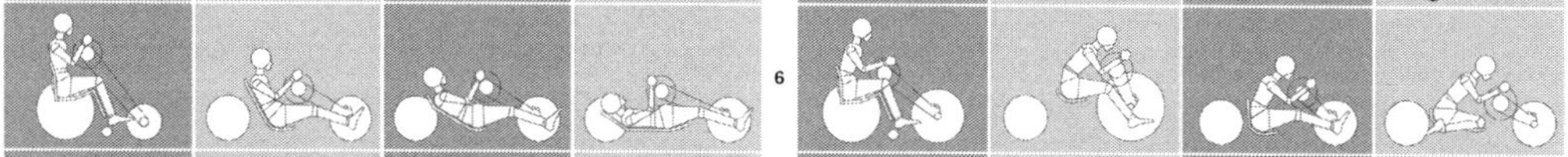

1=class handbike 2=propulsion-type 3=sitting-type 4=trunkposture 5=handbike-type 6=illustration 7=frontal area 8=handbike-use 9=competition-division © Double Performance • Handbike Expertise Centrum

Figure 2.2 Classification of handcycles divided into arm-power and arm–trunk-power models according to Double Performance, a handcycling expertise center in the Netherlands (www.doubleperformance.nl).

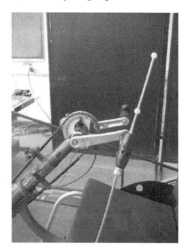

Figure 2.3 Instrumented handle bar with 6 degrees of freedom to measure forces and torques in 3D.

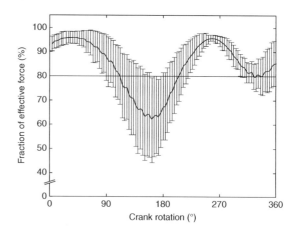

Figure 2.4 Mean and standard deviation of fraction of effective force for handbiking at a mean velocity of 1.39 m/s ($0° =$ top; $180° =$ bottom).

Wheelchair propulsion biomechanics

Propulsion and injury prevention

Understanding propulsion biomechanics is vital to performance and injury reduction, because the propulsive motion in and of itself has been shown to be relatively inefficient. The gross mechanical efficiency (ME) (the ratio between power output and energy expenditure) of everyday handrim propulsion is between 5% and 11%, which is lower than arm ergometry (16%), handcycling (18–21%), and wheelchair racing (15–23%). Sports equipments' geometry, design, and user interface combined with an athlete's conditioning and ability can influence ME.

For the past two decades, researchers around the world have developed methods for analyzing pushrim forces critical to assessing injury mechanisms and propulsion efficiency. For example, researchers at the Department of Veterans Affairs/ University of Pittsburgh Human Engineering Research Labs (HERL) have developed instrumentation to measure kinetics during wheelchair propulsion through a device known as the SmartWheel (Cooper et al., 1997a,b). HERL's studies have found stable pushrim force and moment measures that change with speed, and are also statistically valid metrics (Boninger et al., 1997).

Researchers at HERL have also found wheelchair pushrim forces to be related to nerve conduction variables. Specifically, they have used median nerve conduction studies to diagnose carpal tunnel syndrome and found that when controlling for weight, there were correlations between median nerve function, cadence of propulsion, and rate and rise of the resultant force (Boninger et al., 1999). As a follow-up to this work, longitudinal analysis was completed. This data showed that risk of injury to the median nerve could be predicted by wheelchair propulsion biomechanics (Boninger et al., 2005). For example, 100 individuals who used greater force and cadence during their initial lab visit had greater progression in median nerve damage approximately 3 years later (Boninger et al., 1999). Peak resultant force was also found to be a predictor of the progression of nerve conduction abnormalities. The resulting increased force was found to be highly correlated with the weight-normalized peak resultant force. In another study, researchers found an inverse relationship between median nerve health and range of motions at the wrist (Boninger et al., 2004). Greater range of motion was associated with better median nerve function. They later found that greater wrist range of motion was associated with greater push angles, lower forces, and cadence. Therefore, researchers determined that by taking long strokes, wheelchair users were able to generate greater work without high peak forces.

Additionally, HERL researchers have published many peer-reviewed journal publications on magnetic resonance imaging (MRI) and X-ray imaging studies on people with paraplegia (Boninger et al., 2001). The results of these imaging studies showed a high prevalence of osteolysis of the distal clavicle, which can be a debilitating type of repetitive strain-type injury. However, this study found a much lower prevalence of rotator cuff tears than that reported by Escobedo et al. (1997). The main difference between the two studies was the age of the participating populations. The study by Escobedo et al. focused on an older group with more years since injury. These combined results point to the need for injury prevention, so that the younger populations do not develop these problems later in life.

Because of this work, wheelchair users have been encouraged to use a more forward rear axle position to promote low-frequency, long smooth strokes (larger contact angle) during the propulsive phase. Higher stroke frequencies have been shown to correlate to median nerve injury and lead to increased blood lactate, heart rate, and cardiorespiratory stress. Utilizing a larger contact angle while holding velocity constant enables a person to do the same propulsive work over a longer period of time, loading the handrim less rapidly and potentially reducing the increase in resultant force.

Propulsion efficiency

A properly fit manual wheelchair should offer freedom and efficiency during propulsion. However, defining what that is mechanically and determining the ideal propulsion technique can be complex (Cooper & Bedi, 1990). Work by de Groot et al. (2002) has indicated that the most effective propulsion technique is not necessarily the most efficient propulsion technique from a biological point of view. For instance, when individuals have been trained to apply propulsion forces in a more effective mechanical direction while generating the same external power, gross ME decreases. In essence, because of a fixed arm posture, there is little freedom to optimize force once the hand has grasped the pushrim. Ultimately, the direction of force is likely based on achieving a balance between energy cost and force effectiveness (de Groot et al., 2002). It has also been suggested that during propulsion, both forces and task repetition should be kept to a minimum in order to reduce the risk of injury (Boninger et al., 1999).

Modeling propulsion

Performance modeling addresses the development and application of predictive, reliable, and quantitative models of performance. Human performance modeling considers the human engaged in some goal-directed behavior, in the context of a designed task within a specific environment. In order to evaluate human performance, it is essential to have an appropriate model. The following section will discuss how the power balance model (PBM) and the cyclic concept of propulsion have been applied to the study of wheelchair athletics to improve performance.

Wheelchair propulsion and handcycling are best described as cyclic movements. This means that propulsion is a motion repeated over time at a given frequency (f) to maintain a certain velocity (v). With each push, the rider produces either more or less equal work (A). The product of push frequency and work yields the average external power output (P_o):

$$P_o = f \times A(W)$$

Linking physiological measures (such as energy cost and physical strain) to biomechanical measures (such as power output, work, force, and torque) can be a useful approach in studying the cyclic movements associated with propulsion. For example, work per push can be calculated as the integral of the momentary torque (M) applied by the hands to the handrim over a more or less fixed angular displacement (Q):

$$P_o = f \times \Sigma M \times dQ(W)$$

Torque is defined as the product of bimanual tangential force applied to the handrim and the radius of the handrim. The measurement of angular displacement and the torque around the wheel axle requires specialized experimental techniques for motion analysis and force measurement. In handcycling, energy is transferred from the hands to the crank to go forward. P_o can thus be calculated by multiplying torque applied to the crank with angular velocity. As mentioned earlier, the athlete is the one generating power to propel based on his/her physical capacity. Facts such as upper body muscle force and peak power output must be considered when optimizing the wheelchair to meet the performance needs of the athlete.

Modeling can be particularly useful when studying the performance of a small subject population, which is often the case in wheelchair athletics research. One specific method for the study of cyclic human (sports) performance is through the use of a PBM as proposed by Ingen Schenau (1988). This energy flow model has been used in numerous studies to describe and predict optimal performance in different cyclic sports such as speed skating, cycling, rowing, swimming, and running (Ingen Schenau & Cavanagh, 1990) and in rehabilitation settings such as wheelchair propulsion, handcycling, or walking with an impairment (Groen et al., 2010; Hettinga et al., 2010; van der Woude et al., 2001). PBM gives insight into performance-determining factors of these different modes of cyclic endurance exercise and can thus help to explain performance. For example, it can be used to predict optimal pacing strategy in middle-distance sports such as cycling and speed skating.

Generally speaking, the PBM approach includes the wheelchair and user as a free body that moves with a given speed and encounters drag forces. The athlete is described in terms of mechanical energy resulting in the power balance. While propelling at a constant velocity, the athlete must overcome drag forces and internal friction (F_{int}). Drag forces during propulsion or handcycling are rolling friction (F_{rol}) and air resistance (F_{air}). When going up or down a slope (α), gravitational effects ($m \times g \times \sin \alpha$) also play a role. Accelerations and decelerations are represented by changes in kinetic energy over the race.

The power balance for wheelchair racing and handcycling can thus be described as:

$$P_o = (F_{rol} + F_{air} + F_{int} + m \times g \times \sin \alpha + m \times a) \times v$$

where P_o is the total mechanical power, F_{rol} is the force necessary to overcome rolling resistance, F_{air} is the force necessary to overcome air resistance, F_{int} is the internal force, m is the body mass, g is the gravitational force, α is the angle of inclination, and a is the acceleration of the system.

In daily use, rolling resistance is generally the major resisting force. Rolling resistance can be determined by a coast-down technique or a drag test, and is dependent on floor surface and the characteristics of wheels and tires, since the amount of friction is related to the amount of deformation of tire and floor surface.

However, in wheelchair racing and elite handcycling, velocities are higher; up to 80% of the produced energy is lost to air friction. Factors such as frontal plane area reduction, adaptation of seat position, and orientation of the segments of the body and skin suits will influence the drag coefficient. Energy losses within the wheelchair are very small and are caused by bearing friction around the wheel axles and in the wheel suspension of the castor wheels, and possibly by the deformation of the frame in folding wheelchairs during the force exertion in the push phase.

Performance has been modeled in elite handcyclists using the PBM, which provided indicators of mechanical constraints (air friction, rolling friction), submaximal as well as peak performance, concomitant metabolic cost, and ME. Realistic values for power output and power losses were obtained on an indoor cycling track with all physiological responses occurring as well. Mean gross efficiency was found to be 17.9% ± 1.6%. The empirically derived relationship between velocity and power output, i.e., the PBM, on the track was:

$$P_o = 0.20v^3 + 2.90v \ (R^2 = 0.95)$$

in which 0.20 represents the air friction constant and 2.90 represents the rolling friction force (Figure 2.5). The PBM therefore enabled the simulation of realistic power conditions on a treadmill. In addition, it helped the researchers to understand the magnitude of power production and dissipation during elite handcycling.

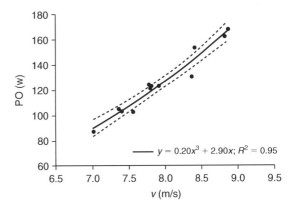

Figure 2.5 The empirically derived relationship between velocity and power output in handbiking. PO, power output.

Wheelchair sports

As mentioned earlier, user interfaces and propulsion biomechanics are vital to performance, injury reduction, and the long-term success of the user. It is also evident that many aspects of everyday wheelchair propulsion, configuration, and user interface translate to the study of wheelchair sports. In the following section, we will examine wheelchair racing, basketball, rugby, and handcycling because of their popularity and status in the Paralympic games. Furthermore, the study of biomechanics and interface of the everyday wheelchair are good starting points in understanding many of the elements of wheelchair athletics. These comparisons must be made cautiously, however, because inherent differences exist between the two. These differences are visible in the speeds and intensity in which activity occur, the tendency toward extreme chair configurations, and, of course, in the conditioning of the athletes.

Wheelchair racing

For optimal performance, racing wheelchairs must be designed and customized to the anatomical features and functional capabilities of each user. A racing chair used in combination with correct propulsion biomechanics can result in an extremely efficient means of movement above and beyond all other handrim sports. Racers have been able to achieve impressive speeds, well in excess of 8 m/s on flat over ground and 9 m/s on a dynamometer. The design of a racing wheelchair optimizes the abilities of each user, incorporating features such as three-wheeled design, high-pressure lightweight tubular tires, lightweight rims, precision hubs, carbon disk/spokes wheels, compensator steering, small handrims, ridged frame construction, and up to 15° of wheel camber. The camber in a racing chair increases its lateral stability and allows the athlete to maintain adequate clearance inside of the arm with the wheel at the bottom of a propulsive stroke. Typical anatomical measurements considered when configuring a racing chair include hip width, chest width, thigh length, arm length, trunk length, height, and weight. In addition, racers position themselves so that paralyzed or weaker portions of the body are brought close to those under voluntary control, which helps increase chair handling, stability, and ultimately propulsion (Cooper et al., 1993).

The frame and seat cage of a racing chair are made to fit each individual, including different disability etiologies and levels. The seat cage upholstery adjustment and rear axle positions are fitted to allow athletes to position their shoulders over the front edge of the pushrims, also creating room to reach the bottom of the pushrims with both arms. Individuals with upper-level spinal cord injury tend to pull their knees up higher toward the chest than do lower-level-injured athletes to further enhance stability, balance, and breathing.

A properly fitted racing chair enables the user to make minor steering adjustments by swinging the upper body or hips. Racers often refer to this maneuver as "hipping" the chair. A racing chair's primary steering, however, is controlled by the upper body's interaction with the front wheel, where pressure can be applied to handle bars, which turn the front wheel from left to right. When racing on a track, athletes use an additional steering component called a compensator that can be engaged with one hand while taking the chair around the curve of a track and then disengaged to accommodate the strait section.

Perhaps the most unique and critical aspect of racing is apparent in the highly specialized propulsive stroke used by the wheelchair athlete. The stroke allows a racer to maintain chair control at high rates of speed for long periods of time. In general, racing propulsion is distinct from everyday or upright propulsion because racers use specialized gloves (Figures 2.6 and 2.7), customize their chairs with large wheels with small handrim diameter, and position their bodies aerodynamically (Cooper, 1990). Racing gloves are available commercially or can be constructed independently by each racer. These gloves are often built using a combination of leather, foam, rubber, and self-molding plastics. Racing gloves promote solid contact between the glove surface and the push ring. This setup allows skilled athletes to productively keep up with the wheel at very high speeds and to deliver more force per stroke to the wheel, minimizing slips and other contact- and release-related inefficiencies. Researchers have found that when velocity increases, the duration of each stroke time decreases, meaning the athlete must apply a greater impulse, applying force over the propulsion phase of the stroke in a shorter push time (Cooper, 1995; van der Woude et al., 1989). A racing glove allows the athlete to match or exceed the speed of the handrim upon contact more precisely without having to actually grip the handrim.

The racing stroke is an involved process taking years to learn. Consequentially, researchers like Cooper (1995) and Higgs (1993) have dissected the stroke into its component parts and phases. Cooper described the racing stroke as a technique where extensive shoulder extension and abduction during the backswing lead to increased hand speed at the impact energy transfer phase. When speed increases, athletes will also demonstrate a shift in contact angle from the top front to top bottom and also execute the drive phase at a faster rate than the recovery phase. There are a total of five phases (see Figure 2.6):

1. drive forward and downward,
2. pushrim contact,
3. pushing through to the bottom of the pushrims,
4. push-off or follow through,
5. elbow drive to the top.

Cooper (1995) determined that the factors relating to injury-free wheelchair propulsion include the proper hand trajectory when approaching the pushrim, the coupling of body segments to effectively

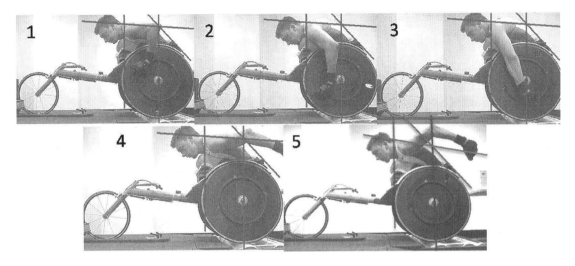

Figure 2.6 Five phases of the racing stroke—(1) drive forward and downward, (2) pushrim contact, (3) pushing through to the bottom of the pushrims, (4) push-off or follow through, and (5) elbow drive to the top.

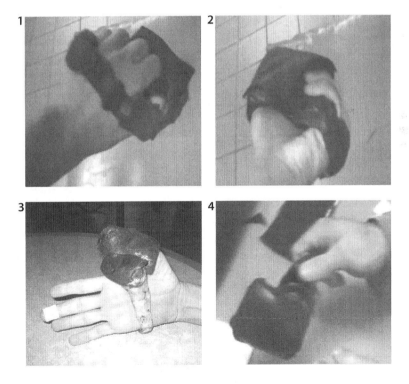

Figure 2.7 (1–4) Variations of the custom-made solid wheelchair racing glove. (2–4) Palmer views of a glove where 3 is designed for thumb catch technique. 2 and 4 are more traditionally designed, where the cuticle region serves as the point of contact.

transfer energy from one segment to another, the angle with which the arms are brought forward and downward so that the prime movers of the upper extremity (UE) are used effectively, maintaining the hand–forearm tangential with the pushrim following contact, and maintaining contact with the rim throughout the propulsion range of motion. Possible causes of inefficiency include the person not being appropriately seated fore-aft, or up-down, the pushrim and wheel size not being appropriate for the person's anthropometry and etiology, and incorrect seat and leg angle, which may restrict motion, or not provide sufficient seating stability and poor temporal sequencing of the torso and upper extremities.

Another critical element of the racing stroke is evident in the use of small-diameter handrims (see Figures 2.6 and 2.8). Van der Woude et al. (1988) have suggested that stroke kinematics is related to push-ring diameter, speed, workload, and fitness of the athlete. Van der Woude et al. (1988) concluded that smaller handrims can reduce cardiovascular stress because a larger handrim requires the athlete to use greater hand speed to achieve an equivalent velocity. However, it is evident that larger handrims can be beneficial when more torque is needed, as in the case of hill climbing or in quick accelerations, but at a metabolic cost. The athlete must ultimately find a handrim diameter that suits his/her overall needs, because only one size is permitted per race. Some elite racers have multiple chairs or wheels with varying sized pushrims: one for track sprinting events (>16 in. diameter) and another for road racing (13–15 in. diameter).

Basketball/rugby

The type of wheelchair used in basketball and rugby is somewhat similar to an individual's personal everyday wheelchair but incorporates other features to enhance maneuverability. These chairs are designed to be lightweight to allow for acceleration from a standstill, and during braking, turning (pivoting), and screening (Vanlandewijck et al., 2001). Rugby, however, incorporates considerable chair-on-chair contact, which can include hitting, picking, and blocking. Consequently, athletes in both sports tend to use a large handrim diameter (see Figure 2.8) that offers the user a higher turning moment. In a study of elite basketball players, Coutts (1992) explained that larger diameter pushrims permit the athlete to generate a more effective force–time impulse, leading to greater increase in velocity and momentum when starting from a speed of zero. Rugby players typically choose a low seat height for improved balance and maneuverability, whereas basketball players determine seat height based on both functional level and team role. For example, guards and forwards make choices based on maneuverability and fast acceleration (outside basketball), whereas center players typically opt for an upright chair favoring a high floor-to-seat height ratio to play in the bucket with more physical presence (inside basketball) (Vanlandewijck et al., 2001).

To compensate for UE impairments, rugby players tend to use extreme wheelchair configurations, in addition to elastic binders, foams, and special tacky gloves all to improve performance. As in basketball, rugby players often become extremely

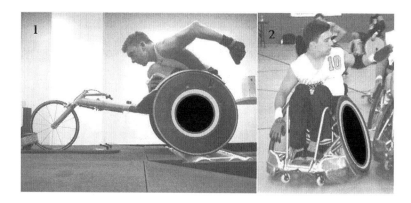

Figure 2.8 (1) a racing chair where the handrim is much smaller in diameter relative to the wheel when compared to the rugby chair's handrim (2).

proficient at adapting their equipment to promote balance and speed. The styles of wheelchairs used in rugby vary considerably depending on each player's preference, functional level, and team role. Players with the most extreme upper body deficits tend to take on more defensive blocking and picking roles and use chairs that have additional length and hardware that enables them to grab other players' chairs. Players with more functional ability are the primary ball handlers and use offensive chairs built for scoring, which requires speed and quick maneuverability similar to basketball. In addition, many ball handlers' chairs are designed to deflect or slide off of other chairs to minimize the likelihood of being stopped or held. Regardless of functional abilities and classification, all rugby chairs have extreme amounts of camber, 16–20°, significant bucketing, and anti-tip bars. The camber provides lateral stability, hand protection, and ease in turning. The bucketing (i.e., knees are high relative to rear end) helps with trunk balance and protection of the ball.

In general, research on wheelchair sports performance is sparse; however, there have been a few studies specific to wheelchair rugby athletes. Goosey-Tolfrey et al. (2006) used arm ergometry to study the aerobic fitness levels of rugby athletes, whereas Abel et al. (2008) used metabolic measures to verify the energy expenditure of wheelchair basketball, tennis, and rugby players.

The following section describes the application of a recently developed activity monitoring technology used in a study to gain knowledge about the speed and distance traveled by wheelchair athletes. It is the hope that technologies like the one described below can not only enhance training and sports performance, but can also record information relevant to injury prevention in a population of individuals reliant on their upper extremities to perform nearly all activities of daily function.

Historically, athletes have used personal feedback monitors to enhance performance. Monitors can measure a variety of variables related to physical output such as force, power, speed, and distance. More athletes with disabilities could take advantage of these technologies during training and competition to improve performance. To date, no published data exists on distances and speeds traveled by rugby or basketball players during game play. In order to collect quantitative data from actual game play, researchers at HERL used miniaturized wheelchair-mounted data logger in a study on athletes at the National Veterans Wheelchair Games. A miniaturized data logger is a device that collects time stamp information that allows for the calculation of velocity, distance, and time when the wheelchair is in motion. Activity time was defined as the sum of time the wheelchair was in motion, and a stop and start was defined as 2 s or more with no wheelchair motion. The average speed was calculated by dividing the total distance by time. Prior to the start of the basketball and rugby tournament at the National Veterans Wheelchair Games, each athlete was fitted with a data logger on his/her sport wheelchair. The miniaturized data loggers were attached to the spokes of the wheelchair in a location that did not interfere with propulsion and game activity (Sporner et al., 2009).

The results showed that over the course of two games, the wheelchair rugby athletes on average traveled 2364.78 ± 956.35 m at 1.33 ± 0.25 m/s with 242.61 ± 80.31 stops and starts in 29.98 ± 11.79 min of play per game. The wheelchair basketball athletes averaged over two games $2679.52 + 1103.66$ m traveled at $1.48 + 0.13$ m/s with 239.78 ± 60.61 stops and starts in $30.28 + 9.59$ min of play per game.

In community-based studies done with miniaturized data loggers, veterans in their everyday wheelchairs traveled 2456.95 ± 1195.73 m/day at a speed of 0.79 ± 0.19 m/s. One should then note the overall intensity of game play found in wheelchair basketball and rugby. The implication of the findings in the Veterans Wheelchair Games is that everyday propulsion is unlikely to adequately prepare a player for competition; therefore, appropriate training techniques need to be further developed and implemented. Data collected from the miniaturized data loggers during game play and practices could be provided to players and coaches and could be used to create training protocols that more accurately reflect game conditions. The ability to quantify how far and how fast athletes travel during practice and actual competitive games may provide beneficial training information for organized wheelchair sports.

Similar to rugby, wheelchair basketball has been described as an activity composed of intermittent intense and medium phases of play and, thus, can be considered an alternating aerobic–anaerobic sport. Coutts (1992) analyzed two basketball players during a 40-min game, and estimated that 64% of the time was spent in propulsive action and 36% in braking activity at both high (>50 W) and low (<−50 W) intensities, with significant amounts of coasting time in between. This equated to roughly 4 min of intense propulsion and 4 min of braking action or positive and negative work. Although not quantified in this study, it was apparent that the athletes spent significant amounts of cardiovascular energy during offensive and defensive actions. Burke et al. (1985) and Schmid et al. (1998) found that during game play, basketball players maintained heart rates close to levels achieved during maximal exercise test. In addition, Sporner et al. (2009) found that with respect to the basketball classification, Class 2 and 3 athletes traveled farther with more starts and stops than the Class 1 athletes. All three classes (National Wheelchair Basketball Association (NWBA) classification system) traveled at roughly the same velocity and played for the same amount of time during a basketball game (Sporner et al., 2009).

As previously mentioned, acceleration and starts from a standstill are important to both rugby and basketball players. In fact, athletes have been shown to achieve 80% of their maximal speed 4.02 m/s within the first three strokes of a sprint (Coutts, 1990). Vanlandewijck et al. (2001) noted that the ability to reach top speeds quickly allows an athlete to maintain a positional advantage, therefore, compensating for lack of speed over longer distances.

The requirements to play rugby and basketball suggest that an athlete should be cognizant of their wheelchair configuration, wheelchair–user interface, body mass, and strength and conditioning. For example, a properly configured chair should minimize wheelchair drag force as much as possible. Aspects of a wheelchair impacting drag include tire pressure, chair alignment, and minimized caster flutter. Camber is an important feature in basketball wheelchairs as well. Camber makes a wheelchair more responsive during turns and protects players' hands when two wheelchairs collide from the sides,

by limiting the collision to the bottom of the wheels and leaving a space at the top to protect the hands. Although wheelchair camber is essential to both rugby and basketball, a study by Faupin et al. (2004) showed that residual torque increased in proportion to increased wheel camber. Coutts (1994) has suggested that athletes performing a simple coast-down race between players of approximately the same body weight (to identify who slows down more rapidly when coasting down from the same speed) can be used to identify wheelchairs that need adjustment when excessive drag is apparent.

The wheelchair–athlete interface, another aspect of performance, is dictated by a number of parameters, including classification of player, level of function, and team position or role. In terms of athlete positioning, the center of gravity (Cg), which is determined largely by the vertical and horizontal position of the rear axle, is a key component related to wheelchair–user interface. A rearward shift of Cg or a more forward axle position tends to decrease the rolling resistance and reduce the inertial rotation torque experienced by the wheelchair and user. A downward shift in Cg or sitting deep in a chair can decrease reaction torque on the trunk and wheelchair and also the vertical distance between the shoulder and axle making pushrim easier to reach. This results in a larger available push angle and allows force to be imparted to the wheelchair pushrim for a longer time, thus decreasing the frequency of propulsion necessary to maintain speed. However, what is ideal for propulsion may not always benefit a basketball player such as a center who needs to sit as tall as possible. As mentioned earlier, each player must compromise in order to maximize both propulsion and role on the court.

Handcycling

Handcycling can be an extremely effective form of exercise for individuals with a broad range of disabilities and can also serve as a useful rehabilitation tool. Not only has handcycling proven to be an efficient means of upper body exercise (high gross ME and increased levels of peak power output), but it has also been shown to place less strain on the upper limbs than other forms of activities like handrim propulsion. The continuous power generation over the full cycle in handcycling results in a greater gross ME compared to handrim propulsion. In addition, cranks and levers in handcycling allow the use of all flexor and extensor muscles around the arm–shoulder joints to actively contribute to external work over the full motion cycle; the latter is in contrast to handrim propulsion where the discontinuous motion allows active work only during 30–40% of the cycle.

The fact that handcycling does not appear to place a person at added risk of developing injury is another benefit of the sport. In fact, a study in 2009 found that patients with tetraplegia were able to improve their physical capacity through regular handcycle interval training, without increased shoulder–arm pain or discomfort (Valent et al., 2009). This is of vital importance because compared to the general population, wheelchair users are at an elevated risk of experiencing UE pain and injury and are less likely to engage in regular physical activity, which can lead to diminished cardiovascular health. It is interesting to note that wheelchair athletes have also been shown to have better psychological profiles than nonathletes.

When set up properly, a handcycle can be an extremely efficient means of propulsion; however, configuring a cycle can be a daunting process. The handcycle offers the user extreme adjustability and component/positioning options. The following factors are crucial when customizing a handcycle: upright versus recumbent or trunk powered positioning, seat angle and position relative to cranks, seat-to-floor height, wheel size and camber, footrest alignment, asynchronous versus synchronous cranking, gear ratios, crank arm length/width, and handgrip style. Upright, recumbent, or trunk powered distinctions refer to the multiple ways the user's body can be positioned. The most primitive types of handcycles are upright cycles and are add-ons that can be attached to a person's everyday wheelchair. The user sits with nearly 90° hip and knee flexion and uses a pivot steer where only the front wheel turns while the cycle remains in an upright position. The benefits of this setup include safer transfers, which makes them popular for new and recreational riders and for those with higher-level disabilities. Upright cycles are less aerodynamic having a high center of gravity, which can

make them susceptible to tips and falls. In contrast, a recumbent handcycle incorporates a reclined back angle that can be fully extended in some cases, with the athlete's legs positioned straight out in front. This setup leads to improved aerodynamics and provides a great deal of support for those without trunk control; the only drawback is that they can be difficult to transfer into. A trunk powered cycle offers the user a body position similar to that of a racing wheelchair, where the rider sits on the shins with the legs tucked up under the torso. This allows for using trunk range of motion when cranking as well as a more aerodynamic profile (see Figure 2.2). Faupin et al. (2008) found that athletes without trunk impairment actually benefited from a sitting style without a backrest. As mentioned previously, in a trunk powered configuration (little to no backrest), the cyclist does not recline against the seat-back as they would in an upright or recumbent-styled handcycle. During trunk powered propulsion, an athlete leans forward with each push and backward with each pull, using the weight of the upper torso to add power to each stroke. This allows riders to more fully utilize abdominal and lower back musculature in addition to the arm, chest, and upper back.

Recent studies have explored how performance is affected by many of these setup and positioning options. For example, van der Woude et al. (2000) found synchronous or in-phase hand cranking to be more efficient than asynchronous cranking, which can lead to higher peak performance. Studies have also shown synchronous handcycling to be more efficient and less strenuous than asynchronous cranking on a motor-driven treadmill. In these studies, cranking occurred at a constant external workload and at the same speed and slope. The lower peak performance and ME in asynchronous cycling is due to the increased muscular co-contraction that occurs in the upper extremities and trunk when one attempts to simultaneously produce power while steering. Synchronous cranking that occurs in the same angular pattern prevents this conflict from occurring.

Another important element of the hand crank configuration includes grip orientation. For instance, Kramer et al. (2009) found that able-bodied subjects were able to generate more power using a pronated handle grip with a fixed orientation of

30°, which is distinct from what can be achieved with conventional handles oriented perpendicular to the ground. Goosey-Tolfrey et al. (2008) found that crank length had a significant impact on ME, where a shorter 180-mm length was more efficient than 200 mm regardless of pedal rate. Power was also shown to improve when crank length to forward reach (FR) ratio was 26% and crank width to shoulder breadth (SB) ratio was 85%. Finally, exercise intensity has been found to influence gross and net efficiency in handcycling. It was concluded that these findings were due to higher relative cost of basal metabolism at lower intensities. Other factors that affect gross efficiency include temperature, pedal frequency, volume, and intensity.

Although the aforementioned results have contributed substantially to the understanding of user interface in handcycling, additional work is needed. For example, van der Woude et al. (2000) have suggested that other aspects of the wheelchair–user interface must be studied in order to generate optimum fitting and design guidelines for different user groups and conditions of use.

Sports biomechanics and the Paralympic amputee

The Paralympic athlete, who has an amputation, raises unique challenges within the discipline of biomechanics. To create an effective "connection" between the individual athlete and their prosthetic device, a complex integration of the purely mechanical prosthesis and the residual musculoskeletal system is required. This results in distinctive biomechanical loads being generated as the athlete conducts daily activities, such as walking, through to the extreme overload situations they create when training for, and competing in, the Paralympic games. To discuss sports biomechanics and the Paralympic amputee, this section is subdivided into two sections that reflect the two scenarios in which the Paralympic athlete competes: (a) sport biomechanics: the amputee with their prosthesis and (b) sport biomechanics: the amputee without their prosthesis. This section ends with a short section on future directions in sport biomechanics for amputees.

Sport biomechanics: the amputee with their prosthesis

For activities such as walking or running, the lower-limb amputee naturally depends on the prosthetic technology to carry out this task. Advances in technology underpin such assistive devices, e.g., the development of the energy-storing prosthetic foot can make a lower-limb amputee's gait more efficient and ambulation faster. Sport biomechanics has identified the kinematic and kinetic parameters of amputee gait, in particular the difference between the anatomical and prosthetic limb of the amputee, as well as comparing these profiles with the typical population. The identification of standard biomechanical measures of range of movement at key joints of the ankle, knee, and hips provides vital knowledge to athlete and coach on what factors that influence performance. A similar scenario is generated when analyzing the angular velocity or angular accelerations at each of these joints. As shown in Figure 2.9, for a unilateral transfemoral Paralympic amputee, when walking the anatomical and prosthetic hip angle are similar, but once the athlete runs, there is a dramatic difference in the anatomical and prosthetic hip angle—creating the complex biomechanical challenge for the sport scientist, athlete, and coach.

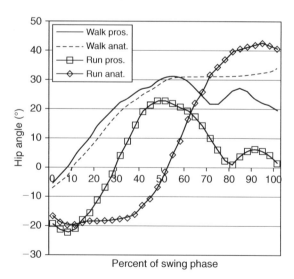

Figure 2.9 Hip angle for transfemoral amputee, comparing anatomical and prosthetic limb when walking and running.

Biomechanical technology such as load cells has allowed the high-frequency measurement of "what forces are actually being developed and transferred" as a consequence of the sporting activity. Classic examples include the impact forces on the foot when running. This scientific knowledge allows modifications made to the sporting equipment, and/or the technique for addressing this issue. Technology in this area has improved the functional performance of machines, or created new devices, such as plyometrics to reduce injury risk and enhance sports performance.

The Paralympic athlete has a greater dependence on this knowledge; due to their disability, any lost function needs to be compensated with support coming from another area. Examples of biomechanical applications in Paralympics include the "functional" design of prostheses for highly active amputees through the energy storing carbon-fiber Flex foot, which is different from the amputee sailor's peg leg. To take full advantage of the energy storing foot, the athlete lands on the prosthetic toe, extending the hip throughout the support phase and achieving maximal deflection of the foot. In other sports, the prosthesis is simply a device to "connect" the athlete with the equipment, such as cycling. For example, if the cyclist has an arm disability, the aerobars may be modified to allow the upper-limb prosthesis to be attached, similarly if the cyclist has a lower-limb amputation the cycling cleat may be fixed directly to the prosthetic limb.

To address the unique requirements within the three field events of shot put, javelin, and discus, athletes may have three sport-specific prostheses built in addition to their everyday prosthesis. For example, the need for support during the rotation phase of the shot put or discus requires different properties in a prosthetic device as compared to the need for stability and linear velocity when running in to throw a javelin. The specific rotation requirements for performing the shot put and discus events have resulted in the development of the J-Leg technology. This prosthesis essentially has a fixed knee unit to provide stability throughout the rotation, and an energy-storing foot has been mounted at 180 to the standard orientation (i.e., toe facing posteriorly). This alignment facilitates extra stability in rotation, and the energy-releasing characteristics of the foot also provide the desired ground push-off before the throw release.

Within the previous Paralympiad, there has been a shift in jumping technique, with transtibial and transfemoral amputees now making the touchdown step with their prosthetic rather than their anatomical limb. According to the principles of projectile motion, a key requirement for this task is maximum velocity at takeoff. Due to the recent advances in prosthetic technology, athletes have found that their prosthetic limbs can absorb and release the ground reaction force more effectively than their anatomical limbs, thus generating higher velocities at takeoff. Prosthetic feet used for running are plantar flexed and do not have a heel to keep sprinters on their toes. The distal posterior pylon is severely bowed, lengthening the foot plate to increase the moment arm for maximal deflection, propelling the athlete's limb into the acceleration phase of swing as the material energy is returned. To take full advantage of this foot, the athlete lands on the prosthetic toe, extending the hip throughout the support phase and achieving maximal deflection of the foot. The three preferred knee system designs for transfemoral athletes are a hydraulic cylinder with a single axis frame that offers athletes a wide range of resistance adjustment and stance control; however, most competitive athletes use a swing-only hydraulic unit because stance control is no longer necessary with athletes who are successful runners; a polycentric axis joint is a favorite for knee disarticulation athletes because of the instantaneous center of rotation capabilities of a four-bar design providing increased toe clearance and greater stride symmetry.

Ambulatory amputee runners have benefited considerably from advances in prosthetic technology. In the International Association of Athletics Federations (IAAF) assessment of Oscar Pistorius, one of the striking biomechanical findings was that the prosthetic limbs developed an energy loss of about 8% during the stance phase, compared to 59% in the human ankle joint. Based on the outcome of this review, the athlete was initially considered to have an unfair advantage over able-bodied competitors, and thus Oscar was not eligible to compete in the Olympic Games. After a subsequent appeal, however, Oscar was allowed to compete, and although he had previously achieved the qualification time, he was not able to repeat this performance after the appeal. Refer to Chapter 5 for additional discussion on this topic.

A factor not considered in a laboratory test of ME is the influence of the stump–socket interface on the prosthesis. This connection is critical to the operation of the prosthesis as any movement of the amputated stump will subsequently swing the prosthetic limb. Furthermore, once the prosthesis makes contact with the ground, it is the stump–prosthesis interface that transmits the load-bearing ground reaction force back to the amputee. The effectiveness of this interface, and the ensuing proprioception, is therefore fundamental for the overall performance of the amputee. Figure 2.10 illustrates the differences in technology and the important connection between residual stump and prosthetic device. Without an effective interface to control the prosthetic device, the potential mechanical efficiency of the technology may not be translated into reality.

As a biological structure, the anatomical stump is influenced by factors such as changes in altitude and local climatic conditions of humidity at the performance environment, which could be different from the athlete's native environment. These factors can influence the volume of the stump, and as the stump is contained in a volume-specific socket, any changes in volume will naturally change the pressure contact points between the stump and socket. This change in volume and subsequent load transfer contact point is also influenced by the altered activities of daily living that athletes may experience while living in the Paralympic village. For example, the immense size of the village can dramatically increase the number of daily steps taken, as athletes are now required to walk from their bedroom down to the dining hall in the Paralympic village for meals, then from the dining hall to the transport zone to train or compete, and then to return. Although no studies have been published yet, this increase in incidental walking within the Paralympic village almost certainly modifies the stump volume and socket interface, a critical factor in the biomechanics for the Paralympic athlete.

The majority of upper-limb amputees generally do not wear their prosthesis for everyday activities as they tend to cope better without the prosthesis. However, when running, sport biomechanics has found wearing an upper-limb "running prosthesis" can minimize the asymmetry when crouched down for the start and provide better arm-to-leg balance when running. An example of a modified upper-limb running prosthesis is shown in Figure 2.11; this device was developed based on biomechanical analysis of the athlete's running performance.

Sport biomechanics: the amputee without their prosthesis

Within the Paralympic games, there are events in which the athlete with an amputation competes without their prosthesis, such as in the sport of swimming. Sport biomechanics has been heavily involved in areas such as analyzing the swimmers start. The lower-limb amputee will naturally have

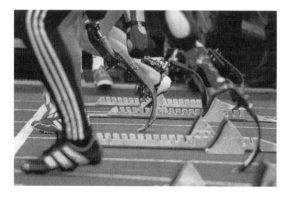

Figure 2.10 Image of the start of the 100-m sprint for transfemoral amputees, highlighting the range of prosthetic technologies utilized by the Paralympic athlete.

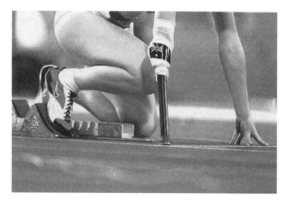

Figure 2.11 Upper-limb running prosthesis.

a unique balance pattern when setting themselves, and the single leg force generation will also require specific analysis. Similarly, the upper-limb amputee balance and "grip" on the start block will be different, particularly for the in-water backstroke start. Once in the flight phase of the start, both the upper- and lower-limb amputee are asymmetrical in body mass distribution, which will therefore influence the trajectory they will travel. Sport biomechanics is fundamental to firstly understanding and then quantifying these relationships; this benchmark data can then be used to determine the effectiveness of any future interventions on the athlete's technique.

Sport biomechanics of the swim start combines the kinematic analysis of segment movements such as rate of arm swing, path of the movement of the head, and the explosive power of the lower limbs. Collectively, this movement pattern is analyzed via the kinetic link chain to determine the summation relationships between timing variables like the drive from the legs, arm movement, and head position. All of these relationships with the human segments then need to be compared with reference to the starting block and water surface. As the swimmer moves their upper limbs, their center of gravity naturally changes; if they are poised with the line of gravity right near the front of the starting blocks, any change in movement pattern will alter the center of gravity relationship and cause the swimmer to lose their balance. When controlled, this can be a benefit to the swimmer as they can then use the natural acceleration forces of gravity to propel them into the water. Some work has been done in this area on the Olympic swimmers start, and is currently being conducted on Paralympic swimmers start. Paralympic swimmers who have reduced balance control, such as lower-limb amputees, can find balancing on the starting block difficult. To understand the relationships, specific understanding of the forces generated on the starting block and the position, velocity, and acceleration of the human segments as they leave the block and enter the water is required. This requires the specific technology of mounting the force plate to the starting block and synchronizing above- and underwater video cameras.

Continuing the sport biomechanics analysis of the swim start, the underwater velocity has been commonly identified as the only variable that distinguishes elite performance. From reviewing the underwater video footage, swimmers who can hold their streamline more effectively tend to generate faster underwater velocity. Athletes with an amputation are naturally asymmetrical and may find it more difficult maintaining balance, tending to oscillate more as they correct their balance, resulting in a less effective streamline position.

The ability to produce force and actual force propulsion may differ due to the loss of energy throughout the kinetic chain, i.e., if there is loss of strength, coordination or range of motion force will be lost or dissipated from the kinetic chain. This loss may increase load on other areas or links in the kinetic chain, potentially leading to injury as a result of change of load on a particular structure or the result of a compensatory strategy. As coaches and athletes know, injury means time out of training which is detrimental to competition performance.

From biomechanical studies, it is well established that asymmetry is common in the general population and as expected greater in unilateral sports. Studies investigating "functional asymmetry" in terms of swimming hand speed and hand path found asymmetric pulling patterns. This asymmetry is higher for the swimmer with an amputation; the task for the coach is to modify this asymmetry for the Paralympic swimmer. For instance, an imbalance in muscular strength, and hence potential force production, may further influence swimming performance. Sport biomechanics has identified that subtle changes in body position in the water can increase either the resistive drag or the propulsive forces of the athlete.

The effect of force symmetry has been identified in front crawl swimmers with particular focus on breathing laterality and symmetry of isokinetic force of shoulder medial rotators. Results showed an increased duration of catch/pull phase of the dominant arm, compared to when breathing on the amputated side. It appears that development of greater strength in the dominant arm and unilateral breathing may lead to asymmetry of stroke and force output.

Qualitative and quantitative techniques are used to analyze swimmers in training and in competition, throughout the year. The type of assessment undertaken depends on the individual swimmer's needs. Video filming is used to provide feedback on starting, turning, and swimming technique. This can be combined with velocity meter analysis, to give information on intracyclic speed fluctuation, streamlining ability, and other performance-related variables. Tethered force analysis provides an insight into the swimmer's stroke-by-stroke force production and anaerobic power.

Velocity meter can measure the instantaneous velocity of the swimmer, continuously and in real time. This biomechanical measure can provide vital feedback to the athlete and coach on the swimming performance. From the sport biomechanics perspective, the objective measures made with this device can guide technique modifications made by the athlete. The swimmer with an arm disability can benefit greatly from this form of analysis, e.g., the influence of kicking or stroking with the amputated limb can be objectively quantified by the sport biomechanist and the informed decisions made on technique modifications for the Paralympic athlete.

In addition to quantifying stroke or kick imbalances in the Paralympic athlete, the velocity meter can also measure streamline ability as the swimmer pushes off from the wall or during the underwater phase of the swimming start. For example, traditionally, a swimmer will maintain an underwater streamline phase for as long as possible before gradually raising up to on top of the water. The Paralympic athlete with a limb amputation may have an impaired ability to hold an effective streamline (arm amputee) or an inefficient single-leg kick (leg amputee). The biomechanical measure of instantaneous velocity will enable the optimum underwater time to be determined for the Paralympic athlete. There are several other applications of this measure, such as monitoring velocity fluctuations within the high drag strokes such as breaststroke. By quantifying the athlete's velocity, the correlation with other biomechanical measures of stroke rate can be investigated. This will enable the optimum stroke rate of the athlete to be determined.

From 2D and 3D video analysis, inter- and intra-swimmer variability in arm coordination can be established. This biomechanical measure quantifies the relationship between arm stroke timing within the complete swimming stroke. From this information, the timing of the swimmer's stroke can be modified, which is particularly important for the arm amputee swimmer. For example, the swimmer's stroke may be quantified as a catch-up stroke, in which the hand of swimmer effectively "catches" up to the opposite hand at the front of the swimmer's stroke. The style of technique generally suits swimmers with a powerful leg kick and/or strong powerful swimming stroke. Swimmers with an arm amputation may need to modify their index of coordination based on the instantaneous swimming velocity biomechanical measured. For further discussion on swimming, refer to Chapter 15.

Future directions in sport biomechanics for amputees

Sport biomechanics for people with an amputation has expanded from the traditional rehabilitative biomechanics that studied the movement patterns of injured or people with disability. One of the key outcomes from these studies has been the modification or development of equipment to retrain the movement pattern. This also includes intermittent mobility devices, such as canes, crutches, walkers, to complete permanent devices, such as prosthesis. The lower-limb amputee will require these devices as part of their rehabilitation (from an acute injury), as well as to correct or modify any existing gait pattern.

An understandable temptation for researchers is to research only "hot topics" that are more likely to be funded through research grants. As the majority of people with disabilities are aged, the development of assistive devices has naturally focused on this market. Paralympic athletes have created a new, albeit small market. Not only are they significantly younger than the traditional aged person with a disability, they are also highly active and as such place far great loads on the assistive devices. This new market demand, in the long term, will result in a better understanding of the relationship between human, activity, and the artificial aid—but there is still a fair amount of ground to cover in this area.

References

Abel, T., Platen, P., Rojas, V.S., Schneider, S. & Struder, H.K. (2008). Energy expenditure in ball games for wheelchair users. *Spinal Cord*, **46(12)**, 785–790.

Boninger, M.L., Cooper, R.A., Robertson, R.N. & Shimada, S.D. (1997). Three-dimensional pushrim forces during two speeds of wheelchair propulsion.

American Journal of Physical Medicine & Rehabilitation, **76**(5), 420–426.

Boninger, M.L., Cooper, R.A., Baldwin, M.A., Shimada, S.D. & Koontz, A. (1999). Wheelchair pushrim kinetics: body weight and median nerve function. *Archives of Physical Medicine and Rehabilitation*, **80**(8), 910–915.

Boninger, M.L., Towers, J.D., Cooper, R.A., Dicianno, B.E. & Munin, M.C. (2001). Shoulder imaging abnormalities in individuals with paraplegia. *Journal of Rehabilitation Research and Development*, **38**(4), 401–408.

Boninger, M.L., Impink, B.G., Cooper, R.A. & Koontz, A.M. (2004). Relation between median and ulnar nerve function and wrist kinematics during wheelchair propulsion. *Archives of Physical Medicine and Rehabilitation*, **85**(7), 1141–1145.

Boninger, M.L., Koontz, A.M., Sisto, S.A., et al. (2005). Pushrim biomechanics and injury prevention in spinal cord injury: recommendations based on CULP-SCI investigations. *Journal of Rehabilitation Research and Development*, **42**(3, **Suppl. 1**), 9–20.

Burke, E.J., Auchinachie, J.A., Hayden, R., Loftin, J.M. (1985). Energy cost of wheelchair basketball. *Physician and Sports Medicine*, **3**(13), 99–105.

Cooper, R.A. (1995). *Rehabilitation Engineering Applied to Mobility and Manipulation*. Institute of Physics Publishing, Bristol, UK, and Philadelphia, PA.

Cooper, R.A. & Bedi, J.F. (1990). Gross mechanical efficiency of trained wheelchair racers. *Annual International Conference of the IEEE Engineering in Medicine and Biology Society*, **12**(5), 2311–2312.

Cooper, R.A., Baldini, F.D., Langbein, W.E., Robertson, R.N., Bennett, P. & Monical, S. (1993). Prediction of pulmonary function in wheelchair users. *Paraplegia*, **31**(9), 560–570.

Cooper, R.A., Boninger, M.L., VanSickle, D.P., Robertson, R.N. & Shimada, S.D. (1997a). Uncertainty analysis of wheelchair propulsion dynamics. *IEEE Transactions on Rehabilitation Engineering*, **5**(2), 130–139.

Cooper, R.A., Robertson, R.N., VanSickle, D.P., Boninger, M.L. & Shimada, S.D. (1997b). Methods for determining three-dimensional wheelchair pushrim forces and moments—a technical note. *Journal of Rehabilitation Research and Development*, **34**(2), 162–170.

Coutts, K.D. (1990). Kinematics of sport wheelchair propulsion. *Journal of Rehabilitation Research and Development*, **27**(1), 21–26.

Coutts, K.D. (1992). Dynamics of wheelchair basketball. *Medicine and Science in Sports and Exercise*, **24**(2), 231–234.

Coutts, K.D. (1994). Drag and sprint performance of wheelchair basketball players. *Journal of Rehabilitation Research and Development*, **31**(2), 138–143.

de Groot, S., Veeger, H.E., Hollander, A.P. & van der Woude, L.H. (2002). Consequence of feedback-based learning of an effective handrim wheelchair force production on mechanical efficiency. *Clinical Biomechanics*, **17**(3), 219–226.

Escobedo, E.M., Hunter, J.C., Hollister, M.C., Patten, R.M. & Goldstein, B. (1997). MR imaging of rotator cuff tears in individuals with paraplegia. *American Journal of Roentgenology*, **168**(4), 919–923.

Faupin, A., Campillo, P., Weissland, T., Gorce, P. & Thevenon, A. (2004). The effects of rear-wheel camber on the mechanical parameters produced during the wheelchair sprinting of handibasketball athletes. *Journal of Rehabilitation Research and Development*, **41**(3B), 421–428.

Faupin, A., Gorce, P., Meyer, C. & Thevenon, A. (2008). Effects of backrest positioning and gear ratio on nondisabled subjects' handcycling sprinting performance and kinematics. *Journal of Rehabilitation Research and Development*, **45**(1), 109–116.

Goosey-Tolfrey, V., Castle, P., Webborn, N. & Abel, T. (2006). Aerobic capacity and peak power output of elite quadriplegic games players. *British Journal of Sports Medicine*, **40**(8), 684–687.

Goosey-Tolfrey, V.L., Alfano, H. & Fowler, N. (2008). The influence of crank length and cadence on mechanical efficiency in hand cycling. *European Journal of Applied Physiology*, **102**(2), 189–194.

Groen, W.G., van der Woude, L.H.V. & de Koning, J.J. (2010). The power balance model: useful in the study of elite handcycling performance. In: L.H.V. van der Woude, F. Hoekstra, S. DeGroot, K.E. Bijker, R. Dekker, P.C.T. van Aanholt, F.J. Hettinga, T.W.J. Janssen and J.H.P. Houdijk. (eds.) *Rehabilitation: Mobility, Exercise and Sports*. IOS Press, Amsterdam, NL.

Hettinga, F.J., Valent, L., Groen, W., van Drongelen, S., de Groot, S. & van der Woude, L.H.V. (2010). Hand-cycling: an active form of wheeled mobility, recreation and sports. *Physical Medicine and Rehabilitation Clinics of North America*, **21**(1), 127–140.

Higgs, C. (1993). Sport performance: technical developments. In: R.D. Steadward, E.R. Nelson & G.D. Wheeler (eds.) *Vista '93—The Outlook, Proceedings of the International Conference on High Performance Sport for Athletes with Disabilities*, pp. 169–186. Rick Hansen Centre, Edmonton, AB.

Ingen Schenau, G.J. (1988). Cycle power: a predictive model. *Endeavour*, **12**(1), 44–47.

Ingen Schenau, G.J. & Cavanagh, P.R. (1990). Power equations in endurance sports. *Journal of Biomechanics*, **23**(9), 865–881.

Kramer, C., Schneider, G., Bohm, H., Klopfer-Kramer, I. & Senner, V. (2009). Effect of different handgrip angles on work distribution during hand cycling at submaximal power levels. *Ergonomics*, **52**(10), 1276–1286.

Schmid, A., Huonker, M., Stober, P., et al. (1998). Physical performance and cardiovascular and metabolic adaptation of elite female wheelchair basketball players in wheelchair ergometry and in competition. *American Journal of Physical Medicine & Rehabilitation*, **77**(6), 527–533.

Sporner, M.L., Grindle, G.G., Kelleher, A., Teodorski, E.E., Cooper, R. & Cooper, R.A. (2009). Quantification of activity during wheelchair basketball and rugby at the National Veterans Wheelchair Games: a pilot study. *Prosthetics and Orthotics International*, **33**(3), 210–217.

Valent, L.J., Dallmeijer, A.J., Houdijk, H., et al. (2009). Effects of hand cycle training on physical capacity in individuals with tetraplegia: a clinical trial. *Physical Therapy*, **89**(10), 1051–1060.

van der Woude, L.H.V., Veeger, H.E., Rozendal, R.H., van Ingen Schenau, G.J., Rooth, F. & van Nierop, P. (1988). Wheelchair racing: effects of rim diameter and speed on physiology and technique. *Medicine and Science in Sports and Exercise*, **20**, 492–500.

van der Woude, L.H.V., Veeger, H.E., Rozendal, R.H. & Sargeant, A.J. (1989). Optimum cycle frequencies in hand-rim wheelchair propulsion. Wheelchair propulsion technique. *European Journal of Applied Physiology and Occupational Physiology*, **58**, 625–632.

van der Woude, L.H., Bosmans, I., Bervoets, B. & Veeger, H.E. (2000). Handcycling: different modes and gear ratios. *Journal of Medical Engineering & Technology*, **24**(6), 242–249.

van der Woude, L.H., Veeger, H.E., Dallmeijer, A.J., Janssen, T.W. & Rozendaal, L.A. (2001). Biomechanics and physiology in active manual wheelchair propulsion. *Medical Engineering & Physics*, **23**(10), 713–733.

Vanlandewijck, Y., Theisen, D. & Daly, D. (2001). Wheelchair propulsion biomechanics: implications for wheelchair sports. *Sports Medicine*, **31**(5), 339–367.

Recommended readings

Wheelchair athletics and training

Cooper, R.A. (1990). Wheelchair racing sports science: a review. *Journal of Rehabilitation Research and Development*, **27**, 295–312.

Fleck, S.J. (1999). Periodized strength training: a critical review. *Journal of Strength and Conditioning Research*, **13**, 82–89.

Harre, D. (1982). *Principles of Sports Training: Introduction to the Theory and Methods of Training*, 1st edition. Sportverlag, Berlin.

van der Woude, L.H.V., Veeger, H.E., Rozendal, R.H. & Sargeant, A.J. (1989). Optimum cycle frequencies in hand-rim wheelchair propulsion. Wheelchair propulsion technique. *European Journal of Applied Physiology and Occupational Physiology*, **58**, 625–632.

Vanlandewijck, Y., Theisen, D. & Daly, D. (2001). Wheelchair propulsion biomechanics: implications for wheelchair sports. *Sports Medicine*, **31**(5), 339–367.

Amputee athletics

American Academy of Orthopaedic Surgeons, Rosemont, IL, USA.

Smith, D.G., Michael, J.W. & Bowker, J.H. *Atlas of Amputations and Limb Deficiencies: Surgical, Prosthetic, and Rehabilitation Principles*, 3rd edition.

Chapter 3
Physiology

Yagesh Bhambhani

Faculty of Rehabilitation Medicine, University of Alberta, Edmonton, AB, Canada

Introduction

The Paralympic Games is the platform for elite sport competition for athletes with physical disabilities. The International Paralympic Committee (IPC) is the governing body for the Summer and Winter Paralympic Games that are held every 4 years in the same cities as the Olympic Games. Currently, individuals of the following five disability groups compete in the Paralympic Games: spinal cord injury (SCI), cerebral palsy (CP), amputation, visual impairment, and Les Autres (i.e., other physical disabilities). These athletes participate in 20 summer sports and five winter sports, some of which are specific to their disability (www.paralympic. org). This chapter will present an overview of several important physiological factors pertinent to Paralympic sport performance in athletes with SCI and CP. From a physiological perspective, there are some unique differences between these two athletic populations that affect their competitive performance. It is anticipated that the information presented in this chapter will provide sport scientists with the necessary information to evaluate the performance of these Paralympic athletes as well as to develop and implement appropriate physical training programs to enhance their performance.

The Paralympic Athlete, 1st edition. Edited by Yves C. Vanlandewijck and Walter R. Thompson. Published 2011 by Blackwell Publishing Ltd.

Spinal cord injury

Anaerobic power, aerobic power, and body composition

Anaerobic power and capacity

Anaerobic power is defined as the maximum amount of power that can be generated using the immediate and short-term anaerobic sources of energy production. Anaerobic capacity is defined as the average power that can be developed over a given period of time using the anaerobic energy sources. In able-bodied subjects, the Wingate anaerobic test is most commonly used to measure anaerobic power and capacity. This 30-s test is performed on either a leg cycle or an arm crank ergometer using a resistance that is proportional to the individual's body weight. The objective is to complete as many revolutions as possible during the 30-s interval. The peak power developed over a 5-s interval (usually the first 5 s) is a measure of the anaerobic power, while the average power generated over the entire 30 s is considered to be an index of anaerobic capacity. The fatigue index (expressed as a percentage) is calculated as the ratio:

$$\frac{\text{Peak minus minimum power}}{\text{Peak power}}$$

In individuals with SCI, the Wingate test has been modified to assess anaerobic power and capacity using arm cranking and specially designed wheelchair ergometers. It is recommended that the latter exercise mode be used to evaluate competitive athletes because of its specificity to sport perfor-mance. Currently, there is no standardized method for determining the appropriate resistance for the Wingate test protocol in individuals with SCI. The resistance applied is considerably lower than that used for able-bodied individuals because of the reduced muscle mass resulting from paralysis. The load setting for wheelchair users performing the Wingate test should be based on the activity limitations resulting from impairment, training sta-tus, and gender of the subjects. Because of the large variation in the functional capacity of the athletes, a resistance equivalent to 2.5–10% of the combined athlete's body weight and the virtual weight of the wheelchair (20 kg) has been used (Van der Woude et al., 1997). The test–retest reliability of the 30-s Wingate wheelchair ergometer test has been well established in wheelchair athletes. In general, ath-letes tend to perform better on the second test due to habituation. It is therefore recommended that athletes be allowed a familiarization trial prior to actual assessment.

In individuals with SCI, the peak anaerobic power and capacity is inversely related to the level of the lesion. This implies that the lower the injury level, the greater the anaerobic fitness is. A well-trained athlete with low-level paraplegia (lesion levels between L4 and S3) can generate peak anaerobic power that is three to four times that of an ath-lete with quadriplegia with lesion level above C6. Competitive wheelchair athletes with high- and low- level paraplegia have significantly higher values for peak power and fatigue index during the Wingate test compared to recreational athletes. Well-trained athletes with low-level paraplegia (lesion at T8 or lower) can attain absolute or relative values of anaerobic power during the Wingate test comparable to those of able-bodied subjects. Gender comparisons indicate that:
• the absolute and relative values of the peak power, mean power, and mean velocity are significantly higher in male compared to female wheelchair athletes;
• the fatigue index is significantly higher in females compared to males, suggesting a greater decline in force output during the test in females;
• there is no significant correlation between peak power and total body mass in either gender, suggesting

that functional muscle mass plays a more important role in this assessment (Bhambhani, 2002).

The indices of anaerobic power (5-s peak and 30-s average) have a moderate to high correlation with the peak power output during an incremen-tal aerobic exercise test. The proportion of the peak power output attained during incremental exercise and the anaerobic power indices range between 17–85% and 14–81% for the peak and average values, respectively. These large variations can be attributed to differences in the lesion levels, testing modes, and fitness status of the subjects. The aero-bic contribution of the wheelchair anaerobic power test is estimated as 30%, which is within the range reported for able-bodied individuals. In wheelchair basketball (WB) players, there seems to be a signifi-cant relationship between the oxygen cost of the Wingate anaerobic power test and functional classi-fication. This implies that muscle mass available for performance plays an important role in developing anaerobic power.

Maximal aerobic power

The maximal aerobic power ($\dot{V}O_{2max}$) is defined as the maximum amount of oxygen that can be uti-lized per unit time. The $\dot{V}O_{2max}$ is dependent on the individual's ability to transport, deliver, and utilize oxygen, and is considered to be the best measure of maximal cardiorespiratory fitness. Mathematically, $\dot{V}O_{2max}$ is the product of the maximal values of the cardiac output ($\dot{Q}$) (central factor) and the mixed arteriovenous oxygen difference $\{(a-v)O_{2diff}\}$, the peripheral factor. $\dot{Q}$ is determined by the product of the maximal values of heart rate (HR) and stroke volume (SV) during exercise. In able-bodied subjects, the $\dot{V}O_{2max}$ is normally assessed using a continuous incremental test protocol to voluntary fatigue on a cycle ergometer or treadmill. These exercise modes are selected because they utilize a large muscle mass and, therefore, it is possible to fully stress the car-diovascular system and attain true maximal values. However, in athletes with SCI, the criteria for $\dot{V}O_{2max}$ are usually not attained and, typically, the peak $\dot{V}O_2$ during the incremental work test is recorded.

The basic principle to be utilized in athlete testing is that the exercise mode should simulate the sport movement as closely as possible. In athletes with

SCI, who are nonambulatory, the peak $\dot{V}O_2$ is assessed using arm crank, wheelchair, rowing, or double poling ergometers. During arm cranking, the subject performs asynchronous cycling exercise with the upper extremities and, therefore, this mode is very suitable for testing handcyclists. In the case of wheelchair ergometry, the subject performs synchronous upper body exercise that is specific to their normal mode of ambulation. This exercise mode is routinely used for evaluating the peak $\dot{V}O_2$ of athletes with SCI involved in wheelchair racing (WR), WB, wheelchair rugby (WRug), and wheelchair tennis (WT). The wheelchair can be mounted on a motor-driven treadmill or frictionless roller system so that the velocity and/or slope of wheelchair propulsion can be regulated. The more sophisticated computer-controlled wheelchair ergometers can quantify power output during exercise. Specific devices such as the SmartWheel® can be attached to the wheelchair so that differences in power generation between limbs can be measured during exercise testing. In Paralympic athletes participating in winter sports such as Nordic skiing (NS) or sledge hockey, a double poling ergometer can be used to evaluate athletes in the sitting or standing position. In Figure 3.1, paraplegic athlete's sit ski was secured to the base of the poling ergometer during testing. This can quantify the power output generated by each limb during the exercise test. When testing

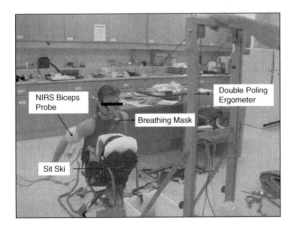

Figure 3.1 Cardiorespiratory and muscle oxygenation measurements being recorded simultaneously on the double poling ergometer in an elite Paralympic Nordic sit skier with low-level paraplegia. The athlete's sit ski was secured to the base of the ergometer during testing.

athletes with SCI on the various types of ergometers, the optimal protocol is to initiate the test at 0 W, and systematically increase the power output by 8–12 W/min in individuals with high-level quadriplegia and 20–25 W/min in individuals with low-level paraplegia, until voluntary fatigue is attained. This protocol is ideally suited for identifying the lactate threshold and the peak $\dot{V}O_2$.

Concept of lactate threshold

The lactate threshold is defined as the lowest oxygen uptake ($\dot{V}O_2$) at which blood lactate increases significantly above resting levels during a continuous incremental exercise test to voluntary exhaustion. The lactate threshold indicates the maximum amount of energy that can be derived from aerobic sources without the accumulation of lactic acid and, therefore, is considered one of the best measures of submaximal aerobic fitness. The lactate threshold can also be determined noninvasively from the respiratory gas exchange responses measured by a metabolic cart during the incremental exercise test. When a significant amount of lactate accumulates in the blood, an additional amount of carbon dioxide, above that formed as a result of aerobic metabolism, is released due to the buffering of lactate by bicarbonate in the blood. The increased carbon dioxide production stimulates the peripheral chemoreceptors, thereby increasing the ventilatory drive. The net result is that the ventilation rate, carbon dioxide production, and respiratory exchange ratio all increase nonlinearly at the lactate threshold. Improved criteria for detecting this threshold from the respiratory gas exchange measurements are a systematic increase in the ventilatory equivalent for oxygen (ratio between ventilation rate and oxygen consumption), without a concomitant increase in the ventilatory equivalent for carbon dioxide (ratio between ventilation rate and carbon dioxide production). In the scientific literature, this exercise intensity is usually referred to as the ventilatory threshold (VT), because the exact physiological mechanism of the relationship between lactate accumulation and the respiratory gas exchange measurements is not completely understood. The validity of detecting the VT using these respiratory gas exchange criteria during the incremental exercise test has been demonstrated in athletes with SCI.

Field tests for predicting peak $\dot{V}O_2$

Because direct measurement of peak $\dot{V}O_2$ requires expensive laboratory equipment and technical expertise for conducting the test and interpreting the results, this testing method is not amenable for testing a large number of athletes on a regular basis. In order to overcome this limitation, some field tests that are commonly used for predicting the peak $\dot{V}O_2$ in able-bodied subjects have been validated in subjects with SCI. The validity and reliability of the Leger and Boucher multistage incremental running test has been established for predicting peak $\dot{V}O_2$ during wheelchair propulsion in male athletes with Class II to V paraplegia (Poulain et al., 1999). The 12-min wheelchair propulsion test has been validated against direct peak $\dot{V}O_2$ measurements in individuals with paraplegia but not with quadriplegia. Stronger correlation coefficients are observed when the peak $\dot{V}O_2$ is expressed relative to body weight, suggesting that body mass plays an important role in determining wheelchair propulsion distance. The strength of the relationship is improved by including other variables such as blood pressure, age, and height of the subjects. In all field tests for wheelchair users, the relationship between test outcome and peak $\dot{V}O_2$ is hampered by the external conditions (e.g., floor surface impacting on rolling resistance and turning capacity), wheelchair configuration (e.g., camber of the wheels impacting on maneuverability), and wheelchair–user interface (e.g., low and backwards oriented center of gravity improves speed and maneuverability).

Body composition

Long-term SCI results in profound changes in body composition due to a variety of factors, including a decrease in the basal metabolic rate, resulting from the muscle paralysis, reduced energy expenditure from lower physical activity levels, and muscle atrophy resulting from disuse. In healthy individuals, the hydrostatic weighing technique has been considered the "gold standard" for measurement of body density (DEN) and for the calculation of percent body fat. However, the underwater weighing procedure poses several practical difficulties for the measurement of body density in individuals with SCI, and, therefore, this technique is not suitable for this population. Body mass index (BMI), which is routinely used to estimate body composition in healthy individuals, provides an index of health risk, and is not suitable for the population with SCI. Other techniques that have been used on able-bodied subjects to evaluate body composition include doubly labeled water (DLW), bioelectrical impedance analysis (BIA), dual-energy X-ray absorptiometry (DEXA), and skinfold thickness (SF). There is limited research pertaining to the application of these measurement techniques to evaluate the body composition of individuals with SCI, including the athletic population. The DLW method has been validated against BIA in sedentary individuals with SCI. However, it is recommended that when using BIA on the population with SCI, the average of all four combinations of hand–leg measurements is used in computing the total body water and percent body fat values (Desport et al., 2000). The DEXA technique is particularly useful because it provides segmental changes in body composition and also measures bone mineral content and density, all of which are of extreme importance in the athletic population with SCI. The SF technique is the simplest, but has problems pertaining to validity because of variations in the way in which SF changes as a result of long-term SCI, particularly below the level of injury. Among the various skinfold sites that are used for estimating body fat, the triceps skinfold has been demonstrated to be the most accurate predictor because it has the least variability when compared to reference values in healthy subjects.

The use of DEXA scans has demonstrated significant differences in segmental body composition in male and female wheelchair athletes. The percentage of body fat is highest in the paralyzed legs when compared to the trunk and arms, while that in the trunk is higher than that observed in the arms. Path analysis indicated that training load was a factor in reducing percent fat in the trunk and arms, and athletic history was a factor in reducing the percent fat in the arms (Mojtahedi et al., 2009). Another DEXA study in female WB and WT players demonstrated a strong tendency for regional differences in bone mineral density when compared to a healthy reference group of females. The bone mineral density in the arms, ribs, thoracic spine, and lumbar spine tended to be higher in wheelchair athletes, while that of the pelvis and legs was higher in the reference group. This suggests that regular physical activity plays an important role in attenuating the loss in bone mineral density in the exercising extremities in athletes with SCI.

Acute physiological responses during incremental exercise

The typical changes in the $\dot{V}O_2$ and HR during an incremental velocity test to voluntary fatigue in elite wheelchair racers with quadriplegia, paraplegia, and CP are compared in Figure 3.2. These athletes completed an incremental velocity test on a roller system during a WR training camp as illustrated in Figure 3.3. Their responses at the VT and at peak exercise are summarized in Table 3.1. The $\dot{V}O_2$ and HR increased in a linear manner during the test until voluntary fatigue. One major difference between individuals with quadriplegia and paraplegia is that the former is unable to attain the

age-predicted maximum HR because sympathetic stimulation to the myocardium is disrupted. As a result, the peak HR that is attainable by individuals with lesion levels above T6 is determined by stimulation of the sinoatrial node. The peak HR that is usually attained in quadriplegics ranges between 110 and 125 beats/min. In contrast, individuals with paraplegia (lesions below T6) have complete stimulation of the myocardium and, theoretically, should be able to attain the age-predicted maximum HR (210–age, years) during upper body exercise. However, in order to attain this maximum HR, it is crucial that the subject is able to recruit as large a muscle mass as possible. Because of the large degree of paralysis of the trunk musculature in high-level paraplegics, it may not be possible for them to attain this age-predicted maximum HR. Generally speaking, the peak HR and $\dot{V}O_2$ attained during exercise is inversely related to the lesion level. In other words, the lower the level of the lesion, the greater are the peak HR and $\dot{V}O_2$, with the opposite being true as well.

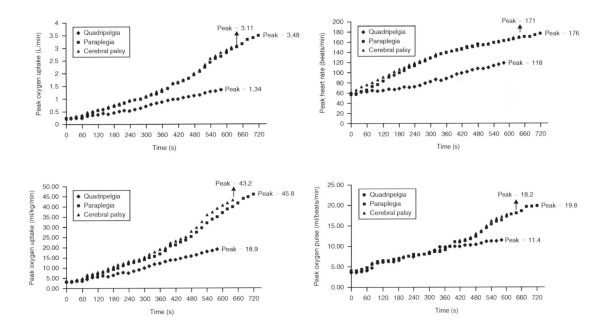

Figure 3.2 Oxygen uptake and HR responses during incremental exercise in elite Paralympic athletes with quadriplegia, paraplegia, and CP. These athletes completed an incremental velocity tests in their competition wheelchair mounted on a frictionless roller system to voluntary fatigue. Cardiorespiratory responses were recorded using a wireless metabolic system.

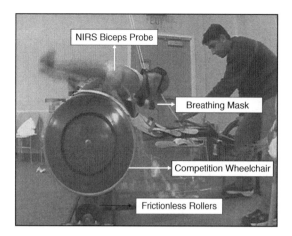

Figure 3.3 Cardiorespiratory and muscle oxygenation measurements being recorded simultaneously during incremental wheelchair exercise to voluntary fatigue in an elite wheelchair marathon racer with low-level paraplegia. The athlete used his competition wheelchair that was mounted on a frictionless roller system.

Table 3.1 Pertinent physiological characteristics of three elite Paralympic wheelchair racers.

Variable	C7 Quadriplegia	L4 Paraplegia	Cerebral palsy
Age, years	37	35	34
Body mass, kg	71	75	72
Body fat, %[1]	16.4	7.4	15.8
Basal metabolic rate, kcal/day[2]	1283	1659	1695
Peak oxygen uptake, l/min	1.34	3.48	3.11
Peak oxygen uptake, ml/kg/min	18.8	45.8	43.2
Peak heart rate, beats/min	118	176	171
Peak heart rate, % age predicted	64.5	95.1	89.2
Peak oxygen pulse, ml/beat	11.4	19.8	18.2
Peak respiratory exchange ratio	1.18	1.23	1.24
Peak blood lactate,[3] mmol/l	9.5	12.8	12.9
Ventilatory threshold, l/min	1.07	2.57	2.05
Ventilatory threshold, ml/kg/min	15.1	33.8	28.4
Ventilatory threshold, % peak $\dot{V}O_2$	80.1	73.8	75.6

[1]Determined from bioelectrical impedance measurements (RJL Instruments).
[2]Predicted from Cyprus software (RJL Instruments) using bioelectrical impedance results.
[3]From finger stick sample taken 2 min postexercise.

There is a large variation in functional capacity among spinal-cord-injured subjects, even at similar lesion levels. The relationship between the International Stoke Mandeville Games Federation functional classification system and the peak $\dot{V}O_2$ of elite athletes with SCI participating in five Paralympic sports, namely WR, NS, WB, WT, and wheelchair fencing (WF), is illustrated in Figure 3.4. It is evident that as the functional classification increases, the peak $\dot{V}O_2$ of the athletes also increases. The peak $\dot{V}O_2$ values ranged from 27.1 ml/kg/min in a WF athlete to a high of 61 ml/kg/min in a WR athlete. The WR and NS athletes had the highest peak $\dot{V}O_2$ values compared to the athletes participating in the three intermittent sports. This is most likely due to the fact that participation in endurance sports places a substantial stress on both the central oxygen transport and peripheral aerobic energy systems, thereby maximizing the increase in peak $\dot{V}O_2$ when compared to participation in intermittent sports that primarily stress the anaerobic energy system (Bernardi et al., 2010).

The VT was identified in these athletes using the following respiratory gas exchange criterion as illustrated in Figure 3.5, Panels A and B: intensity at which there was a systematic increase in the $\dot{V}E/\dot{V}CO_2$ ratio with a concomitant increase in the $\dot{V}E/\dot{V}O_2$ ratio until the peak $\dot{V}O_2$ was attained. It is evident that although the $\dot{V}O_2$ at the VT was higher in the paraplegic compared to the quadriplegic athlete (33.8 vs. 15.1 ml/kg/min), when expressed relative to the peak $\dot{V}O_2$, the trend was reversed (80.1% vs. 73.8%). This anomaly in the VT has been attributed to the loss of sympathetic control to the myocardium and/or loss of central innervation to the intercostals in quadriplegics, which could influence their respiratory response to incremental exercise.

The maximal $\dot{Q}$ during exercise in individuals with SCI is lower than that of age-matched controls because of the lower peak HR that can be attained, and reduced SV resulting from venous pooling in the lower extremities and splanchnic area. The lack of the venous muscle pump significantly reduces the cardiac preload, which diminishes the SV during exercise. Although the respiratory muscle pump is still active in subjects with SCI, it cannot compensate for the reduced preload that results from the paralyzed musculature. The significantly lower peak $\dot{Q}$, referred to as a hypokinetic circulation, is

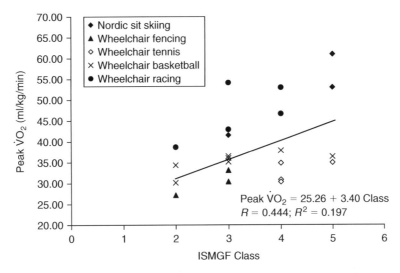

Figure 3.4 Relationship between the International Stoke Mandeville Games Federation classification and peak oxygen uptake in elite Paralympic athletes competing in the following five sports: WR, NS, WB, WT, and WF.

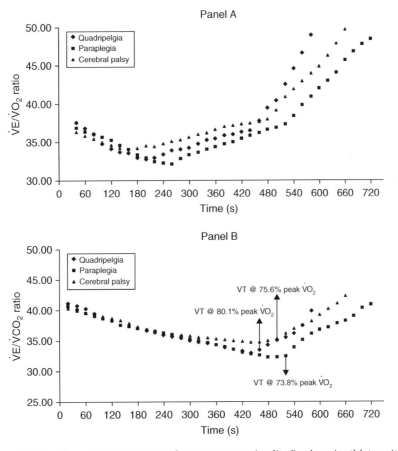

Figure 3.5 Detection of the VT from respiratory gas exchange responses in elite Paralympic athletes with quadriplegia, paraplegia, and CP. The VT was identified as the intensity at which there was systematic increase in the ventilatory equivalent for oxygen without a concomitant increase in the ventilatory equivalent for carbon dioxide.

the primary reason for the significantly lower peak $\dot{V}O_2$ in individuals with SCI. The ability of the muscles to extract oxygen from the blood is dependent on the amount of muscle mass that is available for exercise. This is also inversely related to the lesion level and, therefore, the mixed $(a-v)O_{2diff}$ is usually higher in paraplegics than in quadriplegics. At lesion levels below T10, a large proportion of the trunk musculature can be utilized during upper body exercise, which will result in higher $(a-v)O_{2diff}$ and peak $\dot{V}O_2$ values compared to those with injuries at higher lesion levels, whose ability to utilize these muscles is compromised. Another important factor that has a major impact on the peak responses during exercise is the completeness of the lesion. An incomplete lesion, regardless of its level, usually results in greater functional capacity and, therefore, significantly influences the peak cardiorespiratory responses. With respect to peak blood lactate concentrations during exercise, individuals with quadriplegia generally have lower values because of the reduced muscle mass available for exercise as well as a blunted catecholamine response which significantly affects anaerobic metabolism.

Muscle activation and hemodynamics during wheelchair propulsion

Electromyography studies have demonstrated that recruitment of the shoulder and upper extremity muscles vary considerably during the push and recovery phases of wheelchair propulsion in individuals with SCI. The recruitment of these muscles differs between quadriplegics and paraplegics. In paraplegics, the triceps brachii, antero-middle deltoid, and pectoralis major are more active during the push phase, whereas the postero-medial deltoid, subscapularis, supraspinatus, and middle trapezius are more active during the recovery phase. The extensor carpi radialis and lassitimus dorsi are active during both phases of wheelchair propulsion. In quadriplegics, the activity of the pectoralis major seems to be more prolonged when compared to paraplegics, and the subscapularis demonstrates greater prominence in the push phase. Typically, the contribution of the trunk muscles increases with increasing severity of exercise. The muscles most susceptible to fatigue are the antero-middle deltoid, the supraspinatus, and the recovery muscles.

Hemodynamic changes of the biceps brachii measured optically using near-infrared spectroscopy (NIRS) in elite athletes with SCI indicate that there is considerable variation in the muscle oxygenation and blood volume responses during a maximal velocity wheelchair exercise test to voluntary fatigue. In Figure 3.6, the trends in a representative quadriplegic and paraplegic athlete are illustrated during a maximal wheelchair velocity test. The biceps muscle oxygenation and blood volume were recorded noninvasively using a dual-wave NIRS instrument. Although it is evident that both athletes demonstrated a significant decline in muscle oxygenation (implying greater oxygen extraction), there was considerable difference between the two athletes in the blood volume response. In the quadriplegic athlete, the muscle blood volume declined from the onset of exercise until voluntary fatigue was attained, whereas in the paraplegic athlete, there was a systematic increase in blood volume throughout the exercise test. In the quadriplegic athlete, there was no sign of leveling off in the oxygenation response, implying that the increased oxygen requirement was met primarily by a greater extraction because of the limited blood volume. However, in the paraplegic athlete, there was leveling off in muscle oxygenation approximately 60 s after the test was initiated, which was maintained until the termination of the test. In this athlete, the increased oxygen requirement of the muscle was attained by an increase in the localized blood volume. The application of NIRS to evaluate the hemodynamic responses *in situ* during exercise has important implications for developing appropriate exercise programs for enhancing aerobic fitness of elite athletes with SCI and improving their performance.

Physiological responses during simulated Paralympic sport performance

The overall physiological stress during competitive efforts of Paralympic athletes varies considerably and is dependent on the sport and level of the injury. During distance WR field tests, the HR can approach $90-95\%$ of the peak value attained during an incremental exercise test. Results from simulated racing competitions indicated that recreational athletes with quadriplegia raced at 76% and 86% of their

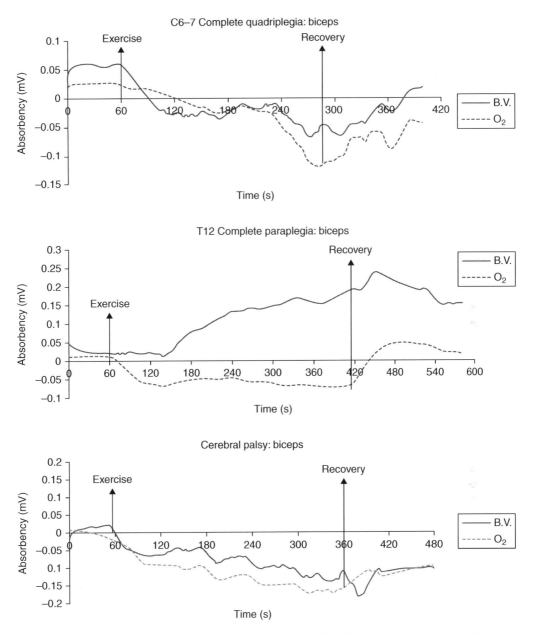

Figure 3.6 Muscle oxygenation and blood volume trends in the biceps brachii during incremental wheelchair exercise to voluntary fatigue in elite athletes with quadriplegia, paraplegia, and spastic CP. Muscle oxygenation and blood volume were recorded from the biceps brachii continuously during the test using dual-wave NIRS. See text for explanation of these measurements (B.V. = blood volume).

peak $\dot{V}O_2$ and peak HR, respectively, while those with paraplegia exercised at 95% of their peak values for both these variables. In male recreational athletes, the energy expenditure during WB and WT training met the minimum requirements (50% of peak $\dot{V}O_2$)

of the American College of Sports Medicine (ACSM) for enhancing aerobic fitness in able-bodied individuals, while those involved in WRug did not meet this criterion. Another study (Bernardi et al., 2010) on elite Paralympians participating in WR, WB, WT,

WF, and NS demonstrated that the intensities were very high with all of them exceeding the maximum range recommended by the ACSM for enhancing and maintaining aerobic fitness. The mean HR response ranged from 79.0% in WT to 94.2% in WR, while the mean $\dot{V}O_2$ values ranged from 73.0% in WF to 84.4% in WR. The absolute and relative values of the HR and $\dot{V}O_2$ during these tests were highest in the NS and WR athletes. This could be attributed to the fact that these athletes participated in sports that continually stressed the cardiorespiratory system and that they incorporated high-intensity aerobic and anaerobic training into the regimens. The three intermittent sports (WB, WT, and WF) elicited significantly lower HR and $\dot{V}O_2$ values compared to the continuous sports, and there were no significant differences for these two variables among these three sports.

Physiological factors predicting Paralympic sport performance

Research that has examined the relationship between the indices of anaerobic and aerobic fitness and Paralympic sport performance is controversial, thereby questioning the validity of using these physiological parameters to predict performance. Generally speaking, average power output during the wheelchair Wingate test has demonstrated a strong inverse correlation with performance during a 200- and 400-m race in elite athletes with a variety of disabilities. However, other evidence indicates no relationship between the arm cranking Wingate test and performance in wheelchair events such as the 400-m race, slalom, and 6-min wheelchair endurance race. The lack of a significant relationship between the measures of anaerobic fitness and performance could be due to the difference in the testing modes: arm cranking versus wheeling. It should be noted that there is considerable variation in Wingate test performance among Paralympic athletes with different disabilities and sports disciplines, which is strongly influenced by the functionality, number of hours of training, and gender of the athletes (Van der Woude et al., 1997).

The relationship between measures of aerobic fitness and endurance performance also appears to be controversial in Paralympic athletes. Some

evidence indicates that the peak $\dot{V}O_2$ in wheelchair athletes was significantly correlated with simulated 5- and 7.5-km race performance. Moreover, the 7.5-km performance time was significantly correlated with the $\dot{V}O_2$, $\dot{Q}$, and SV during the race, but not with the $(a-v)O_{2diff}$, age, and lesion level of the athletes. However, other evidence indicates no significant relationship between the peak $\dot{V}O_2$ and actual WR velocity during a 10-km road race in well-trained athletes with paraplegia. In moderately trained handcyclists, the peak power output and peak $\dot{V}O_2$ during the incremental tests were significantly correlated with performance during a 10-km handcycling race. These observations suggest that aerobic power is important for successful wheelchair distance racing performance in athletes with quadriplegia, and overall oxygen transport plays a more important role than peripheral factors in enhancing performance. A recent study (Bernardi et al., 2010) has demonstrated that the VT is an excellent predictor of performance in elite Paralympic athletes with lesions ranging from high-level quadriplegia (C5) to mid-level paraplegia (T5) in WR, WB, WT, WF, and NS. In each of the sports, the mean $\dot{V}O_2$ measured telemetrically during the simulated field test was closely correlated with the $\dot{V}O_2$ at the VT, stressing the need to improve this measure of aerobic fitness to enhance performance. The fact that three of these five sports were intermittent in nature further highlights the importance of developing this physiological parameter to improve elite sport performance in events that inherently have a strong anaerobic component.

Effects of physical training on physiological fitness

Athletes with SCI who participate in endurance events such as WR and NS have significantly higher peak $\dot{V}O_2$ values compared to their untrained counterparts. Although this cross-sectional evidence suggests that the improved peak $\dot{V}O_2$ is most likely due to the endurance training, two other important factors must be considered when interpreting these data: (a) their aerobic capacity prior to incurring the SCI and (b) their genetic predisposition for aerobic metabolism (e.g., enhanced oxygen transport capacity and the proportion of Type I vs. Type II motor units). Individuals who had high aerobic capacities prior to their injury would most likely adapt more readily to endurance training post injury, which could result in their higher peak $\dot{V}O_2$ values. These factors also influence the VT, which seems to be significantly higher in endurance-trained wheelchair athletes with quadriplegia and paraplegia compared to their untrained counterparts.

A systematic review (Sheel et al., 2008) that examined the effects of upper body exercise training in nonathletic individuals with SCI revealed the lack of well-controlled randomized clinical trials on this topic. These studies have examined a small number of subjects with quadriplegia, paraplegia, or a combination of the two groups. Continuous or interval training in the form of arm cranking or wheelchair ergometry was used in most studies for enhancing aerobic fitness. There is considerable variation in the design of the training programs with respect to the intensity, frequency, and duration of the training. The training intensities were expressed as a percentage of the peak HR, HR reserve, or peak $\dot{V}O_2$. This makes it extremely difficult to draw comparisons among studies to identify the most effective training programs. Despite these limitations, the overall evidence indicates that regular training which meets the minimum ACSM guidelines for training intensity, frequency, and duration induces significant increases in the peak power output and peak $\dot{V}O_2$ of 17.6% $\pm$ 11.2% and 26.1% $\pm$ 15.5%, respectively, in untrained subjects with SCI. In one longitudinal study, which examined the changes in aerobic fitness in athletes with SCI, there was a 30% increase in the peak power output and 26% improvement in the peak $\dot{V}O_2$ following 8 weeks of wheelchair ergometry training performed three times a week at 80% of the HR reserve for 30 min. High-intensity interval training on a wheelchair ergometer (45 min per session with 1-min work: rest intervals at 100% of peak power output) also induced significant improvements in the peak $\dot{V}O_2$, peak oxygen pulse, and the VT in untrained subjects with SCI. Significant reductions in HR and ventilation rate were also observed at the pretraining power output, implying significant adaptations in the cardiorespiratory system. It appears that

circuit training, which combines both endurance and resistance training, induces the greatest improvement in peak $\dot{V}O_2$ in individuals with SCI. Although there is some evidence that endurance training may not be effective in improving the peak $\dot{V}O_2$ in quadriplegics, one longitudinal study on quadriplegic WRug players reported a 40% increase in peak $\dot{V}O_2$ over a 1-year period. Details of the training program during the training season were not provided in the study, making it difficult to fully interpret the findings.

When designing training programs for well-trained athletes with SCI, some additional factors should be considered. First, exercise prescription on the basis of percentage of peak HR may not be valid at low exercise intensities. The validity of this prescription increases at intensities above 85% of peak $\dot{V}O_2$. Second, well-trained wheelchair athletes are able to reliably select specific training intensities based on their perceptual responses. In one study, athletes with SCI were able to consistently select warm-up/cooldown, extensive aerobic training, intensive aerobic training, training in the area of anaerobic threshold, and actual racing intensity based on their perceptual responses. This could be particularly useful to athletes and coaches who routinely rely on this method of training for extended periods. Third, the common practice of wheelchair athletes training at various percentages of their peak racing speed, assuming that it corresponds to training at similar percentage of the peak $\dot{V}O_2$, is not valid.

To date, the phenomena of overtraining and detraining have not been systematically evaluated in athletes with SCI. In order to reach elite status, these athletes accumulate large volumes of training over a period of several years. Some evidence suggests that the incidence of upper respiratory tract infections is higher in athletes with SCI compared to nonathletes, an observation which is consistent with that of the able-bodied athletic population. Mechanical overtraining seems to increase the incidence of shoulder pain and other overuse syndromes of the pectoral girdle in athletes with SCI. Injury and sickness are fairly common occurrences in this population and can interrupt their regular training programs. The rate at which deconditioning takes place in these athletes needs to be researched, so that guidelines for maintaining and restoring fitness during these periods can be developed.

Central and peripheral adaptations resulting from endurance training

The significant increase in peak $\dot{V}O_2$ in individuals with SCI is attributed to significant improvements in central circulation and/or peripheral oxygen extraction. The peak $\dot{Q}$ is enhanced due to increases in peak HR and SV following endurance training. Arm ergometry endurance training performed at 70% peak $\dot{V}O_2$ for 24 weeks significantly enhances SV, but this improvement is not observed after 10 weeks of training at 60% of peak power output. Usually, there is a significant increase in peak HR post-training in paraplegics because of their increased ability to recruit a greater proportion of their non-paralyzed upper extremities and trunk musculature. Because individuals with quadriplegia have a disruption of the myocardium that restricts their peak HR during exercise, the magnitude of the increase in peak $\dot{Q}$ is not as large as that which is attained by individuals with paraplegia post-training. In fact, it is postulated that a majority of the improvement in peak $\dot{V}O_2$ in quadriplegics is due primarily to improvements in peripheral oxidative capacity during exercise. Endurance training is also effective in increasing peripheral oxygen extraction, as evidenced by a widening of the $(a-v)O_{2diff}$. Significant increases in triceps fiber area and oxidative capacity of the slow-twitch motor units have been reported in recreational athletes with SCI following 8 weeks of arm cranking at 80% of peak HR. However, the fast-twitch fiber area and fiber distribution in the triceps were unaffected by the endurance training program.

With respect to myocardial adaptations, some echocardiographic evidence indicates that paraplegic wheelchair athletes have significantly higher left ventricular volumes compared to their untrained counterparts, while other observations indicate no significant difference between the two groups. The left ventricular ejection fraction of well-trained individuals with paraplegia during wheelchair ergometry is comparable to that observed in able-bodied subjects and does not seem to be affected by the level of physical activity in individuals with paraplegia.

Respiratory muscle training in athletes with SCI

Spinal cord injury compromises function of the respiratory muscles, the magnitude of which depends on the level and completeness of the lesion. Cervical and high-level thoracic lesions impair both inspiratory and expiratory muscle function and necessitate the recruitment of accessory muscles to meet the ventilatory demand. While some respiratory muscle function is preserved at lower levels of paraplegia, ventilatory capacity is still compromised because of altered lung mechanics. Resting spirometry tests indicate that the forced vital capacity (FVC), forced expiratory volume in 1 s (FEV_1), FEV_1/FVC ratio, and maximum ventilation volume (MVV) are significantly lower in individuals with SCI compared to their age- and gender-matched healthy controls. Their breathing pattern during exercise is often inefficient as well. A given ventilation rate is usually achieved by a shallow tidal volume coupled with a high breathing frequency. Furthermore, many wheelchair athletes adopt a forward crouching posture during competitions, which restricts air intake into the lungs and further exacerbates the inefficient breathing pattern. Consequently, a larger proportion of the accessory respiratory musculature is recruited during exercise, which will demand a greater than normal increase in blood flow when compared to able-bodied subjects.

Respiratory muscle training (RMT) is a novel method of training that has been used to improve the ventilatory capacity of athletes with SCI in order to enhance performance. RMT programs are designed to increase inspiratory muscle strength and endurance. Inspiratory muscle strength can be enhanced by breathing through specially developed inspiratory resistive or threshold training devices. The athlete usually performs several sets of isometric contractions against a resistance that imposes an inspiratory overload so that inspiratory muscle strength improves over time. The endurance training method, commonly referred to as hyperpnea training, has been advocated to enhance the endurance capacity of the respiratory musculature. Theoretically, this type of training should provide the maximum benefit during endurance events such as WR and NS because of the large amount of respiratory muscle work required. In this type of training, the athlete breathes in and out of a breathing bag connected to a base unit that automatically controls for the carbon dioxide levels. This ensures that the athlete does not rebreathe high levels of carbon dioxide from the system, which could cause nausea and dizziness during training.

Hyperpnea training is prescribed on the basis of either the peak ventilation rate attained during an incremental exercise test or on the basis of the MVV attained during spirometry testing. Typically, training is initiated at an intensity of 60% MVV using a breathing rate between 20 and 40 breaths/min. Training should be performed continuously for 20–30 min, at least three to four times a week for it to be effective. The principle of progressive overload should be adhered to for continual improvements. Figure 3.7 illustrates an elite Nordic sit skier with SCI performing hyperpnea training using a commercially available rebreathing apparatus. The changes in muscle oxygenation of the serratus anterior measured by NIRS during a 12-min RMT session at an intensity of 75% of MVV in two athletes with high- and low-level paraplegia are illustrated in Figure 3.8. In both the athletes, there was a decrease in muscle oxygenation (implying greater oxygen extraction) at the onset of the hyperpnea training, which persisted throughout the test. However, in athletes with high-level paraplegia, there was a leveling off

in oxygenation, whereas in athletes with low-level paraplegia, there was a systematic decline until the test was terminated. In both the athletes, blood volume to the serratus anterior increased continuously as the duration of the training session increased.

Research that has used RMT in athletes with SCI has yielded mixed results. One study which examined the efficacy of hyperpnea training on wheelchair athletes demonstrated significant improvements in lung function and 10-km WR performance (Mueller et al., 2008). However, another investigation reported no improvement in sport performance even though there was a significant improvement in lung function. This could be due to the fact that the forward crouching posture adopted by athletes during competition does not allow the enhanced tidal volume that is observed with hyperpnea training to be utilized and, therefore, their inefficient breathing pattern persists during competition. Therefore, in order to maximize the benefits of hyperpnea training, it is recommended that coaches incorporate appropriate breathing timing techniques into the training regimen of athletes with SCI. It should be emphasized that RMT should not be used as a substitute for the regular aerobic conditioning programs of athletes with SCI. It should only serve as an adjunct to training so as to provide the athlete with the extra advantage that is crucial for performance. Although RMT programs add to the overall training time of the athletes, one advantage is that the training can be done at home without any supervision.

Temperature regulation in athletes with SCI

Thermoregulatory capacity is impaired in individuals with SCI due to disruption of the autonomic and somatic nervous systems that control skin blood flow and sweating below the level of the lesion. As a result, individuals with SCI are at a higher risk for hyperthermia during exercise. The magnitude of their thermoregulatory impairment is inversely related to the level and completeness of the lesion. In a practical sense, individuals with quadriplegia will have a lower heat tolerance than those with paraplegia and able-bodied subjects. Typically, skin blood flow and sweating capacity for a given core body temperature are reduced in spinal-cord-injured

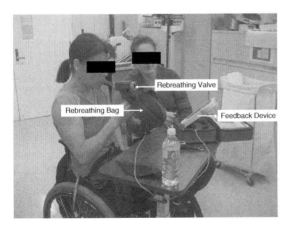

Figure 3.7 Respiratory muscle endurance training in an elite Paralympic Nordic sit skier with low-level paraplegia. The NIRS probe was placed on the serratus anterior, an accessory muscle that is recruited during high-intensity exercise.

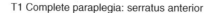

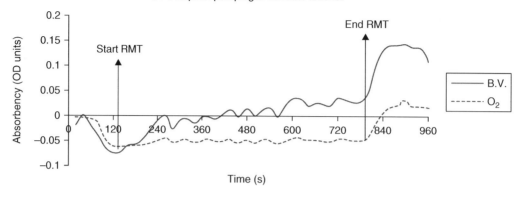

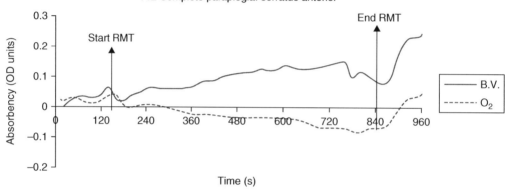

Figure 3.8 Muscle oxygenation and blood volume trends in the serratus anterior during 12 min of hyperpnea training in elite athletes with high- and low-level paraplegia. Muscle oxygenation and blood volume were recorded from the serratus anterior continuously during the test using dual wave near-infrared spectroscopy. See text for explanation of these measurements.

subjects when compared to able-bodied individuals. Athletes with SCI, who compete in endurance events, such as WR, and high-intensity intermittent events, such as WB and WRug, could be at risk for hyperthermic injuries. This risk is greatly increased when the competition is performed in hot and humid environments. The primary physiological reasons for the increased thermoregulatory risk are the failure to stimulate the sweat glands below the lesion and the inability to maintain adequate $\dot{Q}$ during prolonged exercise. Dependency on pharmaceuticals, which can affect bladder capacity and the use of voiding mechanisms by wheelchair road racers, can adversely affect sweating and thermoregulatory function during competition. Although some sweating occurs in the arms and head, this may not be

sufficient to maintain core body temperature within the acceptable range.

Research on athletes with SCI has indicated that passive cooling prior to and during exercise could attenuate the increase in core body temperature that occurs during exercise. Moreover, this attenuation is accompanied by a reduction in the perceptual stress which could translate into improved performance during competition. Localized cooling of the hands by immersion in water at 10C for 10 min is another method that seems to be effective in reducing the postexercise thermoregulatory stress and possibly improving the subsequent simulated WR performance (Goosey-Tolfrey et al., 2008). Localized cooling devices that are worn on the head may reduce HR and esophageal temperature in wheelchair athletes exercising under thermal stress. Besides these techniques, other guidelines that are recommended to minimize thermal stress in able-bodied athletes should also be followed by athletes with SCI including:

• improving aerobic fitness that enhances thermoregulatory capacity during exercise (most researchers agree that training in a cool environment enhances the thermoregulatory responses when exercise is performed at high environmental temperatures);

• avoiding training in environmental conditions above 21°C and 50% relative humidity as this can increase the risk of thermal stress;

• ensuring that adequate fluid–electrolyte balance is maintained during periods of competition;

• refraining from competition during injury or sickness as this can increase susceptibility to heat stress;

• obtaining sufficient rest and sleep when competitions involve travel across different time zones;

• wearing lightweight, loose fitting clothes to enhance evaporation of sweat from the skin surface to facilitate cooling;

• keeping an accurate record of body mass to ensure excessive amounts of fluid are not lost.

Nutritional factors influencing performance

The effects of nutritional supplements on exercise performance in able-bodied athletes have been studied extensively. However, research on this topic in Paralympic athletes is limited (see Chapter 10 for an in-depth discussion of this topic). The available evidence indicates that creatine supplementation (4 × 5 g of creatine monohydrate) over a 6-day period did not significantly reduce the time taken to complete a simulated 800-m wheelchair race on rollers in well-trained wheelchair racers. Also, no significant differences were observed in the peak racing velocity, HR, and blood lactate concentration. It is possible that factors limiting neuromuscular performance at high racing velocities could have masked the ergogenic effects of creatine supplementation. A recent investigation (Temesi et al., 2010) that examined the effects of carbohydrate ingestion on arm cranking performance during a 20-min time trial at 65% of peak $\dot{V}O_2$ in athletes with SCI and complete lesions in the C6 to T7 range

indicated no significant change from the placebo condition. No significant differences were observed between the carbohydrate and placebo trials for the $\dot{V}O_2$, HR, rating of perceived exertion (RPE), lactate concentration, blood glucose, growth hormone, and cortisol concentrations. The lack of improvement in arm cranking performance as a result of carbohydrate ingestion is not consistent with the findings in able-bodied athletes and could be due to altered hormonal factors that regulate carbohydrate metabolism in this population.

Voluntary induction of autonomic dysreflexia (boosting) in quadriplegic athletes

Autonomic dysreflexia is a reflex that is unique to individuals with SCI lesions above the major sympathetic splanchnic outflow (above T6). It is postulated that this response is triggered by nociceptive stimuli distal to the lesion level which result in afferent stimuli that transcend the spinal cord, providing collateral connections to the preganglionic cell bodies of the intermedio-lateral horn, thereby resulting in a massive sympathetic discharge. In individuals with high-level quadriplegia, the magnitude of the amplified discharge is most likely due to:

• denervation hypersensitivity of sympathetic spinal, ganglionic, or peripheral receptor sites;

• loss of supraspinal inhibitory control;

• formation of abnormal synaptic connections resulting from axonal resprouting.

The sympathetic discharge results in peripheral piloerection and vasoconstriction, which is evident in the form of "gooseflesh," shivering, and pallor distal to the level of injury. There is a large increase in systemic blood pressure. In an attempt to buffer the increase in blood pressure, the aortic and carotid baroreceptors are stimulated, which in turn activate the parasympathetic nervous system proximal to the lesion level. However, the descending impulses originating from the vasodilatory center of the medulla are unable to traverse the spinal cord at the level of the lesion, and therefore, peripheral vasoconstriction and systemic hypertension cannot be regulated in the normal manner. The elevated blood pressure can result in several serious conditions such as cerebral hemorrhage, aphasia, blindness, cardiac arrhythmias, and death.

Some athletes with SCI, particularly those who compete in WR and WRug, voluntarily induce autonomic dysreflexia prior to or during the event in order to enhance their performance. Among Paralympians, this is commonly referred to as "boosting." The nociceptive stimuli commonly used to induce boosting are over-distending the bladder by clamping the urinary catheter, sitting on sharp objects, and use of tight leg straps. Research has demonstrated that boosting can significantly increase the peak $\dot{V}O_2$ in athletes with quadriplegia. A 10% improvement in a 7.5-km simulated wheelchair race has been reported in elite wheelchair marathon racers under the boosted condition. Although boosting resulted in an exaggerated systolic blood pressure response, it did not reach levels considered to be dangerous according to the World Health Organization classification for chronic systemic hypertension.

Boosting is considered to be a form of doping in quadriplegic athletes, which is analogous to blood doping in able-bodied sport. The IPC Medical and Anti-Doping Code clearly state that boosting is illegal. Because boosting can be dangerous to health, athletes with SCI who voluntarily induce it prior to competition can be disqualified. Since voluntary boosting cannot be differentiated from the spontaneous occurrence of autonomic dysreflexia, all athletes who demonstrate signs of the condition are subject to medical examination prior to the race. Athletes are routinely checked for visual signs such as increased sweating, skin blotching, "gooseflesh," anxiety, and tremors approximately 1 h prior to competition and at the starting lineup. Repeated blood pressure measurements are taken in athletes who demonstrate some of these signs, and if a systolic blood pressure of ≥ 180 mmHg is consistently observed, then the athlete is prevented from competing.

Cerebral palsy

Neuromuscular deficits resulting from CP

Cerebral palsy is a congenital central nervous system disorder that occurs due to abnormal development or damage in one or more parts of the brain. The condition can be described according to the location of cerebral damage: pyramidal, extrapyramidal, or mixed. Consequently, individuals with CP experience neuromuscular deficits that vary considerably, depending on the location and severity of damage. Damage to the pyramidal tract causes spasticity, defined as an increase in muscle tone, which results in jerky and awkward movements. This is the most common form of CP and accounts for approximately 70–80% of the cases. Damage to the extrapyramidal tract causes two types of dyskinesia that primarily results in uncoordinated movements. Athetoid dyskinesis results in slow, writhing movements that can affect any part of the body including the face, mouth, and tongue. Approximately 10–20% of the cases with CP fall under this category. Ataxic dyskinesis affects balance, coordination, and depth perception. The individual usually has an unsteady gait and has considerable difficulty performing movements that require a great degree of control. Approximately 5–10% of the cases with CP fall under this category. Mixed CP is a combination of the different types of CP, a common combination being spastic and athetoid CP. The following terms are commonly associated with CP:
- quadriplegia implying involvement of all four limbs as well as the head, neck, and trunk;
- triplegia or asymmetric quadriplegia implying involvement of three limbs only;
- paraplegia implying major involvement of only the lower extremities;
- diplegia indicating greater involvement of the lower compared to the upper limbs;
- hemiplegia indicating involvement of upper and lower limbs and the trunk on one side of the body;
- monoplegia indicating involvement of only one limb.

Besides these neuromuscular deficits, many individuals with CP have intellectual, speech, visual, and hearing impairments—all of which could influence physical activity and sport performance.

Measurement of anaerobic power, aerobic power, and body composition

Guidelines for exercise testing

Exercise evaluation of athletes with CP should be based on the functional capacity of their limbs.

Individuals with very mild CP (e.g., Class CP7 or CP8 athletes who are diplegic, hemiplegic, or monoplegic)—who have minimal motor control deficits—can be tested on a treadmill or cycle ergometer with minimal difficulty, provided sufficient care is taken to prevent balance mishaps that can occur during testing. In the more severe cases, individuals with CP who have paraplegia, diplegia, and quadriplegia can be tested using an arm crank or wheelchair ergometer in a way similar to that used for subjects with SCI. It is generally recommended that the testing mode used for evaluating athletes with CP be specific to their mode of ambulation. Regardless of the testing mode, the protocol should be designed to recruit as large a muscle mass as possible so that the maximal physiological responses are elicited within 8–12 min of incremental exercise. In individuals who experience a high degree of spasticity, it may be necessary to strap their hands or feet to the pedals of the arm crank or cycle ergometer during testing in order to obtain a consistent and continuous effort. An accurate record must be kept of the athletes' medications during repeated testing. Many athletes with CP routinely take antispastic medications (e.g., Baclofen or Botox injections) that can influence muscle function and improve performance. The antispastic effects of Botox could last for 6–8 weeks and, therefore, it is recommended that the athletes be evaluated during a period when these effects are nonexistent. The use of anticonvulsive medications, which can influence mental alertness and gross movement patterns, should also be documented during routine athlete testing (Steadward, 1998).

Anaerobic power and capacity

Some cross-sectional studies have demonstrated that the peak anaerobic power and capacity are significantly higher in athletes with CP compared to their nonathletic counterparts. However, the limitations of a cross-sectional design should be kept in mind when interpreting these findings. In one study (Van der Woude et al., 1997), the anaerobic power and capacity of six elite athletes with CP (5 males and 1 female) were evaluated using a 30-s Wingate test performed on a computerized wheelchair ergometer. As was the case for the athletes with SCI, the

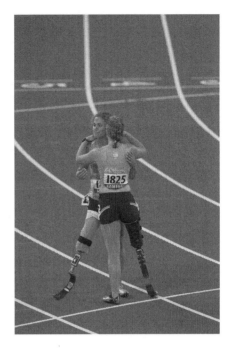

Figure 3.9 Amputee athletes have higher peak 5-s and average 30-s power outputs than athletes with CP. Reproduced courtesy of Lieven Coudenys.

resistance used for testing varied between 2.5% and 10% of the total mass that included the athlete's body weight and the virtual weight of the wheelchair (20 kg). The results indicated a large variation in performance because of the extremely low-power output of two hemiplegic athletes who had a negligible power output on the affected side. Overall, the peak 5-s and average 30-s power output was considerably lower in athletes with CP compared to the track and field athletes with SCI, WB players, and amputees (Figure 3.9). Because of the small number of athletes evaluated, the relationship between anaerobic fitness and sprint performance was not investigated.

Maximal aerobic power and lactate threshold

A comparison of the HR and $\dot{V}O_2$ responses during an incremental wheelchair velocity test to voluntary fatigue in elite athletes with CP, paraplegia, and quadriplegia is provided in Figure 3.2. Unlike individuals with quadriplegia resulting from SCI, sympathetic innervation to the myocardium is not disrupted in individuals with CP. As a result, these individuals are theoretically able to attain their age-predicted maximum HR during incremental exercise to voluntary fatigue. However, localized fatigue can occur before the athlete is able to fully stress the cardiovascular reserve and, therefore, the age-predicted maximum HR may not be attained. This is clearly illustrated in Figure 3.2, where the paraplegic athletes with CP and SCI attained 90% and 93% of their age-predicted maximum HRs, respectively, whereas the quadriplegic athlete with SCI attained only 65% of the age-predicted maximum HR. The peak $\dot{V}O_2$ of the athlete with CP exceeded that of the quadriplegic athlete with SCI, but was 6% lower than that of the paraplegic athlete with SCI. This seems to be a fairly consistent observation in the studies that have reported the peak $\dot{V}O_2$ values in disabled athletes (Van der Woude et al., 2002). Comparison of the peak O_2 pulse, which is considered to be an index of SV, showed that the value of the athlete with CP was higher than that of the quadriplegic athlete with SCI, but lower than that of the paraplegic athlete with SCI (Table 3.1). The lower O_2 pulse in quadriplegics with SCI is most likely due to the venous pooling that occurs in the lower extremities, which tends to reduce the cardiac preload, thereby reducing their SV during exercise. It should be noted that the respiratory exchange ratio exceeded 1.10 in all three athletes, which is one of the criteria for assessing peak aerobic capacity in athletic populations.

The validity of the lactate threshold in athletes with CP is questionable. The nonlinear increase in blood lactate concentration during incremental wheelchair exercise does not coincide with the associated changes in the respiratory gas exchange responses. The reproducibility of the gas exchange responses at the VT is not established. It is hypothesized that these inconsistent responses in athletes with CP could be due to the muscle spasticity which could influence the diffusion of blood lactate from the exercising muscle into the venous blood. It is recommended that when evaluating the cardiorespiratory fitness of athletes with CP, the peak $\dot{V}O_2$ should be used as the criterion measure. The absolute $\dot{V}O_2$ at the VT in athletes with CP is similar during cycle ergometry and treadmill running. However, when the VT is expressed as a percentage of peak $\dot{V}O_2$, the value is significantly higher during cycle ergometry compared to treadmill running, because of the significantly lower peak $\dot{V}O_2$ attained during cycle ergometry. These observations clearly highlight the importance of examining the exercise mode when interpreting these cardiorespiratory fitness data in athletes with CP.

Field tests for predicting the anaerobic power and peak oxygen uptake

In adolescents with spastic CP, the muscle power of the lower extremities can be reliably ($R^2 = 0.94$) measured using a 30-s running test (Verschuren et al., 2007). The individual is asked to complete six 15-m runs at maximal pace, with a 10-s rest between each run. The process is repeated six times in a single session. From these data, the power output for each sprint is calculated using the following equations:

$$\text{Velocity} = \text{m/s} = 15 \text{ m/time}$$
$$\text{Acceleration} = \text{m/s}^2$$
$$\text{Force} = \text{body mass} \times \text{acceleration}$$
$$\text{Power (W)} = \text{force} \times \text{velocity}$$

Many of the field tests used to predict aerobic fitness in able-bodied subjects have also been used in individuals with CP. The 6- and 12-min run-walk test, Astrand–Rhyming cycle ergometer test, and the modified Canadian Aerobic Fitness Test have all been used to predict the peak $\dot{V}O_2$ in this population. However, the validity of these anaerobic and aerobic tests has not been well established in athletes with CP, and there is a lack of normative data for these tests in this population (Figure 3.10).

Body composition

The techniques used to measure the body composition of individuals with CP are similar to those used in individuals with SCI. This includes the use of DEXA, DLW, DEN, BIA, and SF measurements. The use of DEXA and DLW are cost prohibitive and, therefore, are not suitable to test athletes with CP on a regular basis throughout their competitive careers. One investigation, which compared the percentage body fat values in adults with varying degrees of CP using DEXA, DLW, BIA, and SF, reported a strong

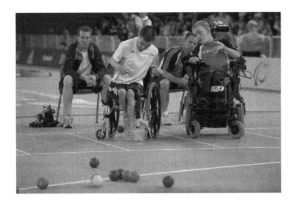

Figure 3.10 There is a lack of normative data for tests of aerobic and anaerobic power in the population of athletes with CP. Reproduced courtesy of Lieven Coudenys.

correlation between the DEXA and DLW methods. However, there was considerable discrepancy between these two techniques and the BIA and SF methods. Another investigation demonstrated a strong correlation between the DEN and SF methods in adults with spastic hemiplegic CP (Hildreth et al., 1997). Although the BIA and SF methods are cost-effective and easy to use, the following factors should be considered when using these techniques to monitor the changes in body composition in athletes with CP. First, the reproducibility of the BIA resistance measurements seems to be influenced by the degree of spasticity in the limbs. It is recommended that sufficient time (15–20 s) be allowed for stability of these measurements to occur and the average of two or three measurements be taken during each evaluation. Second, there are differences in the SF between the paretic and non-paretic sides of subjects with CP in the upper and lower body and the trunk musculature. Therefore, measurements should be recorded on both sides in order to evaluate the changes that occur over time.

Physiological responses during simulated Paralympic sport performance

Quadriplegic athletes with spastic, athetoid, and mixed CP demonstrate significantly higher HRs during power soccer scrimmages and official games compared to those attained by quadriplegic athletes with SCI. One investigation demonstrated that the

difference between the athletes with CP and SCI for the mean and peak HR during the game was 32 beats/min (Barfield et al., 2005). The higher HR in the athletes with CP is most likely due to the fact that sympathetic stimulation to the myocardium is intact, whereas in SCI, quadriplegic athletes' sympathetic stimulation to the myocardium is disrupted. Despite the fact that the athletes were using power (electric) wheelchairs, a majority of them elicited mean HRs that were above the minimum intensity recommended by the ACSM for improving aerobic fitness. The predicted energy expenditure in the athletes with CP was approximately five Metabolic Equivalents (METS), which also exceeds the ACSM criterion for enhancing aerobic fitness. The type of CP—spastic, athetoid, or mixed—did not influence the HR response during the competitions. It is likely that co-contraction of the agonist and antagonist muscle groups contributed to the higher values for the HR and energy expenditure, which resulted in the values being above the minimum ACSM criterion values for enhancing aerobic fitness.

Muscle activation and hemodynamics during wheelchair propulsion

The changes in oxygenation and blood volume of the biceps brachii measured by NIRS in an elite wheelchair distance racer with spastic CP are illustrated in Figure 3.6. This athlete demonstrated a consistent decline in both these variables with increasing velocity of exercise until the test was terminated due to fatigue. This pattern is quite similar to that observed for the SCI quadriplegic athlete but different from that of the SCI paraplegic athlete. The lack of a leveling off in muscle oxygenation in the athlete with CP implies that performance was not limited by peripheral oxygen extraction, which is in contrast to that observed in the paraplegic athlete where peripheral oxygen extraction seemed to reach its limit quite early during the exercise test. The enhanced oxygen requirement in the paraplegic athlete was met primarily by an increase in localized blood volume, whereas in the athlete with CP, the localized blood volume demonstrated a consistent decline from the onset of exercise. These subtle differences in the hemodynamic responses clearly demonstrate that athletes have their independent patterns of meeting the oxygen demands during exercise, and such measurements could be extremely useful in monitoring and designing training programs to enhance athletic performance.

Effects of physical training on physiological fitness

Because CP is a congenital disorder, a majority of the research has focused on enhancing physical fitness in children and adolescents with this condition. There is considerable evidence which indicates that aerobic and resistance training programs induce significant increases in aerobic fitness as well as muscle strength and endurance in individuals with CP. These improvements are accompanied by increases in functional capacity such as faster walking/running speeds, stair climbing ability, and wheelchair propulsion. The enhanced performance may be sustained for several weeks after the training is discontinued. There is some evidence which suggests that resistance training may not enhance the strength of children and adolescents with CP because of co-contraction of the agonistic and antagonistic muscles. However, these observations should be interpreted with caution because the training intensity may not have been sufficient to induce gains in muscular strength and endurance. Regular exercise training does not increase muscle spasticity, reduce flexibility, or induce muscle damage in individuals with CP and, therefore, should not be a deterrent for fitness programming in this population.

There is limited research that has examined the effects of physical training in adults with CP, and more so in athletes with this condition. Cross-sectional evidence indicates that the peak $\dot{V}O_2$ and VT are significantly higher in athletes with CP compared to their untrained counterparts. Comparisons between paraplegic athletes with CP and SCI indicate that the peak $\dot{V}O_2$ is similar or slightly lower in the former group. Longitudinal evidence indicates that untrained adults with CP, who train aerobically for 8 weeks, can significantly increase their physical work capacity and functional performance on a variety of tasks. A 10-week community-based progressive resistance training program can significantly increase leg and arm strength and

improve sit-to-stand performance. Some evidence suggests that regular aerobic training may enhance mechanical efficiency by reducing the gross energy expenditure of functional tasks and improve the self-perception of the participants. These observations have important implications for individuals with CP who are aspiring to become Paralympic athletes. The efficacy of whole body vibration (WBV) training for enhancing muscular strength and endurance in able-bodied individuals has been well documented. One study, which compared the effects of 8 weeks of resistance training with WBV training in adults with CP, demonstrated significant increases in knee extensor strength in both training groups but no improvement in the 6-min walking and timed "up and go" tests. There was no improvement in these functional tasks even though the WBV training group demonstrated a significant reduction in muscle spasticity.

Central and peripheral adaptations resulting from endurance training

The alterations in the central ($\dot{Q}$) and peripheral ((a-v)O_{2diff}) factors contributing to the improvements in peak $\dot{V}O_2$ in individuals with CP have not been investigated. However, one cross-sectional investigation (Oliveira et al., 2007) compared the cardiorespiratory responses and echocardiographic findings between athletes with CP (10 soccer players and 2 sprinters) and athletes with SCI (basketball players and track and field athletes). The athletes with CP had significantly higher peak $\dot{V}O_2$ and VT values when compared to the athletes with SCI, but lower values when compared to able-bodied athletes. However, the echocardiographic measurements, namely the left ventricular internal diastolic dimension, interventricular septum thickness, left ventricular mass/body surface ratio, and left ventricular ejection fraction, were within the normal range observed in able-bodied athletes. These findings suggest that endurance-trained athletes with CP adapt in a way similar to that observed in able-bodied athletes. Therefore, it is assumed that the improvement in peak $\dot{V}O_2$ is most likely due to significant increases in both central circulation and peripheral oxygen extraction (i.e., increased (a-v)O_{2diff}).

RMT in individuals with CP

Individuals with spastic CP have reduced chest mobility, which can reduce their breathing efficiency. It has been reported that RMT can increase the strength of the inspiratory and expiratory muscles and significantly improve the vital capacity in individuals with CP. However, the influence of RMT on ventilatory muscle endurance and functional capacity has not been evaluated in this population. It is possible that the increased spasticity of the respiratory muscles in athletes with CP could increase the energy cost of breathing during prolonged exercise and high-intensity intermittent efforts, thereby adversely affecting performance. While this training modality seems to be effective in athletes with SCI, its efficacy on athletes with CP has yet to be investigated.

Temperature regulation in individuals with CP

Theoretically, a reduced mechanical efficiency (i.e., greater energy cost per unit amount of work) in individuals with CP would increase their thermal stress during prolonged exercise. This could result in thermoregulatory injuries and premature fatigue in athletes competing in long-duration events. The thermoregulatory responses in athletes with CP have not been scientifically studied during exercise. However, one investigation compared the physiological responses in children and adolescents with mild to moderate CP with age- and gender-matched healthy controls during three 10-min intermittent bouts of arm cranking exercise performed at the same relative intensity under two conditions: $21-23°C \pm 1°C$ and $35C \pm 1°C$, 45–50% relative humidity. The results indicted no significant differences between the two groups for the metabolic rate, total heat production, and rectal temperature. However, the rise in skin temperature was significantly lower in the CP compared to the healthy group. The generalizability of these findings to the athletic population is questionable for several reasons. First, the study utilized arm cranking as the exercise mode, which is mechanically more efficient than wheelchair ergometry. Second, the exercise intensity corresponded to approximately 60% of the age-predicted maximum HR of the participants, which is well below the intensity attained by athletes during training and competition. Third, duration of

the exercise protocol was not long enough to induce a substantial thermoregulatory stress. The participants performed three intermittent bouts of arm cranking exercise interspersed with three 10-min recovery intervals. This duration is considerably shorter than the time taken by athletes with CP to complete long-distance races such as the wheelchair marathon. Considerable recovery could take place during the intermittent rest periods of the protocol. Currently, there is a need for research to systematically examine the thermoregulatory responses of athletes with CP exposed to different environmental conditions (hot and cold climates) so that appropriate guidelines for training and competition could be developed.

Summary

There is limited research addressing the physiological aspects of elite Paralympic athletes with physical disabilities. Although techniques such as DLW and DEXA provide more comprehensive information on the body composition, they are not feasible for regular testing of athletes with SCI and CP because they involve invasive procedures and require sophisticated equipment. Additional research is needed to validate the simpler methods such as BIA and SF measurements, so that these techniques can be routinely used to monitor the body composition of Paralympic athletes during the competitive careers. Exercise testing to measure anaerobic and aerobic fitness can be conducted using a variety of exercise modes depending on the functional capacity of the athlete. Researchers have used the treadmill, arm crank, wheelchair, rowing, and double poling ergometers for these evaluations. It is highly recommended that the exercise mode selected for assessing fitness be specific to the exercise mode used in athletic competition. Generally speaking, the findings from the studies published on Paralympic sport physiology need to be interpreted with caution for several reasons:

• There is considerable variation in the load factors used for assessment of anaerobic power and differences in the incremental exercise protocols for measuring peak $\dot{V}O_2$, which makes it difficult to compare the findings across studies.

• The sample sizes within a disability classification are quite small in a vast majority of the studies, thereby limiting the generalizability of the findings to the athletic population under consideration.

• In several studies, descriptive statistics on individuals from different classes or lesion levels are pooled, which makes it difficult to interpret the results.

• The majority of the studies have been conducted on males with a limited database on females. Cross-sectional data indicate that well-trained Paralympic athletes have higher anaerobic and aerobic fitness levels compared to their untrained counterparts.

However, well-controlled longitudinal training studies on Paralympic athletes are very sparse and are urgently needed to confirm the cross-sectional results. Researchers need to make a concerted effort to address these issues in order to improve our understanding of the physiological responses of elite Paralympic athletes, so that physical training programs can be designed on the basis of sound scientific information.

References

Barfield, J.P., Malone, L.A., Collins, J.M. & Ruble, S.B. (2005). Disability type influences heart rate response during power wheelchair sport. *Medicine and Science in Sports and Exercise*, **37**, 718–723.

Bernardi, M., Guerra, E., Di Giacinto, B., Di Cesare, A., Castellano, V. & Bhambhani, Y. Field evaluation of Paralympic athletes in selected sports: implications for training. *Medicine and Science in Sports and Exercise*, 2010, **42**(6): 1200–1208.

Bhambhani, Y. (2002). Physiology of wheelchair racing in athletes with spinal cord injury. *Sports Medicine*, **32**, 23–51.

Desport, J.C., Preux, P.M., Guinvarc'h, S., et al. (2000). Total body water and percentage fat mass measurements using bioelectrical impedance analysis and anthropometry in spinal cord-injured patients. *Clinical Nutrition*, **19**, 185–190. doi:10.1054/clnu.1999.0122.

Goosey-Tolfrey, V., Swainson, M., Boyd, C., Atkinson, G. & Tolfrey, K. (2008). The effectiveness of hand cooling at reducing exercise-induced hyperthermia and improving distance-race performance in wheelchair and able-bodied athletes. *Journal of Applied Physiology*, **105**, 37–43.

Hildreth, H.G., Johnson, R.K., Goran, M.I. & Contompasis, S.H. (1997). Body composition in adults with cerebral palsy by dual-energy X-ray absorptiometry, bioelectrical impedance analysis, and skinfold anthropometry compared with the ^{18}O isotope-dilution technique. *The American Journal of Clinical Nutrition*, **66**, 1436–1442.

Mojtahedi, M.C., Valentine, R.J. & Evans, E.M. (2009). Body composition assessment in athletes with spinal cord injury: comparison of field methods with dual-energy X-ray absorptiometry. *Spinal Cord*, **47**, 698–704.

Mueller, G., Perret, C. & Hopman, M.T. (2008). Effects of respiratory muscle endurance training on wheelchair racing performance in athletes with paraplegia: a pilot study. *Clinical Journal of Sport Medicine*, **18**, 85–88.

Oliveira, J.A., Salvetti, X.M., Lira, E.B., Mello, M.T., Silva, A.C. & Luna, B. (2007). Athlete's heart, oxygen uptake and morphologic findings in paralympic athletes. *International Journal of Cardiology*, **121**, 100–101.

Poulain, M., Vinet, A., Bernard, P.L. & Varray, A. (1999). Reproducibility of the adapted Leger and Boucher test for wheelchair-dependent athletes. *Spinal Cord*, **37**, 129–135.

Sheel, A.W., Reid, W.D., Townson, A.F., Ayas, N.T., Konnyu, K.J., Spinal Cord Rehabilitation Evidence Research Team (2008). Effects of exercise training and inspiratory muscle training in spinal cord injury: a systematic review. *The Journal of Spinal Cord Medicine*, **31**, 500–508.

Steadward, R. (1998). Musculoskeletal and neurological disabilities: implications for fitness appraisal, programming, and counseling. *Canadian Journal of Applied Physiology*, **23**, 131–165.

Temesi, J., Rooney, K., Raymond, J. & O'Connor, H. (2010). Effect of carbohydrate ingestion on exercise performance and carbohydrate metabolism in persons with spinal cord injury. *European Journal of Applied Physiology*, **108**, 131–140.

Van der Woude, L.H., Bakker, W.H., Elkhuizen, J.W., Veeger, H.E. & Gwinn, T. (1997). Anaerobic work capacity in elite wheelchair athletes. *American Journal of Physical Medicine & Rehabilitation*, **76**, 355–365.

Van der Woude, L.H., Bouten, C., Veeger, H.E. & Gwinn, T. (2002). Aerobic work capacity in elite wheelchair athletes: a cross-sectional analysis. *American Journal of Physical Medicine & Rehabilitation*, **81**, 261–271.

Verschuren, O., Takken, T., Ketelaar, M., Gorter, J.W. & Helders, P.J. (2007). Reliability for running tests for measuring agility and anaerobic muscle power in children and adolescents with cerebral palsy. *Pediatric Physical Therapy*, **19**, 108–115.

Recommended readings

American College of Sports Medicine (2010). *Guidelines for Exercise Testing and Prescription*, 8th edition. Lippincott Williams & Wilkins, Philadelphia, PA.

Bhambhani, Y. (2002). Physiology of wheelchair racing in athletes with spinal cord injury. *Sports Medicine*, **32**, 23–51.

Bhambhani, Y. (2003). Principles of fitness assessment and training for wheelchair athletes. In: R.D. Steadward, G.D. Wheeler & E.J. Watkinson (eds.) *Adapted Physical Activity*. The University of Alberta Press, Alberta, Canada.

Goosey-Tolfrey, V.L. & Tolfrey, K. (2004). The oxygen uptake–heart rate relationship in trained female wheelchair athletes. *Journal of Rehabilitation Research and Development*, **41**, 415–420.

Knechtle, B., Muller, G., Willmann, F., Eser, P. & Knecht, H. (2004). Fat oxidation at different intensities in wheelchair racing. *Spinal Cord*, **42**, 24–28.

Litchke, L.G., Russian, C.J., Lloyd, L.K., Schmidt, E.A., Price, L. & Walker, J.L. (2008). Effects of respiratory resistance training with a concurrent flow device on wheelchair athletes. *The Journal of Spinal Cord Medicine*, **31**, 65–71.

Miyahara, K., Wang, D.H., Mori, K., et al. (2008). Effect of sports activity on bone mineral density in wheelchair athletes. *Journal of Bone and Mineral Metabolism*, **26**, 101–106.

Thorpe, D. (2009). The role of fitness in health and disease: status of adults with cerebral palsy. *Developmental Medicine and Child Neurology*, **51(Suppl. 4)**, 52–58.

Williams, H. & Pountney, T. (2007). Effects of a static bicycling programme on the functional ability of young people with cerebral palsy who are non-ambulant. *Developmental Medicine and Child Neurology*, **49**, 522–527.

Chapter 4
Medicine

Stuart Willick[1] and Nick Webborn[2]

[1]Division of Physical Medicine and Rehabilitation University of Utah Orthopedic Center,
Salt Lake City, UT, USA
[2]Chelsea School Research Centre, University of Brighton, East Sussex, UK

Introduction

There are an increasing number of opportunities for individuals with physical disabilities to participate in all levels of recreational and competitive sports. Numerous sports organizations for the disabled now exist, which provide information, resources, and support for nearly all sports and leisure activities. The largest organized events for athletes with physical disabilities are the Paralympic Games. The Paralympics are one of the largest sports events in the world, now second in size only to the Olympics. Since their inception in 1948, originally as the Stoke Mandeville Games, participation in the Paralympic Games has increased dramatically, reflecting an increase in sports participation among individuals with physical disabilities in general. In 1960, 400 athletes from 23 countries took part in the Summer Paralympics in Rome. By 2008, approximately 4000 athletes from 148 countries competed at the Beijing Summer Paralympics. Although earlier Paralympic games included primarily wheelchair athletes, the Paralympics have included ambulatory persons with limb deficiencies since 1976. Today, the Paralympics are an elite sporting event for athletes from different disability groups, including wheelchair athletes, amputees, athletes with cerebral palsy, athletes with visual impairment, and "Les Autres."

Due to the increase in sports participation of individuals with physical disabilities, there has been an increased need for excellent medical care of this population. Despite the growing awareness and popularity of sports for the disabled, there remains a relative paucity of published research on sports medicine specifically for this athletic population. Sports medicine professionals who care for athletes with disabilities should be familiar with the medical and musculoskeletal issues of this unique population. The first part of this chapter reviews general medical considerations for athletes with physical disabilities. The second part of this chapter reviews the literature on disabled sports injury epidemiology. A section on the clinical evaluation of athletes with disabilities during the pre-participation evaluation (PPE) is included. The final part of the chapter discusses special considerations for athletes with disabilities who travel long distances for training and competition.

Medical conditions specific to athletes with a disability

Athletes with physical disabilities can experience the same spectrum of medical conditions as athletes without disabilities. In addition, athletes with physical disabilities can experience some medical conditions that are not seen in able-bodied athletes. These include, but are not limited to, autonomic dysreflexia (AD), orthostatic hypotension, skin breakdown, bladder dysfunction, nerve entrapments,

The Paralympic Athlete, 1st edition. Edited by Yves C. Vanlandewijck and Walter R. Thompson. Published 2011 by Blackwell Publishing Ltd.

and osteoporosis. Disorders of thermoregulation are discussed in Chapters 12 and 13.

Autonomic dysreflexia

Autonomic dysreflexia is a condition specific to individuals with a spinal cord injury (SCI) at or above the level of T6. AD is an abnormal surge of sympathetic output caused by any noxious stimulus below the level of the spinal lesion. Common inciting conditions for AD include an over-distended bladder and musculoskeletal trauma and illness. The untoward sympathetic discharge is a reflex mediated by the spinal cord in the absence of cortical regulation. It results in widespread vasoconstriction, most significantly in the splanchnic vascular bed. Baroreceptors in the neck then mediate a compensatory vagal (parasympathetic) response that results in bradycardia and decreased cardiac output. The decreased cardiac output is not sufficient to offset the abnormal sympathetic surge and hypertension continues. Symptoms of mild and moderate AD include headache, blurry vision, nasal congestions, anxiety, flushing, sweating, and goose bumps. If AD is left untreated and a hypertensive crisis ensues, it can result in stroke and death. For this reason, AD is a medical emergency. Severity and frequency of AD depends on the height of the lesion.

The first-line treatment for AD is to identify and remove the inciting stimulus. This may include emptying an over-distended bladder or treating an acute sports injury. The athlete should sit up in an attempt to cause an orthostatic drop in blood pressure. If hypertension persists or worsens, antihypertensive medication should be given. One safe and effective way to rapidly decrease blood pressure is to apply nitropaste to the skin. Nitropaste is fast acting and can be easily wiped off when symptoms resolve or if hypotension occurs.

Some athletes with high SCI purposefully self-induce AD by providing themselves with an occult noxious stimulus, such as clamping their urinary catheter or sticking themselves with a sharp object in an insensate location below the level of their injury. These athletes try to take advantage of a quasi-controlled sympathetic surge to enhance their sports performance. This technique is referred to as boosting. Boosting may provide the athlete with an unfair competitive advantage and can also pose a serious health risk to the athlete. For these reasons, boosting is a prohibited technique in disabled sports competition. Athletes who are found guilty of boosting are subject to disqualification and long-term sanctions.

Orthostatic hypotension

The same neuroregulatory impairment of the sympathetic/parasympathetic balance can make some individuals with upper thoracic and cervical SCIs prone to orthostatic hypotension. Symptomatic hypotension can occur if an athlete sits up suddenly. It can also occur during intensive sports participation. Symptoms include light headedness, nausea, and syncope. Tachycardia is a compensatory cardiovascular response to the hypotension. Although orthostatic hypotension is generally more problematic during the acute and subacute periods following an SCI, it can sometimes persist even in chronic SCI. There are several treatments available for symptomatic orthostatic hypotension in athletes with high SCI. It is very important for the athlete to maintain proper hydration, nutritional status, and salt balance. Elastic stockings may be beneficial to decrease peripheral pooling of blood. Abdominal binders have been used for the same reason, but are not always well tolerated during athletic activities. If an athlete is experiencing a more severe episode of orthostatic hypotension, he or she should be placed in a supine or Trendelenburg position. In refractory cases, intravenous fluids and sympathomimetic agents may be necessary for blood pressure support. These last two interventions should be used only in an emergency, as they are on the prohibited list of the World Anti-Doping Agency (WADA).

Skin breakdown

Another medical problem seen in athletes with physical disabilities is skin breakdown. Athletes with SCI are prone to pressure sores in insensate areas and they should do frequent pressure releases to avoid skin ischemia. This can be challenging during endurance events and during international travel.

Athletes with severe spasticity are prone to skin breakdown in locations where high muscle tone or contractures cause abnormal or persistent skin friction. Special padding, antispasticity medications, and surgical procedures for tendon lengthening may be required to improve positioning and decrease abnormal skin rubbing. Proper positioning in the athlete's wheelchair is preferred over aggressive use of straps to counter the spastic movements. Athletes with amputations are prone to skin breakdown over the end of their stump and other areas of increased pressure between the skin and prosthesis. Proper prosthetic fit is crucial to decrease the risk of skin problems in these athletes. Other skin problems seen in athletes who use prostheses include verrucus hyperplasia (aka "choke syndrome") and rashes such as tinea and folliculitis. These conditions can limit the individual's ability to participate in athletic activities. Athletes who are at risk for skin problems should perform regular skin checks and seek medical consultation right away if skin breakdown occurs or a rash develops.

Neurogenic bladder

Complications of a neurogenic bladder can also limit sports participation. Many athletes with SCI have a neurogenic bladder that results in an inability to spontaneously void. There are different treatments for neurogenic bladder. In some individuals with SCI, bladder emptying can be facilitated with the use of medications. More commonly, individuals with SCI will require bladder catheterization in order to empty their bladder. This can be accomplished in one of three primary ways. If an athlete has adequate manual dexterity, the preferred method of bladder management is intermittent catheterization every 4–6 h. For athletes with a cervical SCI, who lack sufficient manual dexterity, continuous bladder drainage by way of a Foley catheter attached to a leg bag is the most common form of bladder management. The use of suprapubic catheters has become less common over recent years.

Regardless of the method of bladder management, all individuals with neurogenic bladder are at increased risk of urinary tract infections and other complications. Intermittent catheterization carries a lower risk of urinary tract infection compared with the use of an indwelling Foley or suprapubic catheter. Other complications include the development of bladder sediments and bladder stones, over-distention of the bladder, urethral irritation, and bladder carcinoma.

The inability of elite athletes with neurogenic bladder to spontaneously void has implications for doping control. If bladder management for an athlete is by means of an indwelling catheter that drains to a leg bag, it is necessary to first drain the leg bag completely, discard the urine from the leg bag, and then wait for the production of fresh urine to collect the sample. If bladder management is by intermittent catheterization, the athlete must self-catheterize in order to produce a urine sample. In both of these circumstances, it is challenging to insure the provision of a truly clean urine sample. At the present time, it is not required that athletes catheterize with a new, sterile catheter in order to provide a urine sample for doping control.

Peripheral nerves

Athletes with physical disabilities are also at increased risk of peripheral nerve problems. Athletes with amputations are at risk of getting painful neuromas at the end of their stump. Treatment options include decreasing training time, modification of the prosthesis to unload the painful area, topical treatments, oral medications, and various procedures to either ablate or resect the neuroma. Examples of topical treatments include lidocaine patches and capsaicin cream. Oral medications can include acetaminophen, nonsteroidal anti-inflammatory medications, and neuropathic pain medications. Neuropathic pain medications should be used with caution because side effects include tiredness, which may impair athletic performance. If an athlete is suffering pain that is recalcitrant to noninterventional treatments, attempts at percutaneous ablation of the neuroma with alcohol injection or application of radiofrequency energy may be tried. Surgical resection of the neuroma is considered a treatment of last resort. Neuromas may re-form even after ablation or resection.

Athletes who regularly use wheelchairs or crutches are at increased risk for upper-limb peripheral neuropathies including ulnar neuropathy at the wrist within Guyon's canal, ulnar neuropathy at the elbow within the cubital tunnel, median neuropathy at the wrist within the carpal tunnel, and other more proximal neuropathies. Athletes with below knee amputations are at risk for peroneal neuropathy at the fibular head due to improper prosthetic fit. Underlying neurological conditions such as central and peripheral nervous system injuries and diseases can make it challenging to clinically diagnose a sports-related peripheral nerve injury. Electrodiagnostic testing can be helpful for distinguishing new versus chronic nerve lesions.

Bone density

The medical team should also be cognizant of potential issues related to the athlete's bone density. Athletes with SCI and other neuromuscular conditions such as polio will very often have osteoporosis in the paretic limbs. Low bone density places an athlete at increased risk for fracture with even relatively minor trauma. In the setting of osteoporosis, nondisplaced fractures can be easily missed on plain radiographs. Therefore, the sports medicine practitioner should maintain a high index of suspicion for fracture, even if there was minimal trauma and normal X-rays. Athletes with sensory loss may not report pain even after sustaining a fracture. Magnetic resonance imaging or computed tomography may be necessary to fully assess a possible bone injury in these circumstances.

Young adults with traumatic amputations have been recovering more quickly from their injuries than previously, and are pursuing vigorous activities, earlier in the course of their rehabilitation, with some receiving specially adapted running prostheses as early as 4–6 months after their amputation. Due to case reports of residual limb fractures attributed to osteopenia during competitive running, some have proposed clearance of athletes with bone densitometry prior to initiation of aggressive sports programs. However, this recommendation has not been widely accepted. More investigation into the natural course of bone loss following amputation and SCI, and identification of distal limb bone density reference values, is still required.

Sports epidemiology

Musculoskeletal injury patterns are sport- and disability-specific. Knowledge of alterations in force distribution patterns and compensatory strategies for force generation will help clinicians to better diagnose, treat, and prevent injuries in these athletes. A comprehensive discussion of adaptive sports biomechanics is found in Chapter 2 and will not be repeated here. However, an understanding of the biomechanical concepts related to adaptive sports is very helpful when trying to understand injury patterns.

As mentioned in the introduction section of this chapter, there is a relative paucity of published literature on musculoskeletal injuries in athletes with disabilities. Some of the studies reviewed here focus on athletes with disabilities participating in summer sports and some focus on athletes participating in winter sports. The available epidemiology literature tends to be mostly retrospective surveys with athletes self-reporting medical information. These reports also tend to lack diagnostic specificity with reports limited to the body parts involved, but not the specific diagnosis.

Overall injury rates are the same for athletes with and without physical disabilities. However, injury patterns differ and injuries may carry greater functional consequences for the athlete with a disability. Laskowski and Murtaugh (1992) published data on injuries among skiers with physical disabilities gathered from instructional programs at four ski resorts with large skiing programs for the disabled. Their survey gathered information on total number of injuries, age and gender, type of disability, injury type, location, severity, mechanism, snow conditions, and experience level. They found no significant difference in overall injury rates between able-bodied and disabled skiers (3.7:1000 disabled and 3.5:1000 able-bodied). The types of injuries seen, however, were statistically different with disabled skiers having more abrasions and bruises, while able-bodied skiers sustained more fractures and lacerations. It is noted that there have been substantial technical advances in sit ski equipment since that time, which have likely had an impact on injury rates and types. Prospective data captured during the 2002 Winter Paralympic Games found that 9% of all athletes sustained an injury, with sprains (32%), fractures (21%), and strains and lacerations (14% each) as the most common diagnoses (Webborn et al., 2006). Most of these injuries (77%) had an acute traumatic onset, approximating the percent of acute injuries recorded during the 2002 Winter Olympic Games. Injury rates among Paralympians were higher in sledge hockey (14%) and alpine skiing (12%), and lower in Nordic skiing (2%).

Data on athletes with disabilities competing in summer sports from the Athletes with Disabilities Injury Registry found injury rates of 9.3/1000 athlete exposures (AE). The term "AE" is often defined as one athlete participating in one competition match or practice. This is similar to injury rates in many able-bodied sports: college (American) football 10.1/1000 AE, college (American) soccer 9.8/1000 AE, men's basketball 7.0/1000 AE, and women's basketball 7.3/1000 AE (Ferrara & Peterson, 2000). Nyland et al. (2000) investigated the different types of injuries sustained by athletes with disabilities participating in the 1996 Atlanta Summer Paralympic Games. One notable finding was that athletes with amputations and visual impairment sustained more ankle injuries than athletes with other physical disabilities. The incidence of shoulder pain in all wheelchair users has been variably estimated between 30% and 70%.

Bernardi et al. (2003) retrospectively investigated what they termed "sports-related muscle pain (SRMP)" among elite athletes with various physical disabilities (SCI, amputation, cerebral palsy, and "Les Autres"). Athletes participated in various sports including swimming, basketball, track and field, skiing, fencing, and wheelchair tennis. Fifty-one percent of these athletes reported that they had experienced SRMP during the prior 12-month period. The most commonly involved body regions included shoulder (56%), followed by upper limb (33%) and lumbar spine (13%). Most of the pain was rated as moderate intensity (49%). Self-reported SRMP was generally brief, with 71% reporting that their pain lasted for less than 7 days. Sprinting was the most common cause (33%) of SRMP. Athletic activity was interrupted in 63% of cases. Work activity

was interrupted by these injuries in 11% of cases, highlighting the more global impact sports injuries can have on athletes with disabilities. This study also showed that athletes with SCI and amputation were more prone to SRMP than athletes with other types of physical disabilities. Other factors statistically associated with SRMP included training more than 7 hours per week and higher body mass index (BMI).

A study performed by Ferrara and Peterson (2000) looked at different injury patterns in wheelchair and ambulatory athletes. In contrast to wheelchair athletes who primarily experience upper-limb injury, ambulatory athletes (amputee, visually impaired, and cerebral palsy) more commonly experience lower-limb injury. Among amputees, athletes with upper-limb deficiencies tend to have more cervical and thoracic spine injuries, whereas athletes with lower-limb deficiencies have more lumbar spine injuries. Klenck and Gebke (2007) speculated that the greater incidence of thoracic and cervical injuries among upper-limb amputees was due to balance issues, while the greater incidence of lumbar injuries among lower-limb amputees was due to excessive lumbar spine lateral flexion and extension. Although injury prevention and outcome studies have not been published, it is possible that the incidence of spine injuries among athletes with amputations might be decreased with training programs that emphasize balance, proprioceptive training, core strengthening, and maintaining flexibility about the hip and knee.

Osteoarthritis (OA) of the hips and knees is another concern in athletes with lower-limb amputations due to altered loading patterns. Studies have demonstrated that amputees have an increased prevalence of OA in the contralateral knee (primarily medial and anterior compartments) compared with able-bodied persons (Melzer et al., 2001). However, whether or not participation in sports increases this risk is not known.

This limited body of epidemiologic literature informs us that injury prevention programs should include careful monitoring of volume, progression and type of training (e.g., hours per week), and BMI. There is also a need for better protection of areas of high impact and stress in disabled athletes. Two examples of this include protecting the lower limbs from direct trauma during sledge hockey (Figure 4.1) and protecting the upper limbs of skiers from excessive torque when using outrigger poles. Changing

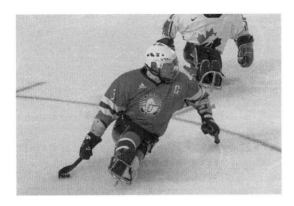

Figure 4.1 Protecting the lower limbs from direct trauma during sledge hockey reduces the risk of injury. Reproduced courtesy of Lieven Coudenys.

patterns of sports participation and advances in wheelchair and prosthetic design will require ongoing study as they will change biomechanics, adaptive mechanisms, and injury patterns. The International Paralympic Committee has instituted a long-term injury surveillance system designed to characterize athlete injuries in detail, with a focus on identifying risk factors for injury and implementing injury reduction strategies.

Clinical evaluation

There are no specific guidelines for PPEs of the disabled athlete. Preferably, the PPE should be conducted by the team of medical professionals that will be involved in the longitudinal care of the athlete and who understand the individual's baseline functioning. Some of the many factors that should be considered include the athlete's current health status, level of competition, environment in which the activity will occur, requirements of the position played, adaptive and protective equipment, technical aspects of the sport, psychological maturity, and understanding of the inherent risks of injury by the athlete, family, and coach.

The PPE should parallel that of an able-bodied athlete and include a detailed history, review of symptoms, and physical examination. Evaluation of the current state of health must include general and disability-related health issues. Complete neurologic, musculoskeletal and cardiopulmonary, and skin assessments should also be performed.

Muscle tightness or contracture is not uncommon, especially in the hip flexors. Tightness of the hip flexors can lead to increased lumbar lordosis and resultant low back pain. Also, for those wanting to participate in competitive sports, a detailed assessment of other musculoskeletal impairments is necessary for correct sport-specific classification. Finally, as with all athletes, a full evaluation of other medical issues should be performed. Paralympic athletes tend to be older than their able-bodied counterparts. Cardiac testing may be considered depending on the level of desired activity, age, and cardiovascular disease risk factors.

In those with congenital limb deficiencies, it is important to realize that they may have other deficiencies in muscles, bones, soft tissues, and ligaments that are not readily apparent. For example, individuals with congenitally short femurs may have anterior cruciate ligament (ACL) deficiencies as well and can be misdiagnosed with an acute ACL tear based on clinical laxity.

Athletes with certain physical disabilities may take medications to treat symptoms of the disability. These medications and their side effects may not be familiar to health-care providers who do not regularly take care of the disabled population. Examples of such medications include medications to control spasticity and movement disorders, medications for neuropathic bladder and bowel function, and medications for neuropathic pain. For a further discussion on this topic, refer to Chapter 10.

A keen understanding of potential implications that an injury may have on the activities performed by the athlete is essential for both the clinician and the athlete. This applies not only to the athlete's sport participation but also to their ability to perform specific activities in daily life. For example, a lower-limb amputee with Achilles tendinopathy that suffers a rupture of the tendon will have a much greater impact on specific activities in comparison to an able-bodied athlete with the same injury.

Travel considerations for athletes with a disability

The act of traveling long distances can have various consequences that can impact on health for anyone.

However, for an athlete with a disability, there may be additional factors that increase the risk of becoming ill. To ensure that the athlete with a disability arrives for any competition in the best condition, there are several things that need to be done in preparation and planning. Both injury and illness can impact on wellness so strategies need to be in place to help prevent, or just overcome problems that athletes will inevitably face. In this section, the author (Webborn) writes in the fairly unique position of having been a sports medicine practitioner traveling with and looking after elite athletes, and also having been a competitive athlete with a disability traveling to competitions around the world.

Although much can be learnt from the literature related to able-bodied athletes in relation to athlete illness and injuries, the health-care team has to think slightly differently because of the unique nature of the individual disability of the athlete. Health risks are dependent on the individual's susceptibility. Any pretravel risk assessment must be based on a sound knowledge of the athletes and their medical condition. Depending on the disability, it is possible that the same medical problem will have an impact on some athletes which is different in some respects from able-bodied athletes. Some conditions can actually have a significant impact on "health" but little impact on performance. For example, wheelchair racers who have a fracture of their paralyzed leg may not see that as a significant limitation to performance if they do not experience any pain. In an able-bodied athlete, this would be seen to have a massive health and performance impact. However, a problem that might seem relatively minor to an able-bodied athlete might significantly impair the health of an athlete with a disability. For example, a small blister caused by skin chafing on the knee would be considered relatively minor in health terms, but if this was where a prosthetic limb rubbed and caused pain during running, then it would have an important limitation on performance. The important lesson is that athletes must be thought of as individuals and perform individual risk assessments to help them stay healthy during travel so that they can train and compete optimally. A physician or therapist traveling with a team will need the necessary skills, experience, and equipment to optimize medical conditions

based on this risk assessment. Oftentimes athletes with disabilities travel unaccompanied by medical staff. The approach outlined below can be utilized by athletes or accompanying coaches as an aide-mémoire to planning for long-haul travel.

Paralympic athletes learn to cope and live in their home environment, adapting to the environmental conditions, developing support services, such as doctors, physiotherapists, or others on the health-care team. Athletes are familiar with their home accommodation, methods of travel, training environments, and by familiarity and adaptation learn to cope with any limitations. However, traveling to training camps and competitions away from home can present many challenges that athletes will have to adapt to and manage. Having local knowledge and people to liaise with can be very useful, but one cannot always rely on a complete understanding of their needs. On face value, what appears to be acceptable to the local provider does not meet the needs of many Paralympic athletes. An example might be an "accessible" room with a door to the bathroom that is too narrow to take a standard size wheelchair. It is important to try to check out these requirements in advance where possible, for accessibility to rooms, dining, transport, and training facilities. For example, it may be necessary for athletes to take essential equipment such as sliding boards or nonslip bath mats. It is also prudent to consider what foods will be available in the destination country. Some athletes may prefer to take foodstuffs they are familiar with to ensure adequate carbohydrate replacement after exercise. Taking some carbohydrates, with or without additional protein, in powder form may be a good option for some athletes. Consultation with a nutritionist is suggested before an athlete decides to "experiment" with food substitutes.

Planning the journey

From the health-care aspect, there are general issues applicable to all and disability-specific issues that will require additional attention. The following discussion addresses the major issues facing athletes with a disability preparing for a competition that requires them to travel. Table 4.1 provides a checklist of these important points.

Table 4.1 Checklist for athletes traveling to competitions.

Checklist:
Passport valid ☐ Visa required? ☐
Immunizations needed? ☐
Antimalarias needed? ☐
Get repeat prescription of medicines/catheters/dressings ☐
Letter from doctor re-medications ☐
Travel insurance ☐
Medical kit ☐
Sunscreen/hat/fan ☐
Flight socks (compression stockings) ☐
Snacks for journey ☐

Immunizations

Each country will have its own requirements for immunization (vaccination) status for entry into the country. Some of these will be essential and others optional but recommended for the individual's well-being. It will also depend on the country of origin (e.g., a yellow fever endemic area will require proof of immunization against yellow fever). It will also depend on where the athlete will be traveling to in the country being visited (e.g., the risk of Japanese encephalitis may be minimal in a large city, but if traveling into the country areas after the competition, then this might be advised). Athletes should check with their own doctor or by using a variety of websites, including the one from the World Health Organization (WHO) on "Travel and Health" (www.who.int/ith/en/) for current requirements. In these days of H1N1 flu (swine flu), and also normal seasonal flu, the coming together of many people from all over the world, often in cramped living conditions, is an ideal environment for the spread of infectious disease. Encourage athletes to discuss with their doctor the possibility of immunization against flu, which should take into account their particular disability that may make them more susceptible or more vulnerable to the effects, should they contract the disease. Everyone should take the following standard health precautions to avoid developing or spreading infection:

• cover the nose and mouth with a tissue when coughing or sneezing;

• throw the tissue in a waste bin after use;

• wash hands often with soap and water (or an alcohol-based hand rub, avoid touching the eyes, nose, or mouth);

• avoid close contact with sick people and stay in the dormitory room if the athlete is unwell and seeks medical help.

Athletes and staff will need education with regard to infection control. Medical staff should also consider how to isolate infected athletes within the accommodation that is available at the destination. Athletes need to plan the timing of their immunizations well in advance to complete the course and to consider implications for training or competition schedules. There may be muscle soreness in the shoulder afterwards, which may interfere with wheelchair propulsion or transferring, and some athletes develop a mild "flu-like" reaction to some immunizations when training hard.

Prescription medicines

Many athletes will require prescription medications for a variety of health conditions. It is essential that athletes take their own supply of medications for the duration of any trip. For this, they will need to contact their doctor well in advance to ensure there is enough time to obtain an adequate supply. At the same time, they should ask their doctor for a letter confirming the medications they are taking. This is important when bringing medications into some countries, as the medication needs to be confirmed to be for their personal use. It is especially important to check whether there are restrictions on importing certain medications, such as narcotic analgesics like morphine, into some countries. Check with the embassy of the relevant country before departing if there is any doubt. A jail sentence may be applicable if ignored in some countries. If athletes use syringes and needles (e.g., for diabetics), then they should have a letter from their doctor confirming their diagnosis and stating that they need to take these as carry-on luggage in the aircraft. In these days of enhanced security, sharp items will be confiscated unless supported by evidence. Air crew can keep medications, such as insulin, refrigerated during the flight, but it is best to inform the airline in advance if this service is required. Taking the insulin in a cool bag with an ice pack is also a good option. As a general rule, if going west (e.g., from the United Kingdom to United States), the usual advice is to increase the time between injections and adjust the dose upwards by 3% of the total daily insulin dose for each hour of time zone shift. If going east (e.g., from the United Kingdom to Australia), decrease the time between injections and decrease the amount of insulin given by 3% of the total daily insulin dose per time zone crossed. However, this is best discussed in advance by the athlete and the doctor.

Athletes will also need to ensure that they have adequate supplies of any catheters, urine collection bags, gloves, or dressings that they may use. Make sure that athletes pack enough supplies in their hand luggage to last for a few days in case their luggage goes missing. It may not be possible to get the same type in the country they are visiting. There should be a similar product available, but it may take a few days to find a supplier.

In addition to any regular prescribed medicines, it is useful for individuals to have their own first aid kit, particularly if there is little medical support traveling with the team. This should include items such as simple painkillers, antidiarrheal, antacids, cream for insect bites, and a few plasters for small cuts. An antiseptic hand wash is a useful addition to any traveler's bag to help prevent infection. Hygiene standards are not always optimal when traveling and washing facilities in toilets are variable. It is not uncommon to find that all the paper towels have run out or there is one dirty, damp hand towel to use; an ideal source of transferring infection. It is possible for athletes to contaminate their hands and subsequently their catheter, by pushing a wheelchair around dirty streets or into a dirty toilet, which may subsequently cause a urinary infection. It is good practice to use an antiseptic hand wash before handling the catheter and after disposing it. Remind athletes that they cannot take anything liquid in their hand luggage larger than 100 ml on to an airplane, and this will need to be put in a clear plastic bag. Advise to have a small bottle in their carry-on luggage and a larger one packed in their suitcase.

Malaria

Malaria is caused by a parasite that is transmitted via the bites of infected mosquitoes. The parasites then multiply in the human body, in the liver, and infect red blood cells. Symptoms of malaria include fever, headache, and vomiting, and usually appear between 10 and 15 days after the mosquito bite. Malaria can quickly be life threatening and, in many parts of the world, the parasites have developed resistance to a number of malaria medicines. Malarial parasites and the mosquitoes that transmit it are prevalent in many different countries throughout the world, predominantly in Central and South America, Africa, Middle East, the Indian subcontinent, and Southeast and Far East Asia (see the WHO website for further information). The risk may vary according to the time of year and altitude, and the type of malaria may vary too, along with the degree of drug resistance. It is important for athletes to consult their doctor to determine if they are at risk and what medication they may need to take to prevent contracting malaria. The first main step is to try and prevent getting bitten by the mosquitoes, and the standard advice would be to cover the legs and arms during dawn and dusk and to use insect repellents and nets. The second step is to take the malarial preventing medicine advised by a doctor. There are several different medications used for the prevention of malaria, but all will require starting to take the medication before travel, continuing taking the medication during the period of the trip, and carrying on for a period of time after the return. The duration of these will depend on the medicine used, but make sure athletes understand the instructions and follow them. Warn them that if they develop a feverish illness after returning from a malarial zone, then they must let any treating doctor know where they have been abroad.

Therapeutic use exemption

Any prescribed medications should be checked against the World Anti-Doping Association prohibited list. Athletes may be required to take certain medications for their health, but these may appear on the prohibited list. They may apply for a therapeutic use exemption (TUE) (see Chapter 10) through their national anti-doping organization if the medication is essential for health, does not give any additional competitive advantage, and there are no suitable alternative medications that are permitted.

Visa and insurance

Athletes will also need to establish whether a visa is required for the country being visited. This can take some time to process and so check this well in advance. At the same time, try to find out about the health-care system in the country and see whether they have any reciprocal agreement for treatment with the athlete's own country. This may cover them for emergency treatment, but they will still need travel insurance for other medical problems and particularly if they need to be flown home on medical grounds. For nationals from the European Union, the European Health Insurance Card (EHIC) allows nationals to access state-provided health care to cover any necessary medical treatment due to either an accident or illness in all European Economic Area (EEA) countries and Switzerland at a reduced cost or sometimes free of charge. Try to establish the nearest hospital or medical facility to the athlete's accommodation or training area. There may be a local pharmacy where additional medical supplies can be purchased. Different countries will have different regulations regarding medical practitioners and their ability to acquire medicines in that country. Establishing a partnership with the local clinic or hospital in advance is ideal.

Climate

Training and competing in a hot environment (see Chapter 12) provides an additional challenge to certain disability groups, particularly those athletes with an SCI who have impaired thermoregulation and so it is important to prepare properly. Advise athletes to take appropriate clothing including a wide-brimmed hat. Sun screen is important for health reasons, but also getting sunburned delays acclimatization to the heat. Simple items to take include a hand-held fan or a water-mist spray. Athletes who use ice vests or limb cooling methods will need to look at how they will access ice or freezers at the destination.

Pollution

Exposure to a polluted environment (see Chapter 12) is unhealthy and may trigger respiratory conditions such as asthma. Athletes who suffer from asthma may experience an exacerbation in a polluted environment and should consider increasing any inhaled anti-inflammatory medication prior to and during the period of exposure. Athletes will need to ensure that they have sufficient supplies of relieving medication. Documenting an athlete's "normal" lung function prior to departure is useful, so that any change in lung function may be more objectively assessed on exposure to the new environment. Simple protective face masks have little value in reducing the effects of pollution.

Deep vein thrombosis

It is well recognized that long-haul travel is associated with an increased risk of deep vein thrombosis (DVT). In one study, the risk of developing an asymptomatic calf vein thrombosis was 10% in long-haul flights over 8 h. People who take the combined oral contraceptive pill and who have factor V Leiden mutation are at particular risk of thrombosis, with 1 for every 200 patients developing a symptomatic DVT after long-haul flights. Factor V Leiden is a variant of the protein Factor V that is needed for blood clotting. People carrying the Factor V Leiden gene have a five times greater risk of developing a thrombosis than the rest of the population. If athletes have a strong family history of DVT, then screening for factor V Leiden mutation should be considered. Medical guidelines for airline travel state that those with a lower-limb paralysis have a moderate risk of DVT and should consult their doctor about using graduated compression hose (flight socks) and the use of low-dose aspirin, if there are no contraindications, although the evidence for the use of aspirin is limited. Advise all the athletes and staff to purchase flight socks prior to travel. This may require some additional assistance as athletes with abnormal limb lengths or shapes may not suit standard "off-the-shelf" compression hose.

Epilepsy

The stress of flying and the mild hypoxemia at altitude can precipitate seizures in people with epilepsy. Athletes with epilepsy should be advised that they need to take their medications relative to the time zone changes to ensure that they do not have low blood levels, which may further exacerbate the problem. Ensure that they are carrying with them treatment to manage any seizure that occurs, or warn any accompanying medical staff that they will need to have this medication available to them during the flight.

Respiratory problems

It is possible that some athletes in more severe impairment groups may use supplementary oxygen intermittently. It is possible to take supplementary oxygen on board an aircraft with prior agreement with the airline.

Time zone changes

Long-haul travel reduces the ability to keep a regular sleep/wake schedule through a normal pattern and in itself causes sleep loss and fatigue. However, world travel can also bring challenges to adapting to new time zones for journeys crossing three time zones or more. In general, traveling westward is less arduous than traveling eastward because the internal body clock tends to run slightly longer than 24 h, making it easier to adapt to a longer day. In general, the literature suggests that it will take approximately 1 day for each time zone crossed to recover to one's normal pattern. The impact of jet lag is discussed later, but there can be some strategies that can put in place prior to travel, which may help to minimize the effect. It may be possible to start some time zones shifting prior to travel by making the going to bedtime or waking time slightly later or earlier, dependent on the direction of travel. On arrival, exposure to sunlight, or restriction of exposure to sunlight, may help the body to re-synchronize. For further details on this aspect, see the website www.bodyclock.com.

Travel

Boarding the aircraft can be stressful and also a potential source of injury for athletes, if lifting and handling is performed carelessly. In general, anyone

Table 4.2 In-flight checklist for the traveling athlete.

In-flight:

Careful transfer to seating to avoid injury ☐

Put flight socks on ☐

Drink plenty of water ☐

Avoid alcohol and caffeinated drinks ☐

Adjust watch to time zone of destination ☐

Snacks for journey ☐

Take medications at correct times ☐

requiring additional assistance will be asked to arrive early at the airport and the departure gate. People requiring assistance will also board first but get off last and so they will be on the airplane the longest period of time. If an athlete requires assistance transferring onto the aircraft aisle chair and lifting into the seat, it is possible that the staff may not fully understand their disability. Make sure that they are informed how they would like to be lifted and the athlete controls the procedure. It is important to make sure that they do not scrape any part of their body in the transfer that might cause skin breakdown. If the athlete does not have normal sensation, then it would be advisable to use their normal wheelchair cushion on the aircraft seat if possible. It is generally easier to put on their flight compression stockings prior to getting onto the aircraft because of limited space but should be completed before takeoff. See Table 4.2 for a checklist of in-flight precautions.

In general, it is advised that watches be adjusted to the time zone at the destination on departure of the aircraft so that a new behavior that is appropriate to the new time zone is started. This should include eating habits and exposure to light if possible. Athletes will also need to adjust the timing of when they take their medications. During the flight, advise that they should try and drink nonalcoholic drinks regularly to maintain their hydration. The cabin air is air-conditioned and has reduced water vapor content, which means that they will lose more water through breathing. There is sometimes a temptation to reduce fluid intake to decrease the number of toilet visits by those athletes who require physical assistance to the toilet or do not pass urine normally (e.g., require use of the catheter). Although this seems like a practical solution, this is not a healthy one as it increases the likelihood of urinary tract infections, stones in the kidney and bladder, increases the likelihood of DVT, and impairs general well-being. Advise to avoid the temptation to have alcohol and to keep caffeinated drinks to a minimum. Both act as diuretics and can cause dehydration.

Airline food is not particularly noted for its high level of cuisine and there will usually be limited choice. To be on the safe side, advise athletes to take some familiar healthy snacks such as cereal bars and fruits. The change in air pressure with altitude will also tend to cause gas to expand and can produce some abdominal discomfort, particularly if already constipated. Advise athletes to try to ensure that they open their bowels on the day of departure if possible.

During the flight, athletes who are capable need to get up and move around to encourage movement of the circulation in the lower limbs. If athletes are unable to use their legs, it may be possible to do some self-massage to their calves. If an athlete wears prosthesis on a limb and removes it during the flight, they may notice a change in the size of the residual limb over the duration of the flight, which makes it more difficult to fit the prosthesis on arrival. Be careful not to chafe the skin on putting on shoes or prosthesis at the end of the journey.

Sitting for long periods in cramped aircraft seats is uncomfortable at the best of times. Athletes who already experience pain as a result of their disability will need to ensure that they have suitable amounts of painkillers available to them to use in flight. Advise athletes to try and get as comfortable as possible using any appropriate cushions or neck pillows. Inflatable neck pillows are available that are easy to carry in their hand luggage. For athletes with a high SCI who are subject to getting AD, it is possible that this can be induced by the prolonged sitting in an uncomfortable position. Athletes who get dysreflexia should ensure that they carry any appropriate treatment medication (e.g., nifedipine capsules to use if required), and any accompanying medical staff should be aware of the athlete's condition.

Similarly, it may be uncomfortable for athletes who suffer from marked muscle spasm (e.g., cerebral palsy), and they may wish to increase the amount of antispasmodics for the period of the journey. However, this may impact on muscular control as some ambulant athletes with cerebral palsy will be utilizing the muscle tone for stability also. Simple analgesics may be preferred.

Arriving at the destination

On arrival at the destination, although people will be fatigued from the long journey, there are several key health checks that athletes need to make when getting to their accommodation. First, they need to consider their hydration status by looking at their urine color and volume. If the urine is dark and the volume is small, then this is an indication of dehydration. In a well-hydrated state, the urine should be a light straw color. There are other ways of assessment that sports scientists or doctors may use, such as measuring urine, osmolality, or specific gravity. This can be particularly useful if athletes are taking vitamin B supplements that can color the urine, thereby making the urine color alone an unreliable indicator of hydration status. There are some foods, such as asparagus and beets, that can also make the urine darker.

Next, advise athletes of the need to check their legs for swelling. If they are unable to move their legs, it is more likely that they will have edema (swelling in the tissue under the skin) as they are not able to use the calf muscles as a pump to help with circulation. Tell the athlete that edema is present— if they press on the skin with their finger, it will create a dimple, which will slowly fill up again. Wearing flight compression socks may reduce this but may not eliminate it entirely. Lying with the legs elevated above hip level will help to reduce the swelling. They can also place a pillow under their ankles when in bed at night. If one leg is more swollen than the other, it may indicate that a DVT has developed. If the athlete is able to feel normal pain sensation, then the calf may also be tender to the touch at the back of the calf in the midline. There may also be some increased redness of the skin. Advise the athletes that if they are in any doubt, it would be better to seek medical advice at an early stage as DVT can lead to more serious consequences such as pulmonary embolus, causing chest pain, and shortness of breath.

Finally, if they do not have normal pain sensation in their skin, then they should check the pressure areas (e.g., buttocks and feet and ankles) for any evidence of skin breakdown. A small pocket mirror can be used for this purpose. They should also check out the skin in a residual limb if they wear a prosthesis as this may also have swollen during the flight and may cause increased rubbing or chafing of the skin. This might be exacerbated by having to do long walks through the airport.

Athletes should have already changed their watch to the new time zone when they boarded the aircraft, but advise them to check that they have done this on arrival. Part of the process of adapting to the new time zone is from changing their meal types and times, daylight exposure, and sleep time to the new time zone. Suggest that if they are really tired and do need to take a nap during the daytime, then try to limit it to about 45 min. If they take longer and get into a deep phase of sleep, they will not feel refreshed and will slow their adaptation to the new time zone. Their nights may well be disturbed finding that they are lying awake unable to get back to sleep. It is important that they stay in the dark environment to help their acclimatization. Advise athletes not to switch on the lights, particularly if they are sharing a room with a colleague who is sleeping. They should also try not to stimulate their brain by watching the television or a video but remain in bed, perhaps listening to some music or an audio book on headphones. They will probably need to get up during the night to pass urine as their body will not have made adaptations yet to its hormone mechanisms. Normally at nighttime, we secrete antidiuretic hormone (ADH) that reduces the amount of urine produced at night through the kidney and so we can sleep undisturbed. This cyclical release of ADH is put out of phase by the time zone change and will take a few days to adapt. It is suggested that athletes accept that this is likely to happen but perhaps to agree with their rooming partner that they will not flush the toilet during the night if they are asleep to avoid waking them. Exposure to daylight at appropriate times will also help to speed adaptation (see www.bodyclock.com).

Athletes will also need to become familiar with the new environment in terms of accessibility, but this is probably more important for those athletes with a visual impairment who will have to learn to cope with their new habitat. Try to ensure that any trip hazards or low hanging objects that could cause

a collision are removed where possible or warnings given. A familiarization tour is a good idea for all.

Athletes will also need to acclimate to the new environment. For colder environments, there are short-term physiological changes that take place to try and reduce heat loss (vasoconstriction), but wearing appropriate layers of clothing and minimizing cold exposure are the most important (see Chapter 13). If there is a significant wind, this will also speed the rate of heat loss. Protecting the head, hands, and feet is particularly important, especially if athletes cannot feel temperature properly as in the case of someone with an SCI. These athletes will be particularly susceptible to cold exposure.

For hot temperatures (Figure 4.2), humans make some adaptations in the short term that help them cope better, which relate to changes of an elevated heart rate and increased circulating plasma volume (see Chapter 12). This is why it is particularly important to remain hydrated in these early stages. It is in these early days that athletes are most susceptible to heat illness, particularly light-headedness and feeling faint. This has an important impact on the ability to train hard, and so one would generally recommend reducing the length and intensity of training sessions in the first few days in a hot and humid environment. Athletes should also try and choose cooler times during the day to undertake their training. As time goes by, over 7–10 days, the body starts to make increases in the amount of sweat produced by the skin, which causes evaporation

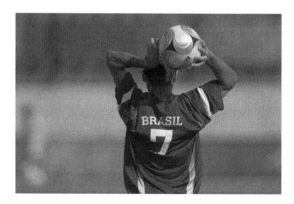

Figure 4.2 Competition in a hot environment requires special caution on behalf of the athlete from the medical staff. Reproduced courtesy of Lieven Coudenys.

and cooling. Athletes start to sweat earlier and also reduce the amount of sodium (salt) that is produced in sweat to help conserve it. Kidneys also start to conserve more salt to compensate for the increased amount lost in sweat.

Practical preparations for exercising in a hot environment include choosing appropriate lightweight, breathable clothing, keeping well hydrated, wearing a hat to limit sun exposure to the head, using a fan and/or water-mist spray, choosing shaded areas for recovery, using precooling methods such as ice jackets or cold water hand or foot immersion. It is particularly important to include a warm-down period after training or competing, otherwise circulating blood can temporarily pool in the legs causing fainting. A slow warm-down period after completion of training or competition will also reduce the chance of a sudden drop in blood pressure due to blood pooling in the periphery. This can be achieved by gradually diminishing low-intensity exercise in the sport-specific environment over 5–10 min.

Athletes should discuss with their coach adapting their training in the early stages after a long journey. This may be due to a combination of travel fatigue, jet lag, and different climatic environments. The body has a cyclical release of certain hormones that allow athletes to feel better and perform better at certain times of the day. If the athlete's body is out of synchronization with this cycle because of the change in time zone, they may not be able to exercise at the same intensity during a training session as they would back home or in the early part of their trip. Heart rate responses may be higher than the same intensity of exercise performed when fatigued and at a different time of day. If athletes are traveling for a competition, they will want to practice competing at the same time of day that their competition will take place, but this may not be appropriate initially.

There is also the temptation when traveling abroad for a training camp or competition, to train at every opportunity. Some athletes may not be training twice a day in their home environment, perhaps because of work commitments, and wish to "catch up" for lost training. Sudden increases in training volume are one of the most common causes of overuse injury. Therefore, changing training from 8 to 12 sessions in 1 week, for example, is a 50% increase in training volume. Encourage

athletes to discuss with their coach prior to traveling what the agreed progression in training intensity, frequency, and duration will be and that it is a graded increase rather than a sudden one.

Return travel

At the end of a long training camp or competition period, athletes are always eager to get home. Sometimes in this eagerness, athletes forget all the good things they did to keep healthy on the return trip back. It is just as important to arrive home healthy. The time zone change will be reversed and they will experience jet lag once again. In general, it takes about 1 day to recover for each time 1 h zone difference, for any time zone changes above 3–4 h. Athlete's sleep may be disturbed and this may limit return to normal training patterns. They need to return any medication to the normal time of taking. If returning from a malarial zone where they have been taking antimalarial tablets, they must continue to take them on their return home for the period advised by the prescribing doctor. This varies according to the type of medication.

Long-haul travel is an inevitable part of international competition in Paralympic sport at an elite level. It is important for all athletes to understand the challenges, to acquire the skills to combat those challenges, and to put in place individual strategies to combat different situations. It is a learning experience and a necessary part of becoming a champion, but perhaps more important is an acquired skill of learning how to stay healthy when challenged by different environments.

Conclusions

Athletes with physical disabilities may present to the sports medicine practitioner with all of the same medical and musculoskeletal problems that affect athletes without disabilities. Members of the sports medicine team must also be aware of the particular disability-specific medical issues that affect disabled athletes. Overall, the injury rates among disabled and nondisabled athletes are approximately the same. Injury patterns differ, however, and are sport- and disability-specific. An understanding of the injury patterns and causative factors of injuries seen in adaptive sports will enable members of the sports medicine team to better diagnose and treat musculoskeletal injuries. Athletes with disabilities may need to take certain precautions when traveling long distances for training or competition.

References

Bernardi, M., Castellano, V., Ferrara, M.S., Sbriccoli, P., Sera, F. & Marchetti, M. (2003). Muscle pain in athletes with locomotor disability. *Medicine and Science in Sports and Exercise*, **35**(2), 199–206.

Ferrara, M.S. & Peterson, C.L. (2000). Injuries to athletes with disabilities: identifying injury patterns. *Sports Medicine*, **30**(2), 137–143.

Klenck, C. & Gebke, K. (2007). Practical management: common medical problems in disabled athletes. *Clinical Journal of Sport Medicine*, **17**(1), 55–60.

Laskowski, E.R. & Murtaugh, P.A. (1992). Snow skiing injuries in physically disabled skiers. *The American Journal of Sports Medicine*, **20**, 553–557.

Melzer, I., Yekutiel, M. & Sukenik, S. (2001). Comparative study of osteoarthritis of the contralateral knee joint of male amputees who do and do not play volleyball. *The Journal of Rheumatology*, **28**(1), 169–172.

Nyland, J., Snouse, S.L., Anderson, M., Kelly, T. & Sterling, J.C. (2000). Soft tissue injuries to USA Paralympians at the 1996 summer games. *Archives of Physical Medicine and Rehabilitation*, **81**(3), 368–373.

Webborn, N., Willick, S. & Reeser, J.C. (2006). Injuries among disabled athletes during the 2002 Winter Paralympic Games. *Medicine and Science in Sports and Exercise*, **38**(5), 811–815.

Recommended readings

Stocker, D.J., Marin, R., Stack, A.L., Goff, B.J. & Pasquina, P.F. (2007). Amputee bone density evaluation for competitive sports (running) clearance. *American Journal of Physical Medicine & Rehabilitation*, **86**(4), 329.

Webborn, A.D.J. (2000). Medical considerations associated with travelling with athletes with disabilities. *Your Patient and Fitness*, **14**(1), 10–16.

Webborn, A.D.J. (2006). The disabled athlete. In: P. Brukner & K. Kahn (eds.) *Clinical Sports Medicine*. McGraw-Hill. Columbus, OH USA.

Webborn, A.D.J., Price, M. & Crosland, J. (2009). The travelling athlete. In Goosey-Tolfrey, V. (ed.): *Wheelchair Sports*. Human Kinetics. Champaign, IL USA

Yekutiel, M., Brooks, M.E., Ohry, A., Yarom, J. & Carel, R. (1989). The prevalence of hypertension, ischemic heart disease, and diabetes in traumatic spinal cord injured patients and amputees. *Paraplegia*, **27**, 58–62.

Chapter 5
Philosophy

Steven D. Edwards and Mike J. McNamee

Department of Philosophy, History and Law in Healthcare, School of Human and Health Sciences,
Swansea University, Swansea, UK

Introduction

Paralympic sport, representing the pinnacle of sporting excellence for sportsmen and women with disability, is a relatively new phenomenon. The first systematically organized games for persons with disabilities occurred in the United Kingdom in 1948, and when joined by Dutch athletes 4 years later, the Paralympic Movement began. Over time, the Paralympic Games have become parallel games and not merely as somehow lesser to their longer-standing and illustrious counterpart, the Olympic Games. Today, new sports forms are being devised to test and perfect the athletic skills and character of athletes with a disability. While there is much that unites the different sports forms, and their athletic contestants, there are genuine and interesting aspects of Paralympic sports that—if they are to be properly mined—require attention to conceptual and ethical issues characteristic of philosophy, and the philosophers robust and focused attention to argument, clarity, and coherence. To date, there has been relatively little philosophical or ethical attention in the world of disability sports, generally, and Paralympic sports particularly (Jespersen & McNamee, 2009) while the philosophy of sport has taken as its paradigm a narrow model of able-bodied Olympic sport.

The Paralympic Athlete, 1st edition. Edited by Yves C. Vanlandewijck and Walter R. Thompson. Published 2011 by Blackwell Publishing Ltd.

In able-bodied sports, the nature of contests, their organization, rules, and classification systems have evolved over thousands of years from their Western roots in ancient Greece. Paralympic sport, by contrast, is a relative newcomer to the world of elite sports. It is yet to probe, let alone resolve, many of the conceptual and ethical issues that arise therein. These issues relate across the whole spectrum of Paralympic sports, from the organization of events, their marketing, and promotion to the more obvious dimensions of participation and officiating in them.

The contrast ought not to be thought of as too sharp, especially in the light of the magnificent Beijing games of 2008 (Figure 5.1). This is not to say that conceptual and ethical issues are absent from the Olympic Games. Cheating, doping, and foul play are everywhere to be found in just about all sports at elite levels. There is no reason to think that Paralympic sports will be an exception, human nature being what it is. Moreover, there remain thorny legitimacy issues regarding sex verification that give athletes, administrators, medics, and philosophers problems. Nevertheless, these represent rather minor exceptions to the general business as usual of Olympic sports. It is, however, often far from clear at times who should be competing against whom in the Paralympic Games as in disability sports in general. In Olympic sports, contestants are typically divided according to sex (e.g., athletics, field hockey, and football), but also sometimes according to weight (e.g., boxing, judo). Why this is so is partly historical and partly logical. Sometimes the rationale is clear and justified while

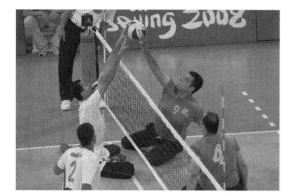

Figure 5.1 Athletes competing in the 2008 Beijing Paralympic Games. Reproduced courtesy of Lieven Coudenys.

at other times it is not. At times, sex-segregated sports are organized on grounds of prevention of harm, and at times this argument extends to competitions with same sex contestants. At other times, sex is irrelevant to the performance of activity (e.g., equestrianism) where sex differences are thought not to offer unfair opportunities to win the contest (Figure 5.2). In Paralympic sport, by contrast, disputes as to who should compete against whom are almost ubiquitous. In this philosophical contribution, we therefore spend considerable time and attention marking conceptual distinctions as to the nature of disability, the arising issues of eligibility and classification that are at the center of Paralympic sport, and then discuss three, among many, key ethical issues regarding doping, therapeutic use exemptions (TUEs), and health-care rights for Paralympic athletes.

Issues of classification and eligibility

It is clear that all Paralympic athletes, in order to compete in the Paralympic Games, must have a disability. It is sometimes reported that around 10% of the world population may be considered disabled. Clearly, however, an appreciation of this statistic begs questions as to the criteria for what constitutes "disability" itself. Without a fairly clear understanding of the concept and its criteria, any ensuing discussion may be misconceived or, worse,

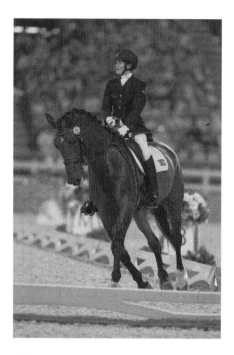

Figure 5.2 Gender is not relevant in the classification system for equestrian. Reproduced courtesy of Lieven Coudenys.

plain meaningless. Thus, before we may consider any of the many ethical issues that surround Paralympic sports participation, it is necessary to consider some basic conceptual issues regarding who may be considered a "Paralympic athlete."

The International Paralympic Committee (IPC) states that a necessary condition of being eligible to compete in Paralympic sports is that the athlete must have an impairment. Moreover, the impairment must "lead to a permanent and verifiable activity limitation" (IPC, 2007, p. 10). This statement of eligibility employs key concepts—"impairment/activity limitation"—that are central to the very idea of Paralympic sport. In this section, their meanings are unpacked.

Readers familiar with attempts to taxonomize disability in general will recognize the terms "impairment" and "activity limitation" as deriving from a specific theoretical perspective. To appreciate the full significance of these terms, however, it is necessary to understand alternative and sometimes competing ways that scholars and scientists have tried to capture the meaning and experience of disablement in ways that are theory-laden. The first systematic attempt to taxonomize disablement was undertaken by the World Health Organization (WHO) in 1980.

The International Classification of Impairment, Disability, and Handicap (WHO, 1980)

According to this early taxonomy, it is observed that disease can lead to impairment, which can lead to disability, which can lead to what was then described as a handicap. This is represented in a schema presented below, which illustrates the sense in which impairment, disability, and handicap are conceived of as *consequences* of disease:

> "disease >>impairment >>disability
> >>handicap" (p. 11)

Impairment, as noted above, is a central component of this schema. It is defined as follows:

> "Impairment: In the context of health experience, impairment is any loss or abnormality of psychological, physiological or anatomical structure or function" (WHO, 1980, p. 27).
> Impairments are said to arise at the level of "parts of the body" (WHO, 1980, p. 28).

Thus, the Paralympic athlete Oscar Pistorius (OP) satisfies this definition of impairment because, due

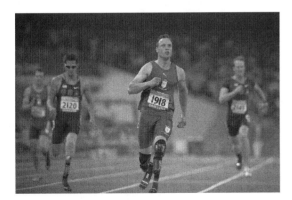

Figure 5.3 Paralympic athlete Oscar Pistorius (OP) was born without fibulae. Reproduced courtesy of Lieven Coudenys.

to a congenital disease, he was born without fibulae (Figure 5.3). Consequently, his legs were amputated just below the knee when he was 11 months old. Since lacking fibulae counts as an abnormality of anatomical structure, it is an impairment according to the WHO definition. Moreover, it is an impairment that stems from a disease, namely the genetic anomaly, which caused the absence of fibulae. Thus, the impairment of the athlete matches the schema captured in the diagram above in which impairments are construed as consequences of disease. It should be noted that, according to the schema above, OP is not yet classified as disabled.

The next key term in the schema is that of disability. Recall that impairments are said to be consequences of disease, and disabilities consequences of impairments. The definition of disability offered is thus:

> "Disability: In the context of health experience, a disability is any restriction or lack (resulting from impairment) of ability to perform an activity in the manner or within the range considered normal for a human being" (p. 28).

Whereas impairments arise at the level of "body parts" such as organs, disabilities are said to arise at the level of the whole individual (WHO, 1980, p. 28). Thus, impairments are properly attributed to body parts and disabilities are properly attributed to persons. Consider further the example of OP. His relevant body parts include his legs but if one was to attribute disability to OP, this would occur at the level of the person—namely OP himself—as opposed to one (or more) of his impaired body parts. Thus, one would say it is the person OP who is disabled, not his legs, shins, nor any other part of his body.

In what respect should we consider OP disabled? The most obvious (if contentious) answer would appear that he is disabled with respect to the normal human function of walking. Thus, without prostheses, OP lacks an "ability to perform an activity in the manner or within the range considered normal for a human being" (WHO, 1980, p. 28). As with impairment, the definition of "abnormality" (and normality itself for that matter) is a biostatistical one. This understanding is often called, rather loosely, "the medical model." The medical model of disability is predicated on the belief that there is a causal relationship between a person's impairment and his/her disability; it is therefore an outgrowth of the biomedical model of health. In a series of essays, widely regarded as classics in the philosophy of medicine, Christopher Boorse (1975, 1977) famously argued that health was conceptually the equivalent to "normal functioning." Health, within his theory, is understood as "species typical functioning" that occurred normally in the absence of disease or impairment. His account is deeply sympathetic to the medical profession's dominant self-understanding, techniques, and ideologies. Moreover, it is positivistic in spirit. For Boorse, normal functioning is a matter of fact.

The WHO schema is in sympathy with the medical model and Boorse's general theory. Thus, persons are considered normal or abnormal in relation to a reference class (all human beings) who are conceived of as a class with a normal distribution. That is to say, one cannot evaluate normality without a baseline description prior to the evaluation. One implication of this understanding, central to the classification cited earlier, is that in comparison with all humans of the same developmental level, OP has a disability if he is unable to perform an activity typical of the human species. As walking is such an ability, OP's inability to walk without prostheses renders him disabled. Hence the schema above: disabilities are consequences of disease, disease leads to impairment, which leads to disability.

The fourth category in the International Classification of Impairment, Disability, and Handicap (ICIDH), namely that of "handicap," is defined as:

> "Handicap: In the context of health experience, a handicap is a disadvantage for a given individual, resulting from an impairment or a disability, that limits or prevents the fulfillment of a role that is normal (depending on age, sex and cultural factors) for that individual" (WHO, 1980, p. 29).

As mentioned, impairments are properly attributed at the level of "body parts," and disabilities at the level of "persons," so it is said that handicap is attributed to the higher level of "social phenomena." In contrast to the other two consequences of disease, this category makes explicit reference to social and cultural factors. The category "disability" involves statistical comparison with other humans, but not with reference to specific social or cultural factors. Although the term "handicap" is still used nowadays around the world, in the English language it is considered politically incorrect. The promotion or endorsement of any particular linguistic hegemony is not promoted here, so having noted this widespread perception of "political incorrectness," some words are necessary to explain its more widespread use and the widespread deployment of WHO's schema.

It can be claimed that a disability (in the example of OP) "limits" in the sense of 'hinders' "the fulfillment of a role that is normal . . . etc." Thus, for example, it may be more difficult to obtain paid employment if one has a severe disability, e.g., if one is unable to walk or see. Thus, the disability is said to lead to a handicap—e.g., to hinder one's chances of obtaining employment.

Of course, in some parts of the world, much has been done to modify the social environment to render it more accessible or functional to persons with disability. Thus, many public buildings can be accessed via ramps; public transport has been modified to make it easier for people who use wheelchairs to board them, and so on. So it is less clear that being unable to walk limits one's opportunities to the degree it once did. But, nonetheless, one can see the point that is being made in the WHO definition; those who cannot walk are thought to be handicapped in some way. Also, as with the other components in their taxonomy, recall the "consequences of disease" schema. Hence, the handicap would result from the disease which results from the impairment which is a consequence of disease.

Nevertheless, there is much that is controversial in the WHO taxonomy, and some things are unclear. Take, for example, the expression "fulfillment of a role that is normal," this was explained earlier in terms of paid employment, but not everybody is in paid employment. They may be doing something else, such as raising children, and this surely counts as a role which is normal. Also, it was said in the earlier analysis that OP is unable to walk but this is untrue. OP is able to walk, with the use of artificial aids or prostheses. Also, recall that the expression in the definition of disability refers to the inability to perform an activity in the manner or within the range "considered normal for a human being." Due to the lack of legs below the knee, OP is unable to walk, it may be claimed. But suppose "the kinds of activity considered normal" refers instead to "being able to get from one location to another" (i.e., instead of referring to what we would usually consider as our abilities, such as walking, talking, hearing, and seeing). A wheelchair user might say that they can easily get from one place to another and hence ought not to be classified as disabled.

Some initial difficulties with the ICIDH taxonomy have been raised, which have been instrumental in the development of Paralympic sports organizations. Stronger critics have rejected completely the idea that disability and handicap are "consequences of disease." Commentators who promoted what became known as a "social model" of disability argued against the medical model that the causes of disability lie in the social environment and not in the individual person, as the WHO said (or seemed to say) in its ICIDH.

If all that prevents a person with paraplegia from working is the absence of ramps to public buildings and wheelchair-friendly public transport, then one can see the plausibility of the claim that the cause of disability or handicap lies in the social environment, not in the individual (Oliver, 1990). In the same vein, the Union of the Physically Impaired Against Segregation (UPIAS, 1975, p. 3) states, "it is society which disables physically impaired people."

Before moving on to discuss the most recent WHO approach, it is worth pointing out that the "social model" of disability has itself been subjected to criticism (Harris, 2000; Shakespeare, 2006). Critics complain that just as the ICIDH may have overemphasized factors internal to the individual person to the neglect of social factors, in the causation of disability, the social model makes the opposite mistake; namely, by overemphasizing social factors and neglecting the significance of individual impairments. One might add, also, that it is difficult to see how the social model can easily encompass severe intellectual and sensory disabilities.

The International Classification of Functioning, Disability, and Health

In response to criticisms of their earlier ICIDH, the WHO produced a subsequent version, which attempted to address some of the problems of the earlier one, and uses noticeably different terminology. The newer version is the *International Classification of Functioning, Disability, and Health* (ICF) (WHO, 2001).

This new development should not be seen as a total rejection of the previous schema. One key similarity between the old and the new lies in its definitions of three of its main categories. The old threefold classification of impairment, disability, and handicap is replaced with impairment, activity limitations, and participation restrictions. As previously cited, impairment (e.g., an abnormality in anatomical structure) led to disability (e.g., inability to walk), and finally to handicap (e.g., inability to work). New nomenclature includes impairments, activity limitations, and participation restrictions. The schema retains the part-whole-societal structure (ICF, p. 188), though the simplistic causal connection that someone found in the ICIDH is now explicitly rejected in favor of a "bio-psycho-social" approach.

The three basic categories in the ICF are as follows (impairment is presented in almost exactly the same terms as before):

"Impairment is a loss or abnormality in body structure or physiological function (including mental functions). Abnormality here is used strictly to refer to a significant variation from established statistical norms (i.e., as a deviation from a standard population mean . . .)" (ICF, p. 190).

So, as was the case with the ICIDH, OP would qualify as having an impairment according to this definition for the same reason.

The disability dimension of the ICIDH, the "person level" dimension, is defined thus:

"Activity limitations are difficulties an individual may have in executing activities. An activity limitation may range from a slight to a severe deviation in terms of quality or quantity in executing the activity in a manner or to the extent that is expected of people without the health condition" (ICF, p. 191).

Note that the explicit reference to "activities within the range considered normal for a human being" is now deleted. But of course it is still there implicitly in the reference to "people without the health condition"; though this can now be considered more specifically in terms of people within the social context of the person as opposed to human beings *per se* as is indicated in this quote: "Limitations or restrictions are assessed against a generally accepted population standard" (ICF, p. 21). Note also that reduction in the quality of performance of an activity is mentioned explicitly within the definition. So, if one is capable of shooting an arrow in an archery contest, but, due perhaps to a condition that leads to muscular atrophy or loss of motor control (e.g., multiple sclerosis or cerebral palsy), one can do this only unsteadily, then one would also qualify as having an "activity limitation." By way of summary, then, in the new definition, the term "disability" is now dropped and the dimension of the phenomenon of disablement previously referred to by that term is now referred to by the term "activity limitation." It is this term, in addition to "impairment," which is employed by the IPC in their literature (IPC, 2007). Although the IPC uses the term, their definition is stated more briefly than that of the WHO. According to the IPC, an activity limitation refers to "difficulties an individual may have in executing activities" (IPC classification code, November 2007). Thus, as mentioned earlier, one might hold that OP manifests an activity limitation since, without his prostheses, he has difficulty walking.

Returning to the ICF, it is noteworthy that the term "handicapped" is no longer included, and is replaced by the term "participation restriction," which is defined thus:

> "Participation restrictions are problems an individual may experience in involvement in life situations. The presence of a participation restriction is determined by comparing an individual's participation to that which is expected of an individual without disability in that culture or society" (ICF, p. 191).

So, as with the ICIDH category "handicap," it appears that a "participation restriction" is determined by reference to the kinds of activities typically engaged in by one's peers, who become the reference class. If one is restricted from engaging in such activities, due to "impairments" or "activity limitations," one is considered to suffer from a "participation restriction."

Building on the critics of the "Medical Model," the authors of the ICF make it clear that disablement should not be conceived of solely as a problem of the individual (i.e., their anatomical structure and functioning). The role of environmental factors is explicitly referred to: "A person's functioning and disability is conceived as a dynamic interaction between health conditions (diseases, disorders . . .) and contextual factors" (p. 10). To signal this, it is made explicit that the ICF involves a rejection of a Medical Model of disability, without embracing a social model. Instead, a model that recognizes a role for both kinds of factors is adopted. As the ICF declared by using the Medical Model, "a 'biopsychosocial' approach" is used (p. 28) in this case. In other words, their approach—encapsulated in the definition—takes into account factors at each of the three levels of analysis identified earlier. The new definition makes redundant the old terminological progression of impairment, disability, and handicap.

It is interesting to illustrate how the newer taxonomy is supposed to apply in the context of intellectual disabilities. A person may have an impairment such as the loss or abnormality of psychological function. This impairment may be associated with an activity limitation such as in problem solving or some other function of cognition "learning and applying knowledge" (ICF, p. 19). This activity limitation may in turn be associated with a participation restriction. Certain activities typical in one's peer social group may not be accessible, such as playing chess, competing in complex motor-skilled activities like sports, or perhaps the concept of a "relay race" might be impossible for a person with a severe intellectual disability because of the timing component.

Summary of the main differences between the ICF and the ICIDH

The ICF "provides a multi-perspective approach to the classification of functioning and disability as an interactive and evolutionary process" (p. 25). It takes into account the person themselves, their body, and their views, understood in the context of their physical and social environments. The ICF alleges that it "is based on an integration of [the medical and social] models. In order to capture the integration of the various perspectives of functioning, a 'biopsychosocial approach' is used" (p. 28). This, by implication, concedes that the ICIDH placed insufficient emphasis on "nonmedical" factors generally.

Impairment is not now the fundamental category in the ICF (Bickenbach et al., 1999). Again, by implication, this suggests that impairment *was* the "fundamental category" in the ICIDH. Though as indicated in our discussion of the ICIDH earlier, this may stem from an unsympathetic reading of it. "Disability" now has very broad usage: "Disability is an umbrella term for impairments, activity limitations and participation restrictions. It denotes the negative aspects of the interaction between an individual (with a health condition) and that individual's contextual factors (environmental and personal factors)" (WHO, 2001, p. 190, see also p. 3).

This chapter has thus far focused primarily on the taxonomy of disability produced by the WHO, together with an important criticism of it advanced from the standpoint of the "social model" of disability. However, it is important to signal the fact that disability is itself a hotly contested concept. This can be illustrated well by providing a brief description of the theory of Professor Lennart Nordenfelt (1983, 1993). Statistical norms play a key function in both WHO definitions. Nordenfelt is critical of such biostatistically based approaches because they fail to do justice to the values and priorities of the individual person.

To illustrate this, consider again OP. According to reports, OP (Edwards, 2008) refuses to park in parking spaces reserved for disabled people. This is because he does not consider himself disabled. Nordenfelt's theory of disability lends some weight to OP's claim. His theory is that persons are disabled when they are unable to do things which are important, things which Nordenfelt labels "vital [personal] goals." Thus, if leading a very active or athletic lifestyle is of great, or even paramount, importance to disabled people and they are able to do this, in addition to do all those activities required to do so (e.g., drive to training venues and shop for food), they can fulfill their vital goals. And insofar as they are able to do this they are not, on Nordenfelt's influential analysis, to be thought of as disabled. On this, more radical account, OP would not be characterized as disabled.

According to Nordenfelt (1983, 1993), disabilities typically stem from a combination of internal factors (such as impairments) and external factors (such as wheelchair-unfriendly public transportation systems). Thus his account is not open to the kind of criticism to which the ICIDH account seemed vulnerable. But in allowing that disability is not wholly and exclusively caused by the social environment, he manages to avoid an implausible implication of the rival social model approach, too.

Time and space do not allow a full account of Nordenfelt's approach, but the description just given is sufficient to illustrate the central way in which it differs from the WHO approaches. Specifically, as indicated, it would certainly do justice to the kind of attitude voiced by OP, and many others who would be classified as "disabled" (by virtue of having impairment, as well as an activity limitation together with a participation restriction) according to the WHO definitions.[1] As noted earlier, according to the eligibility criteria of the IPC (2007) clause 5.2, "an athlete must have an impairment that leads to a permanent and verifiable activity limitation" (Figure 5.4).

A first point to note is that if one considers someone such as OP, it is not obvious that he has an activity limitation at all, still less a permanent one. As is well documented, he is capable of achieving highly respectable times in some track events by the standards of national-level athletes without impairments. And if one thinks of wheelchair races, again it is not obvious that medal winners in these events suffer from activity limitations relevant to that kind

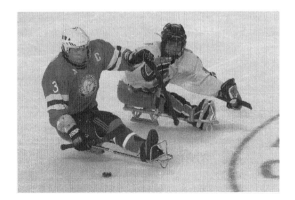

Figure 5.4 The IPC Classification Code indicates that the athlete must have an identifiable impairment. Reproduced courtesy of Lieven Coudenys.

of event. The world records for wheelchair marathon events are notably quicker than those run by able-bodied athletes. This might raise the question as to whether co-participation between able-bodied and wheelchair athletes might be permitted and also questions regarding the very nature of the activities of "wheeling" (or "rolling") and running. Much would hang on how the conceptual nature of the sporting contests at hand was articulated, and what was considered fair and unfair advantages in the technologies used to cover the distance. So perhaps the point here is, as is implied in the WHO definition of activity limitations that the activities referred to are unaided. Thus, it would indeed be the case that OP has an activity limitation if this refers to an activity such as "walking unaided."

A second point of interest is the reference to the permanence of the activity limitation. This is further emphasized in clause 5.4 of the IPC Classification Code which states,

> "If an athlete has an activity limitation resulting from an impairment that is not permanent and/or does not limit the Athlete's ability to compete equitably in elite sport with Athletes without impairment, the Athlete should be considered ineligible to compete" (IPC, 2007).

So the permanence of the impairment is a vital component of the IPC framework. It is a necessary condition of an athlete's proper entitlement to compete in Paralympic activities. It seems clear, though, that this is too strong a requirement. Many athletes might be rendered ineligible to compete for no reason other than the march of progress in medical and prosthetic technology. Equally, developments in genetic and nanomedicine raise the possibility of growing, missing, or repairing, damaged tissues can be grown or transplanted (e.g., nerve tissue or bone). If this is the case, then many severe impairments will in fact not be permanent (i.e., irremediable) because there is the possibility of remedies for the impairment becoming available.

Before moving on from issues of classification, it is interesting to consider briefly the possibility of integrating Nordenfelt's (1983, 1993) theory of disability with the IPC/WHO account of activity limitations. Recall that, according to Nordenfelt, one is only disabled if one cannot, due to impairment, pursue one's vital goals. If it is the case that many athletes competing in the Paralympics are indeed pursuing their vital goals perfectly satisfactorily as they themselves see it, then—perhaps paradoxically—it follows that they are not disabled according to Nordenfelt's theory. Thus, the general impression that Paralympic sport is synonymous with disability sport would need to be abandoned. Instead, one would need to focus more on the notions of impairment and activity limitation, where the latter is understood—perhaps arbitrarily as the OP case shows—to involve unaided activity.

Ethics and Paralympic sport

Among the different subdisciplines of philosophy that are discussed by philosophers of sport, the subfield "ethics of sport" has seen the most growth and activity over the last decade (McNamee & Tarasti, 2010). The term "disability" itself is a contested one. The word "ethics," while in everyday use, is even more problematic. While it is both difficult and undesirable to police language and to prescribe usage in order to minimize conceptual confusion, it is necessary to make some remarks more generally about ethics and the ethics of sport before moving on to raise some ethical issues in Paralympic sport.

The words "ethics" and "morality" (and their counterparts in non-English languages) have been used interchangeably in everyday discourse. Many mainstream philosophers have come to question the concept of "morality" as a peculiarly Western convention that seeks to universalize our understanding of right conduct. The idea that morality refers to principles to which all reasonable persons ought to conform has come under assault from various groups of philosophers who think that it is either too restrictive (often being reducible to the notion of "respecting persons") or the product of a Western modern bias. They have argued, *inter alia*, that a broader notion of ethics should be embraced. This would include a wider range of norms, rules, values, and concepts that inform good character and living as well as right actions. The precise nature of these debates need not detain (Rachels, 2002), except to note that readers are unlikely to find universal assent for an ethics of Paralympic sport which concluded in specific courses of action that could neatly be classified as right, wrong, or praiseworthy but not obligatory, is overly optimistic.

Instead, this chapter will focus on three ethical issues that are prominent in Paralympic sports. The selection of these issues is an attempt to recognize that there are issues in Olympic sport which are also problematic in Paralympic sport with little difference; but there are also issues that, while not unique to Paralympic sport, take on a rather different texture and importance. The issues to be discussed are fair opportunity and fair play; doping, health-care rights, and TUE certification; and the mis/use of technology.

Equality, fair opportunity, and fair play in Paralympic sport

All sports share the same "gratuitous logic" in that they challenge athletes to overcome what are unnecessary obstacles (Suits, 1978, 2005). The overcoming of these difficulties or obstacles, which are created and preserved by the rules, is what gives sports their point and players enjoyment. The underlying structure is that of a test which is shared by contestants in the form of a competition (Kretchmar, 1975). The rules that shape each sport are of two kinds: constitutive and regulative. Constitutive rules define the activity (the size of the playing area, the duration of the activity, the composition and weight of playing equipment, and so on), whereas the regulative rules lay down what manner of means may be employed by contestants.

There is much dispute as to whether the rules alone create a structure of fairness, within which contestants engage in a mutual quest for victory (Simon, 1991), or whether rules are also necessarily reinforced by the ethos or prevailing set of unwritten norms as to how the activity should be engaged in (McFee, 2004). Clearly, both written and unwritten rules contribute to the fairness of the contest.

There are issues of equality that go beyond the nature of sports contest themselves. These relate to the treatment of individuals. Much has been made of the inequalities between Paralympic and Olympic sports. Athletes in the former tend to be less well financially supported, have less sports medicine and

science support, and are remunerated less (Howe, 2009). Their media coverage, though it witnessed very significant enhancement during the Beijing games of 2008, also falls far short of the Olympic Games and this has immediate consequences for the founding of Paralympic sports and the profile of their participants.

A further inequality that occurs outside of the Paralympic contest is found in the equipment to which Paralympians have access. Clearly, athletes from more economically advanced countries and/or those with strong state support for Paralympic sport will enjoy preferential access to more expensive and efficient technologies (Figure 5.5). This will allow them an advantage in their training and performance. It is an open question whether and to what extent Paralympic sport should model itself on, e.g., Formula 1 motor racing, where there are relatively tight parameters on equipment specification. In many technology-dependent sports, policy makers will have to determine the parameters of equipment not merely on grounds of fairness, but also in terms of harm minimization (or prevention) and also to ensure that talent and training win out over mere technological advances afforded inequitably to athletes from more privileged backgrounds. Clearly, as with all sports, it is both undesirable and practically impossible to make all background conditions homogeneous.

In terms of fair play and fair opportunity to contest victory, it should be noted that the diversity of

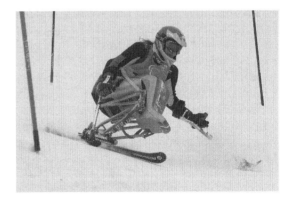

Figure 5.5 Athletes from more economically advanced countries enjoy preferential access to more expensive and efficient technologies. Reproduced courtesy of Lieven Coudenys.

classifications for Paralympic contests is intended to ensure that like athletes compete against like athletes. This is not always possible and the history of Paralympic sport records these disputes. Nevertheless, it is worth recording the incident which led to the expulsion of athletes with intellectual disability. During the 2000 Paralympic Games in Sydney, Spain won gold in the basketball competition. It was subsequently found that 10 of the 12 players were not intellectually disabled. Clearly, the possibilities for cheating—intentionally gaining an unfair advantage by means of deception—are more widespread in Paralympic sport for those with intellectual disabilities, because it is harder to determine their classification in comparison to athletes with structural impairments. The basketball case in Sydney was the trigger for an in-depth evaluation of the eligibility system for athletes with an intellectual disability, which proved to be invalid. For this reason, the IPC took action against the whole class of athletes with intellectual disabilities by banning them from the Paralympic Games. This decision has recently been overturned and athletes with disabilities will be able to compete in the London Games of 2012, though they will have to prove eligibility via a new "sports intelligence" test, the precise contours of which are yet to be determined (BBC, 2009).

A final example of fair opportunity to perform arises when Paralympic athletes and Olympic athletes co-compete. There have been many instances where athletes with a disability have competed on equal terms with Olympic athletes, though in that context they were simply viewed as athletes (DePauw, 1997). Notably, DePauw cites Liz Hartel (post-polio), who won a silver medal in the equestrian dressage at the 1952 Olympics, and Jeff Float, a deaf swimmer, who won a gold medal in swimming at the 1984 Los Angeles Games. Similarly, a wheelchair archer, Neroli Fairhall, also competed in the 1984 Olympic Games; however, her disability became an issue as her alleged stability advantage was questioned by traditional upright archers. If the fair opportunity to perform (Loland, 2009) is an important principle across all sports, then the stability of the base of the archer will be important to determine to see if a significant unfair advantage accrues between contestants.

A similar (though more high profile) case arose when professional American golfer Casey Martin won the right to play on the highly lucrative United States Professional Golf Association (USPGA) tour (Pickering-Francis, 2007). Martin required the use of a buggy (motorized cart) to move between shots. The USPGA argued that this gave him an unfair advantage. It was argued that Martin did not have to undergo the same physical test as able-bodied golfers and therefore would be less fatigued, thus gaining an unfair advantage. This problem in the ethics and philosophy of sport became the subject of a legal dispute in US employment law. In 2001, the Supreme Court in the United States held, by seven votes to two, Casey's legal right to use the golf cart between shots. The extent to which this ruling provides a policy precedent for Paralympic/Olympic competition is not clear. This issue will be discussed further in relation to technology in the final section of this chapter.

Doping, rights and responsibilities, and TUE certification

As noted earlier, there exists a dual structure to the rules of all sports, Paralympic or otherwise, and that these are classified according to their function: those that constitute the sport and those that regulate action within it. It has also been argued that there are auxiliary rules (Meier, 1985) which are a special set of regulative rules that determine how contestants may prepare themselves. Rules regarding the use of performance-enhancing drugs (often referred to simply as "doping") are of such a nature.

It is recognized in Paralympics and Olympic sport that the right to fair opportunity to perform in sport is subservient to the more basic right to health care. There arise in sports occasions where the need for medication for a medically authorized condition, which is also performance enhancing, supersedes the fair contest rights. Contestants must ensure that there are no alternatives that are suitable treatments which are not on the banned list of the World Anti-Doping Agency (WADA) (see Chapter 10). They must also have a TUE certificate to legitimate their use of the banned substance. It is the athlete's responsibility to ensure that the TUE is up to date and that, for example, in the obtaining of new inhalers that their contents or delivery systems for the medication do not offend the list which is regularly updated. This responsibility is in effect a duty of care that the athlete must undertake to train and present themselves in competition in a manner consistent with the rules of Paralympic sport.

It has been the subject of some controversy whether only performance-enhancing substances should be included on the banned list. WADA's current policy is that a substance may be considered for the banned list if it meets two of the following three criteria:

- performance enhancing;
- harmful (or potentially so);
- against the spirit of sport.

The presence of cocaine on the list has long been controversial because it is not performance enhancing, and the evidence based on its harmfulness has been questioned in relation to other recreational drugs such as alcohol which are not proscribed. Moreover, athletes must also be aware of the condition of strict liability. In doping cases, antidoping agencies are not required to prove guilt or the intention to dope. The mere presence of a banned substance suffices to constitute a doping offense and subsequent suspension from participation (McNamee & Tarasti, 2010). Take for example the case of Canadian Wheelchair Paralympian, Jeff Adams, who won gold in the 2000 Paralympic Games. Adams was found to have committed a doping offense despite his protestations that a stranger in a nightclub had put cocaine into his mouth and that he had ingested it unknowingly, he was found guilty of a doping offense.

Ethics, fairness, and technology in Paralympic/Olympic sport

In the section on classification and eligibility, the example of the South African runner OP was used extensively. While he is far from alone in creating controversy in the history of Paralympic sport, his case provides an interesting and contemporaneous focal point for a consideration of whether and how technology may alter or even undermine the nature and goods (i.e., those inherent aspects thought to be of value) of Paralympic contests and in his particular case, the possibility of shared competition between Olympic and Paralympic athletes (Edwards, 2008).

During the period prior to the 2008 Olympics in China, there was a considerable debate over whether or not OP should be allowed to compete, were he to make the required qualifying time for inclusion into the South African Olympic team. The main concern centered on whether or not OP's running "blades" (prostheses) gave him not simply an advantage over other competitors, but an unfair one. To substantiate or refute any such claim presupposes a robust definition of what counts as an unfair advantage and that proved very difficult to produce. Moreover, although the debate took place in the context of consideration of his desire to compete in the Olympics, some cogent points can be raised in relation to his competing in the Paralympics too (e.g., if it is true that the blades give OP an unfair advantage in comparison to nondisabled runners, which excludes him from competition in the Olympics, perhaps it should follow that he should be ineligible to compete in the Paralympics too).

The kinds of advantages that OP's blades were claimed to produce were as follows: For mechanical reasons, there may be advantages to OP due to the special properties of the blades. They may be lighter than natural legs, more aerodynamic, and have reduced contact area with the ground when compared to natural legs. They may also give greater "spring" than natural legs, thus leading to a longer stride. All these properties, it may be claimed, give OP an unfair advantage over athletes with natural legs.

But even if one conceded that advantage exists, one can still claim that it does not constitute an unfair advantage. Suppose, for the sake of argument, then that the blades do indeed confer an advantage. If this were so, would that be sufficient grounds upon which to exclude him? It is plain that advantages abound in sport. Current rules of competition do not exclude competitions in which some athletes have an advantage over others. For example, there are advantages which stem from the natural and social lotteries. These are not "deserved," in that they are not earned. They are matters of historical accident. Thus an athlete brought up in the high plains in Ethiopia might have an advantage over other athletes raised at sea level. An athlete raised in wealthy countries might be said to have an advantage over athletes raised in much poorer countries.

So, some athletes are advantaged in relation to others because of factors over which they have no control—e.g., the geography and economic conditions that prevail in their birthplaces. The arguments do not distinguish the kind of advantage (allegedly) possessed by one competitor from the advantages possessed by other athletes and regarded as unproblematic—such as those regarding athletes from the high plains of Africa, or wealthy countries. For just as the "blades" might not be available to other athletes, so being born and brought up in a wealthy country is not available to other athletes. And of course, strictly speaking, the blades could be available to other athletes, were they prepared to have their lower legs amputated.

Conclusion

In this chapter, a number of related but conceptually distinct accounts of disability that inform understandings of the nature of Paralympic sports have been established. It should be stressed that none of those mentioned has universal acceptance, and the differences between the WHO definitions upon which the IPC rely and others such as that devised by Nordenfelt (1983, 1993) are profound. This illustrates to the reader the highly problematic nature of what might seem to be a straightforward concept, namely "disability."

Following attention to the conceptual boundaries of disability as they inform Paralympic sports, the examination of a number of ethical issues in Paralympic sport, such as equality, fair opportunity, doping and TUEs, and the impacts of technology for fair competition, was explained. These issues are examples of how conceptual and ethical issues are interwoven. They are also illustrative of debates in need of pressing attention by athlete's representative bodies, coaches, and Paralympic sports organizers, as much as by policy makers and philosophers attempting to develop a coherent approach to Paralympic sports.

Note

1. The definitions of disability and handicap given by Nordenfelt are these: "A disability, as well as a handicap, is a nonability—given a specified set of circumstances—to realize one or more of one's vital goals (or any of its necessary conditions)" (1993, p. 22).

References

BBC (2009). Intellectual disability ban ends. Available at: http://news.bbc.co.uk/sport1/mobile/other_sports/disability_sport/8323369.stm (accessed on November 21, 2009).

Bickenbach, J.E., Chatterji, S., Badley, E.M. & Üstün, T.B. (1999). Models of disablement, universalism and the ICIDH. *Social Science & Medicine*, **48**(9), 1173–1187.

Boorse, C. (1975). On the distinction between disease and illness. *Philosophy & Public Affairs*, **5**, 49–68.

Boorse, C. (1977). Health as a theoretical concept. *Philosophy of Science*, **44**, 542–573.

DePauw, K. (1997). The (in)visibility of disability: cultural contexts and "sporting bodies". *Quest*, **49**, 416–430.

Edwards, S.D. (2008). Should Oscar Pistorius be excluded from the 2008 Olympic Games? *Sports, Ethics and Philosophy*, **2**(2), 113–124.

Harris, J. (2000). Is there a coherent social conception of disability? *Journal of Medical Ethics*, **26**(2), 95–100.

Howe, P.D. (2009). An Accessible World Stage: Human Rights, Integration and the Para-Athletic Program in Canada. *Cambrian Law Review*, **40**, 23–35.

International Paralympic Committee (IPC) (2007). *IPC Classification Code and International Standards* (November 2007). International Paralympic Committee, Bonn, Germany. Available at: http://www.paralympic.org/Sport/Classification/index.html (accessed on January 13, 2010).

Jespersen, E. & McNamee, M.J. (eds.) (2009). *Ethics, Disability and Sports*. Routledge, London.

Kretchmar, R.S. (1975). From test to contest. *Journal of the Philosophy of Sport*, **II**, 23–30.

Loland, S. (2009). Fairness in sport: an ideal and its consequences. In: T. Murray, Maschke, K., & Wassuna, A. (eds.) *Performance Enhancing Technologies in Sports*, pp. 160–174. Johns Hopkins University Press, Baltimore.

McNamee, M.J. (ed.) (2010). *Reader in Sport Ethics*. Routledge, London.

Meier, K.V. (1985). Restless sport. *Journal of the Philosophy of Sport*, **XII**, 64–77.

Nordenfelt, L. (1983). *On Disabilities and Their Classification*. University of Linkopping, Linkopping.

Nordenfelt, L. (1993). On the notions of disability and handicap. *Social Welfare*, **2**, 17–24.

Oliver, M. (1990). *The Politics of Disablement*. Macmillan and St. Martin's Press, Basingstoke.

Pickering-Francis, L. (2007). Competitive sports, disability, and problems of justice in sport. *Journal of the Philosophy of Sport*, **XXXII**(2), 127–132.

Shakespeare, T. (2006). *Disability Rights and Wrongs*. Routledge, London.

Simon, R. (1991). *Fair Play*. Westview Press, Boulder.

Suits, B. (1978/2005). *The Grasshopper: Games, Life and Utopia*, 1st and 2nd edition. Broadview Press, Toronto.

Union of the Physically Impaired Against Segregation (UPIAS) (1975). *Fundamental Principles of Disability*. UPIAS, London.

WHO (1980). *International Classification of Impairments, Disabilities and Handicaps*. WHO, Geneva.

WHO (2001). *The International Classification of Functioning, Disability & Health*. WHO, Geneva.

Recommended readings

Edwards, S.D. (2005). *Disability: Definition, Value, and Identity*. Radcliffe Press, Oxford.

Jespersen, E. & McNamee, M.J. (eds.) (2009). *Ethics, Dis/ability and Sports*. Routledge, London.

McFee, G. (2004). *Sport, Rules and Values*. Routledge, London.

Rachels, J. (2002). *The Elements of Moral Philosophy*, 4th edition. McGraw-Hill, New York.

Chapter 6
Sociology

P. David Howe

School of Sport, Exercise and Health Sciences, Loughborough University, Loughborough,
Leicestershire, UK

Introduction

Debate and discussion surrounding the social scientific exploration of the Paralympic Games center around two key sociological concepts—structure and agency. The first of these concepts refers to the social structure of society and is employed to refer to features of social organizations or mechanisms, including institutions, roles, and statuses, which are believed to ensure the continuity of patterns of behavior and group relationships over time. Agency however highlights the ability of individuals to affect social change, make independent and autonomous choices, and act in self-determined ways. Therefore, structure is seen as static, rigid, and unchanging, whereas agency is flexible and the degree to which it is applied is ever-changing. Social scientists such as Pierre Bourdieu (1977) and Anthony Giddens (1979), and their numerous followers have used the relationship between structure and agency in the past to good effect when exploring the social world.

A fair amount of high-quality social scientific research into Paralympic sport balances the role of the structure of society against the desire of individuals to transform the Paralympic Movement. In other words, small changes instituted by the International Paralympic Committee Governing Board have the possibility of altering the direction of the movement but often not to the extent to what might be imagined since the structure of the organization has a stabilizing quality, which means that the pace of social change may be slower than expected. In this chapter, a number of issues are emphasized that contemporary social scientific research into the Paralympic Movement considers of importance in the hope of encouraging more scholarship in this fascinating field of endeavor. The Paralympic Movement began in the United Kingdom in 1948. It is an umbrella term that refers to the desire to achieve social reform for individuals with a disability through the practice of sport. At the structural level, this chapter will focus on the issue of integration of athletes with disabilities into "mainstream" sports and the sociological interpretation of athlete classification. Paralympic bodies will be the focus of the second part of the chapter because it is at the level of the individually impaired body where we are best placed to explore issues of agency. Specifically, issues related to severe disability, gender, and technology will be highlighted. Before discussing these issues, the chapter begins by exploring the relevance of disability studies to Paralympic research.

Disability studies and Paralympic research

It is only in the last decade that social scientists of sport, who have chosen disability as the focal point of their research, have actively embraced the

The Paralympic Athlete, 1st edition. Edited by Yves C. Vanlandewijck and Walter R. Thompson. Published 2011 by Blackwell Publishing Ltd.

extant literature in the field of disability studies. This corpus of work, which is a direct product of a political movement led by people with disabilities themselves, has given researchers—whose focus is the Paralympic Games—an ability to explore more deeply the importance of the disability sport movement. Early work on the Paralympic field was little more than a description of various adapted physical activity practices that became part of the Paralympic Games. Over the last decade, social scientific research on the Paralympic Movement has been transformed largely by the adoption of more critical conventions used in the field of disability studies which owes part of its roots to sociology. For example, it has been widely accepted within disability studies circle that a "person first" approach should be adopted when addressing persons with a disability. That is to say, it is more appropriate to refer to *athletes with disabilities* than *disabled athletes*. Some of the quotes taken from the work of scholars in the field used to highlight points below adopt the latter term *disabled athletes*. These quotes have been left as written and as such they should be seen as part of the social historical record of changing attitudes toward disability. Within the field of disability studies, the choice of words used to discuss individual athletes who engage in Paralympic sport is also seen to have political relevance. When the phrase "sport for the disabled" is used instead of "disability sport," it becomes clear that sporting provision for the disabled is part of what might be labeled a "disability industry." Therefore, because Paralympic sport is run largely by the "able," the phrase "sport for the disabled" seems appropriate. While some familiar with this field of study may see the use of the term "sport for the disabled" as outdated to properly explore scientifically the Paralympic Movement, it is vital that researchers and readers alike are reminded of the social hierarchy that is at play in all cultural contexts.

Disabled activists and theorists make the distinction between impairment, an acquired or born trait, and disability, the wider impact of the social context of these impairments and the sociological literature on Paralympic sport has increasingly adopted this approach. The view that disability is a social construction is known in the field of

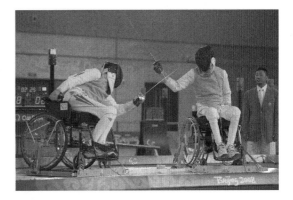

Figure 6.1 The "social model" of disability is seen as being in direct opposition to the "medical model," which focuses on the "disability" rather than "ability." Reproduced courtesy of Lieven Coudenys.

disability studies as the "social model" of disability. This model is seen as being in direct opposition to the so-called medical model that highlights disability as a medical problem (Figure 6.1). To those who advocate the social model, impairment is a functional trait, or in lay terms what is "wrong with a person," which often has consequences as to whether the persons' body is seen as "normal." It has been suggested that "[i]mpairment does not necessarily create dependency and a poor quality of life; rather it is a lack of control over the physical help needed which takes away people's independence" (Morris, 1996, p. 10). By extension, it appears that sport for the impaired might be a more appropriate term than "sport for the disabled," yet the former lacks the overt political connotation that is culturally relevant within sociological approaches to Paralympic sport. The difficulty in sociological interpretations of Paralympic sport is that the practice of sport for the disabled is closely linked to medical taxonomic systems.

Medical taxonomic categories were the foundation for the classification system established by the International Organizations of Sport for the Disabled (IOSDs). This federated group is made up of a number of disability-specific federations that remain an integral part of the Paralympic Movement and these are the Cerebral Palsy International Sport and Recreation Association (CP-ISRA), International Blind Sport Association (IBSA), International Sports Federation for Persons with Intellectual Disability

(INAS-FID), and the International Wheelchair and Amputee Sport Association (IWAS). IWAS is a federation that was launched in September 2004 at the Athens Paralympic Games. It is the result of a merger of two federations, the International Stoke Mandeville Wheelchair Sports Federation (ISMWSF) and the International Sport Organization for the Disabled (ISOD), that have been part of the Paralympic Movement since the mid-1960s. The IOSD developed their own classification systems to facilitate what they felt was equitable participation between their athletes. These classification systems are no longer seen as appropriate to the International Paralympic Committee (IPC), but they set the initial standard from which all future systems would be judged.

The development of Paralympic sport through the IOSDs, which have a charitable mandate, has negatively impacted certain impairment groups. It was the IOSDs and their predecessors that helped to organize the Paralympic Games from 1960 through 1988. The fact that these games were staged at all is a testament to the commitment of those involved with the IOSDs. For example, athletes had to raise substantial sums of money for the opportunity to compete in the Paralympic Games in 1988. Those who could not raise the funds were replaced by athletes who may be less proficient in their chosen sports but better fund-raisers. Athletes as well as officials went cap in hand to other charitable organizations in order to fund their involvement in the games (Brittain, 2010). Early Paralympic Games as a result placed less emphasis on high performance and more on the opportunity for international participation. This is not to say that elite athletes were not involved, but that participation was the main imperative. This ethos of participation has been difficult for many of the IOSDs to move away from, and hence has added tension to their negotiations regarding classification and IPC programs. As a result, there has been a reluctance to devolve power to the IPC, fearing that their athletes will lose the opportunity to participate in the Paralympic Games and IPC world championships (Brittain, 2010). The charitable ethos of the IOSDs led the Paralympic Movement to celebrate participation over performance, and as such is still a central component of Paralympic culture. Even today, while the IPC has

international corporate sponsors, the International Olympic Committee (IOC) has, since 2001, become one of the largest financial supporters of the Paralympic Movement. Today, the Paralympic Games is a high-performance spectacle and should be celebrated as such, but from a sociological perspective, it is important that we remember how and why the games were organized in the past. This chapter will now turn the sociological interpretation of integration in sport before turning attention toward the classification of Paralympic athletes.

Integration and sport for the disabled

The integration of athletes with a disability, which is being undertaken by mainstream sporting organizations in many western nations, is seen as important if an inclusive society is to be achieved. Integration, broadly speaking, is the equal access and acceptance of all in the community. Some scholars have distanced themselves from discussion of integration since the concept implies that the disabled population are required to change or be normalized in order to join the mainstream (Ravaud & Stiker, 2001). In other words, the concept of integration requires members of the disabled community to adopt an "able" disposition in order to become members of the mainstream. However, other scholars working within the social scientific investigation of Paralympic sport have adopted a concept of integration that is useful in the current overview of this field. Sorensen and Kahrs (2006), in their study of integration of sport for the disabled within the Norwegian sport system, developed a "continuum of compliance" that aims to explore the success of their nation's inclusive sport system. Within this study, integration, where both athletes with disabilities and those from the mainstream adapt their cultural systems, is referred to as *true* integration. Athletes with a disability who are forced to adopt the mainstream culture without any attempt at a reciprocal action are seen as assimilation. On the continuum, the least integrated model is seen as segregation, where neither group is willing to transform its core cultural values in spite of being jointly managed within the sport system.

Those working and researching in Paralympic sport would be most content if integration was *true* in the sense discussed earlier. If sport, and by extension society, is going to become more inclusive, "it is necessary for existing economic, social and political institutions to be challenged and modified. This means that disabled people [sic] are not simply brought into society as it currently exists but rather that society is, in some ways, required to change" (Northway, 1997, p. 165). In the long term, this might ultimately mean that the IPC and the IOC become equal partners, as this would be an overt indication that *true* integration had taken place. This conceptualization of integration reflects recent work, which argues that integration can be effectively understood as an outcome of an inclusive society. More specifically, it is argued that "[i]ntegration occurs through a process of interaction between a person with a disability and others in society" (van de Ven et al., 2005, p. 319). In other words, it is the process of interaction between an individual with a disability who possesses their own attitude toward integration, strategies, and social roles and others in society who adopt certain attitudes and images of people with disabilities. As a result, factors that influence the success of the integration process are both personal and social, and also include an element of support provision that will be distinct depending on the severity of the individual's disability.

It is possible, for example, to see *true* integration as a literal intermixing that entails the culture of both groups adapting to a new cultural environment. Dijkers (1999) uses the term community integration to articulate a similar conceptualization as *true* integration. According to Dijkers community integration:

"is the acquiring of age, gender, and culture-appropriate roles, statuses and activities, including in(ter)dependence in decision making, and productive behaviours performed as part of multivariate relationships with family, friends, and others in natural community settings" (Dijkers, 1999, p. 41).

True integration, therefore, is "a multifaceted and difficult process, which although it could be defined at a policy level rhetoric, [is] much less easy to define in reality" (Cole, 2005, p. 341). The difficulty when exploring the success of integration policies is that the balance between the philosophical position and the reality (in this case a sporting context) is not always clear. Simply exploring the policy landscape means that any interpretation of the sporting context is devoid of explicit cultural influences though all policy is a cultural artifact. This being said, the ultimate aim of integration should be to allow people with disabilities to take a full and active role within society. The ideal would be:

"[a] world in which all human beings, regardless of impairment, age, gender, social class or minority ethnic status, can co-exist as equal members of the community, secure in the knowledge that their needs will be met and that their views will be recognised, respected and valued. It will be a very different world from the one in which we now live" (Oliver & Barnes, 1998, p. 102).

Within the context of high-performance sport, this aim is hard to achieve. By its very nature, elite sport is selective as Bowen suggests, "Within professional sport, though, all but the super-able 'suffer' from 'exclusion or segregation'" and "sport isolates individuals, but only those who are *super-able*. The rest *are* left to the realm of the minor leagues, masters' leagues, local tournaments, or backyard pick-up games" (Bowen, 2002, p. 71). This understanding of sport makes it difficult to address the issue of integration. It is believed to be important, however, that international sporting organizations achieve *true* integration at the high-performance end of the spectrum in order to send a clear message regarding the positioning of people with disabilities within wider society.

Classifying bodies in disability sport

Categorizing the body of athletes with a disability based on the degree of functional difference places it on a continuum, where one trait may make an individual less marginalized than someone else who exhibits another different trait (Figure 6.2). While categorization is often seen as unproblematic

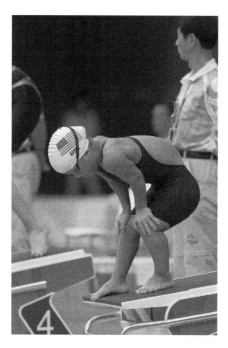

Figure 6.2 Categorizing athletes with a disability on the degree of functional difference may make that person more or less marginalized based on a single or multiple traits. Reproduced courtesy of Lieven Coudenys.

within the Paralympic Movement, it has negatively impacted the wider disabled community by placing various impairment groups in a hierarchy of acceptability where some impairment is more marginal than others. The notion of the categorization of impairments that leads directly to a marginal position in society stems from the work of Erving Goffman (1963). *Stigma: Some Notes on the Management of Spoiled Identity* was one of the first studies that drew attention to the nature of the problem of the stigmatization for people with impairments. Some critics of disability research have argued that the role of studies of stigma was an attempt to "medicalize" disability in order to classify it with respect to the predominate views that are expressed by society as large. For this reason, Goffman's work on stigma is useful when exploring the categorization or rather classification of athletes with a disability within Paralympic sports.

A complex disability-specific classification system, which is the result of the historical development of sport for the disabled, made it initially difficult for the IPC to attract the desired media attention. Since the establishment of the IPC, there has been constant pressure to remove the IOSDs from decisions about classification in order to streamline Paralympic programs. The IOSDs were on the front line offering expertise (in 1989) when the IPC was established. Many of the first officials of the IPC had previously held posts within these founding federations. Consequently, there was initially carte blanche acceptance of the IOSD's classification systems in the early days of the Paralympic Movement. According to Steadward (1996, p. 36), "the potential benefit of decreasing classes by using a functional integrated classification system is that it may simplify the integration into the rest of the sports world." Such a functional integrated classification system was developed in some sports such as swimming and downhill skiing. In this system, athletes are classified according to what they can and cannot achieve physically rather than by the severity of their disability, as is the case with the disability-specific classification system. The use of the functional integrated classification system reduced the number of classes for a group of athletes by focusing on functional ability rather than disability and, ultimately, leads to an increase in the number of viable events at major championships. This system is no longer in fashion within the IPC, but the use of integrated functional approaches can be seen as a step taken toward the development of ever more rigorous practices in classifying bodies with disabilities for sport.

Classification in Paralympic sport is simply a structure for competition similar to the systems used in the sport of judo and boxing where competitors perform in distinctive weight categories, except for the fact that athletes are able to diet themselves out or eat themselves in to such categories. Within Paralympic sport, competitors are classified in an attempt to minimize the impact of impairment on the outcome of competition. Therefore, it is important that the classification process is robust and achieves equity across the Paralympic sporting practice and enables athletes to compete on a "level playing field." As Sherrill (1999, p. 210) suggests, one of the "basic goal[s] of classification is to ensure that winning or losing an event depends on talent, training, skill, fitness, and motivation rather than unevenness among competitors."

The practice of classifying for sport is largely a medical one that can lead to stigmatization and alienation because it ultimately creates a hierarchy of bodies. It creates a hierarchy of impact of impairment on activity limitations or on competitive outcome. Such hierarchies may have a negative impact on the identities of people with disabilities involved in sport and throughout life more generally (Deal, 2007). There is a problem with seeing people with disabilities as being entirely marginalized, since this suggests that the social position of the disabled community hinges upon the type and severity of impairment, but the culture of Paralympic sport is not so clear-cut. In this regard, the work of Hall (1996) is important in unpacking the position of athletes within the social environment of Paralympic sport because key to identity formation is the ability to identify with others. Hall (1996) suggests that:

> "… identification is constructed on the back of a recognition of some common origin or shared characteristics with another person or group, or with an ideal, and with the natural closure of solidarity and allegiance established on this foundation" (Hall, 1996, p. 2).

In other words, identification is a social construction, which is never a completed process. The establishment of a disabled identity is not something that is concrete. It will be continually transformed. Identification is important since through the process of classification that all athletes undergo within the practice of the Paralympic Games, they will be forced to accept their place within the organizational structure of the sport and begin to draw similarities and differences between themselves and those individuals both inside and outside their categorization. Hence, athletes with a disability are controlled by the process of classification that is a requirement for the participation within the sporting practice.

While the athletes may be seen to be controlled through classification, it is important to note a number of key factors in establishing a complete sociological picture. First of all, the process of classification "belongs" to the sport. Only a few sports are still under the umbrella of the IPC; hence, the IPC cannot control all systems in place. Secondly, many sports, such as swimming, are not disability based. The IPC also has recently developed the classification code to make the classification process as consistent as possible. The IPC suggests, "The classification code will aim to synchronise all sport specific classification processes and procedures, in much the same way that the World Anti-Doping Code has done for international anti-doping rules and regulations" (IPC, 2004, p. 11). In this manner, the classification code has acted as a catalyst for various sports to make their classification system more robust. In the sports that it does maintain like athletics, the IPC has a role to play in policing the fair use of the classification system though it did not have a direct hand in developing the systems themselves. Perhaps most significantly, IPC recently accepted a position stand on evidence-based classification system, whereby the purpose is stated unambiguously and empirical evidence indicates that the methods used for assigning class will achieve the stated purpose. Importantly, this position is not disability based.

The culture that surrounds the practice of Paralympic sport and the knowledge participants have of their bodies and their self-identity means that to work toward achieving goals on an individual level is just as important as the work done through and by institutions, such as the IPC. Through work on and with the body, athletes experience, establish, and extend their limits and abilities, while placing them in the context of a number of rules and styles that make up social circumstances. This is not simply a matter of doing exercises, but of monitoring and refining, keeping training records and making confessions, giving and taking up different behaviors.

In this regard, the world of contemporary Paralympic sport is indistinguishable from the sporting mainstream except for the impact of the process of classification. This is, in part, why classification may be seen as central to a sociological investigation of Paralympic sport. While other sporting practices have forms of classification, such as age and weight, because the general population varies across the categories, they are less restrictive than the protocols established within Paralympic sport. Classification within Paralympic sport has been one of the disagreements between the IOSDs and the IPC, since the latter feels that the integrated functional classification system advantages some impairment groups over others. Critics of this system suggest that some impairment groups may be at a systematic disadvantage and in some cases may no longer be able to compete. Specifically, the system may be more difficult to classify because of the need to consider a great number of impairments simultaneously and many of the tests used have not been statistically validated. A decade ago, there was even fear that athletes would "cheat" the system by fooling the classifiers because the classification tests have not been validated statistically. According to Wu and Williams (1999), this has been a problem within the sport of swimming:

> "Misclassification is an interesting and perennial problem in disability sport. As with many others, it is the root cause of much frustration and anger (a) among swimmers who feel they have been disadvantaged by losing to a competitor who should be in a higher class and (b) among coaches and swimmers who may believe that they have been disadvantaged by being placed in a higher class than their impairment warrants" (Wu & Williams, 1999, p. 262).

Perhaps more importantly, athletes may be penalized for enhancing their own performances as the training of an elite athlete is central to the culture and identity of the majority of Paralympians. If athletes train and improve their technique in swimming (or any sport that adopts an integrated functional classification system), they may be reclassified based on their new ability. This is a key concern, as Vanlandewijck and Chappel (1996) have pointed out:

> "The concept of athletic excellence can only be fully appreciated when the performance is related to the functional physical resources available to the athlete in competition. These resources represent the athlete's performance potential. Whether such a potential is fully utilized by the athlete is one crucial determinant of excellence. An acceptable classification system would allow the definition and measurement of performance potential.

The definition of *potential* in this way is the cornerstone of the classification process" (Vanlandewijck & Chappel, 1996, p. 73).

This quotation highlights some of the sociological conundrums in investigation classification. The International Classification of Functioning, Disability and Health (ICF) terminology was not used at the time of the publication of this statement and, therefore, the concept of functional potential is not defined in these terms. In the current era with the IPC classification code, an evidence-based approach, and ICF terminology, the problems highlighted in swimming above can be eliminated and not be simply replaced by other matters of concern. In practice, the determination of sporting potential is almost impossible to achieve through any classification system. Yet, the aim of achieving as fair a competition as possible is still the goal of the classification process, and the place one's body occupies within a category may impact significantly on identity.

Processes of classification within Paralympic sport for the disabled create distinctive classes for athletes depending on their physical potential. It is the intention of classification that by classifying athletes in this manner will create an equitable environment for competition where successful athletes in each class have an equal chance of winning. In reality, however, there are a number of factors that impact on the accumulation of capital (both physical and cultural) in various classifications. The first factor is the number of athletes within a particular event. If there are only a handful of athletes, then the amount of capital that can be accumulated in most cases is limited. In some classes, there may be only six athletes from four countries (the IPC minimum for eligible events), which means winners are less likely to receive the same kudos as an athlete who defeats 20 athletes. Another important factor in terms of whether winners ultimately gain capital from their involvement in sport is the nature and degree of their impairment. A component of the culture of Paralympic sport illuminates a hierarchy of "acceptable" impairment within the community of athletes where the most "able" are seen as superior to the more severely impaired (Sherrill & Williams, 1996). The chapter now turns its attention to Paralympic bodies with discussion regarding severe disability, women, and the role of technology.

Paralympic bodies

In the first half of this chapter, some of the institutional structures within Paralympic sport, most notably classification, were addressed. Because the Paralympic Movement is relatively young, the changes and transformations that are ongoing within the classification system are a normal state of affairs. The aim, after all, is to provide fair competition. It is hoped that the evidence-based approach to classification will be an improvement on previous systems (Figure 6.3). It must be remembered, however, that any system will have consequences (both positive and negative) upon Paralympic sport. The second half of this chapter will explore issues related to agency by using the bodies of Paralympians as a vehicle to explore how individual athletes may be affected by the social world surrounding contemporary Paralympic sport.

The bodies of impaired athletes have continually been judged in relation to an able-bodied "norm," and the standards of play and performance are compared with those of mainstream competitions. This can have an adverse effect on participation rates within sport for the disabled as these bodies do not match up to the able-bodied norm.

> "It is through the study of the body in the context of, and in relation to, sport that we can understand sport as one of the sites for the reproduction of social inequality in its promotion of the traditional view of athletic performance, masculinity, and physicality, including gendered images of the ideal physique and body beautiful" (DePauw, 1997, p. 420).

Sport is an embodied practice and as such many people who possess less than normal bodies may shy away from the masculine physicality associated with sport. In sociological terms, the bodies of athletes can be seen to take center stage in their lives. Following Seymour, "embodiment is our life-long obsession. Eating, sleeping, washing, grooming, stimulating and entertaining our bodies dominate our lives" (1998, p. 4). For sportsmen and women with a disability, the manner in which they are embodied often marks them out for "special" treatment in society as their bodies highlight these individuals in

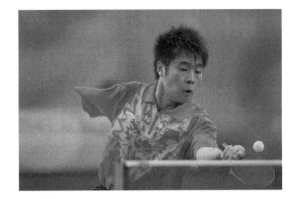

Figure 6.3 An evidence-based approach to classification will lead to fair competition.

a meaningful way as imperfect and, therefore, inadequate. This is because a lack of a physical impairment is seen as normal. The imperfect body highlights the opposite—a lack of normality.

In the context of Paralympic sport, there are two broad types of bodies that are of concern, those with either congenital or acquired impairments. Both broad types of bodies will have traveled different roads before they got involved in Paralympic sport. Individuals with congenital impairments traditionally would have attended what in the west are commonly referred to as "special" schools. Congenitally impaired Paralympians would have perhaps gotten their first exposure to sport through adapted physical activity classes at their school. These early experiences will have been instrumental in shaping the sporting experiences of these individuals. Today, in many cases, congenitally impaired individuals are schooled in inclusive environments, but depending on the nature of the impairment they may or may not engage in a segregated physical education environment. Regardless of the type of access they have to organized sport, the socialization of these young people will be distinct from those who attended special schools.

Those who come to Paralympic sport as a result of a traumatic accident, such as a car crash, are often socialized differently than congenitally impaired individuals. If the traumatic injury occurred in their youth, these individuals may also have attended a special school or had adapted physical activity classes as their introduction to sport. If the traumatic injury happens after the age when young people attend school, there is bound to be a period of transition to the new bodily circumstances. These individuals, regardless of age, go through a process of rehabilitation where their bodies need to be retrained often in the most basic tasks such as the management of daily hygiene regimes. After these individuals have relearned the basic tasks or perhaps alongside these activities, they in essence become re-embodied, i.e., learning some of what their "new" body can and cannot do in an adaptive physical activity setting where sport will be featured.

Both congenitally and acquired impaired bodies that make up the major subgroupings within the Paralympic games can be further subdivided into athletes with a severe disability. In 2005, the IPC Athletes with a Severe Disability Committee (ASDC) produced a revised definition that includes a specific list of sport classes where persons with a severe disability compete. The current definition is: "An athlete who requires assistance during competition, based on the rules of the sport and/or an athlete who requires support staff in the sport environment, including for daily living functions, travel/transportation, transfers, etc." (IPC, 2005, p. 10). The ASDC was established to increase involvement of the most severely impaired athletes in the Paralympic Movement. For these athletes, the sports in which they compete have to be the most adapted and their physical prowess is the least acknowledged within the Paralympic Movement. This should not be a surprise because even Paralympic sport is ultimately about physicality. In an environment where the body is essential such as sport, imperfection becomes evident. DePauw (1997) examines how sport marginalizes the disabled and argues that the sports need to reexamine the relationship between sport and the body as it relates to disability.

> "Ability is at the centre of sport and physical activity. Ability, as currently socially constructed, means 'able' and implies a finely tuned 'able' body. On the other hand, disability, also a social construction, is often viewed in relation to ability and is, then, most often defined as 'less than' ability, as not able. To be able to 'see' individuals with disabilities as athletes (regardless of the impairment) requires us to redefine athleticism and our view of the body, especially the sporting body" (DePauw, 1997, p. 423).

This is a laudable goal. However, to redefine athleticism would require an overhaul of sport itself. The point that DePauw makes is an important one in relation to the ASDC and this is only one of the key issues for the IPC—to ensure that these athletes are celebrated for the physical prowess.

It is not just the ASDC athletes that are marginalized through the practice of sport because as DePauw (1997) suggests masculinity, physicality, and sexuality are integral aspects of sport and each of these is a social construction. Social constructs are generally understood to be the by-products of countless interactions between humans instead of laws resulting from divine will or nature. Therefore, these three components have socially ascribed definitions and together these elements marginalize bodies that do not fit into society's definition of sport. Athletes that are the remit of ASDC athletes have traditionally been marginal to the practice of sport.

Women have also been traditionally marginalized in the context of sport and, therefore, it is not surprising that the IPC has a committee to give voice to female Paralympians. Paralympic female athletes (Figure 6.4) are not unlike their able-bodied peers who have also been marginalized in the context of sport (DePauw, 1997). In the Paralympic Games, in particular, low numbers of women competing in events are seen by some as a result of the double bind that women with disabilities must face. As Seymour (1998) suggests, because of the connotations with masculinity, it is a strong male body that resonates with the re-embodied image of a high-performance athlete.

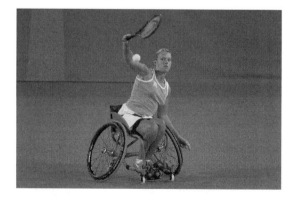

Figure 6.4 The IPC has a committee to give voice to female Paralympians. Reproduced courtesy of Lieven Coudenys.

"A winning wheelchair athlete is seen as the epitome of rehabilitative success. The vision of the strong male bodies competing for honours on the sports field is an image that has currency in the able-bodied world. Bravery is overcoming the catastrophe of a damaged body is a quality everyone can admire" (Seymour, 1998, p. 119).

Of course, not everyone can match up to this image. Even a male who has used a wheelchair all his life does not have the heroic tale to go with his achievement in the same way as someone impaired in an accident might. Those with more severe impairments may never be able to achieve the image of the successful wheelchair hero and as a result such images can be counterproductive to the equitable treatment of people with disabilities as not everyone can achieve this form of re-embodiment. The use of role models with a particular physicality due to spinal cord injury "may disenfranchise the very people who most need its services. The creation of sporting heroes as rehabilitative triumphs obliterates from view the many severely damaged people for whom such activities will always be an impossibility" (Seymour, 1998, p. 120). In other words, social issues like gender and degree of impairment are subjects of concern that in a more detailed sociological account should not be treated in isolation (Brittain, 2010).

The muscularity that makes the highly functioning male wheelchair body cause for celebration will lead some women with the same physique to be seen as lacking femininity. Pressure for those with severe impairments to conform to able-bodied norms is great but they also have a gendered component. A physical or intellectual impairment can be seen as a threat to masculinity. Some gender scholars have suggested that control over senses and physical and mental toughness are attributes that have traditionally lead to hegemonic masculinity (Connell, 1995). Hegemonic masculinity implies that more often than not men are in positions of control within society, which is a reflection of their strong masculine identity. The presence of impairment undermines this social order. According to Connell, "the constitution of masculinity through bodily performance means that gender is vulnerable when the performance cannot be sustained—for instance as a result of physical disability" (Connell, 1995, p. 54).

Since sport embodies hegemonic masculinity, it has been popular with men with disabilities as a vehicle for reclaiming and re-embodying themselves. Like men, women can regain body function through rehabilitation regimes that may have sport as a constituent part but "such activities do not have the same powerful effect for women as they do for men since such bodily attributes are associated with masculinity and are considered to be contradictory aspects of femininity" (Seymour, 1989, p. 114). This is in part because women are influenced by the dominant gender ideology that, though some may perform in sport at a high level, many women with disabilities choose to avoid sport because of its close association with masculinity and the nonathletic images of desired femininity.

"The insistent focus on the body in commodity culture exaggerates the anxieties that disabled women feel about being 'normal' and 'feminine'. In Western societies, there is a particularly high value placed on youthfulness and the aesthetics of physical perfection and slenderness, and the disabled body can easily become a source of embarrassment. Like able-bodied women many disabled women have very low self-esteem and hatred for their bodies and self-images. They experience a very personal fear of body display, which keeps them out of sport" (Hargreaves, 2000, p. 187).

The centrality of the perfect female body in western societies has sparked an increase in physical activity and fitness regimes, particularly among young, able-bodied women, and when these activities are commodified, a great majority of women with disabilities are discouraged from becoming involved as a result of the understanding of how a healthy female body should look. Some women with disabilities do reshape their bodies through exercise regimes generally and participation in sport more specifically.

It must be remembered that these women fall into the broad categories of acquired and/or congenitally disabled as highlighted earlier. For the former, some may consider themselves too old to reinvent themselves after a disabling injury, while the latter may not have been actively encouraged into physical activity in the home or school settings where they were socialized. Notably, sport for the disabled has mirrored the gender inequalities that have been inherent in modern sport since its inception in the 19th century. It is heavily male dominated, with fewer female participants than male and a lower portion of women than men in the senior administrative roles. Ultimately, both disability and gender can be seen to negatively impact and limit choices and opportunities for disabled women and girls to participate in sport. These problems may arise because Paralympic sport is isolated from politics.

> "Sport is separate from disability politics. Disabled sportswomen are not connected with politics and disabled organisations are not interested in sport—the primary issues are jobs, health and housing, etc. So there is no support from disability organisations—I mean those run by disabled people who are tuned in to the political debates about disability and are making demands about equality in other areas. ... We need to politicize sport—we're doing it in other areas, like the arts and theatre, but sport tends to be run by non-disabled people along the lines of non-disabled sport. And that's probably not appropriate for most disabled people—and certainly not for most disabled women" (Hargreaves, 2000, p. 195).

Sport for the disabled could benefit from a more radical presence of advocate athletes, and if this was supported by the wider feminist movement, the gendered nature of Paralympics would be more readily highlighted. This is a difficult end to achieve because the advocacy-driven disability movement that led to the development of radical disabled politics does not focus on bodies and, therefore, sport is seen as irrelevant. One of the ways the IPC is dealing with this issue is to establish the Women in Sport Committee, and this must be seen as a positive development. One of the women's committee's chief mandates is the active encouragement of participation from grass roots to elite performance. At the Paralympic Games, the value of women as role models should not be underestimated according to some.

> "Elite performers transform the stereotypes of disabled women as weak, inactive victims into incredible, dynamic sports performers, blurring the able-bodied/disabled body divide. The female stars of disabled sport signal an identity which is resistant to being reduced to 'the Other'. They also symbolize a challenge to ableist ideology, a reinvention of the (dis)abled body and a redefinition of the possible. Disability sport is tied to the cultural 'politics of difference' and can be seen as a site of resistance, a freeing—specifically of disabled women—from the constraints of culture and ideology" (Hargreaves, 2000, p. 199).

Some high-profile sportswomen with disabilities have begun to exhibit the ability to empower themselves by embracing the narratives of "ability over disability" each time they compete. These women Paralympians can exhibit the aesthetics of high performance—the skill, strength, and coordinated movement that come from a highly trained athletic body. There are an increased number of women with disabilities using the agency of their bodies in a confident manner, which suggests they understand themselves in relation to the culture of Paralympic sport and their own identity. Of course, not all women with disabilities are in a position to challenge the widely held views that disability precludes women's involvement in sport. A majority of disabled women lack power in their interactions with able-bodied women and men with disabilities.

This is a situation that the IPC is well aware of and their mission statement includes the following: *To develop opportunities for women athletes and athletes with high support needs at all levels and in all structures.* With this firmly on the IPC agenda, it is clear that more sociological research surrounding both women and athletes with severe disability can be prioritized by sociologists in order to more fully explore what is limiting participation among these groups. This chapter now turns its focus toward technology as this is something from which all bodies—able and disabled—can benefit. It is the sociological importance of movement technologies that interests us here.

Technology in sport

Development of mobility technologies that are specifically designed for sport is a response to the desires of the athletes to perform with greater proficiency. Today, many of the top athletes work with leading wheelchair and prosthesis suppliers to ensure that their future success is based not only on their detailed and comprehensive training regimes but also on the synergy between their bodies and the competitive technologies (Figure 6.5). Athletes who use mobility technologies such as racing chairs and prosthetic limbs are largely the public face of the Paralympic Movement. These technologies have traditionally been symbols of weakness, dependency, and neediness, but when they are used in a sports context, they transcend these notions and celebrate power, speed, and muscularity. To the outside world, the Paralympics are celebrated for the cyborg athlete, i.e., the marriage of human and machine that is embodied in figures like Chantel Petitclerc and Oscar Pistorius. Because of the high-profile nature of these athletes, technology may be seen as literally pushing the Paralympic Movement forward. As Charles (1998) suggests:

> "Technology and kinesiology are symbiotically linked. They have a mutually beneficial relationship. As technology advances, so does the quality of scientific research and information accessible in the field. As kinesiology progresses and gains academic acceptance and credibility, technology assumes a more central role in our field. The more scientific the sub-discipline, the more we can see technology at play" (Charles, 1998, p. 379).

Following this statement, it is clear that the field of high-performance sport (of which Paralympic sport is a subset) has benefited from an increase in technologies that have been developed to harness the power of the human body (Davis & Cooper, 1999). This is most self-evident in the Paralympic Movement by developments in technologies associated with mobility, namely, the wheelchair and prosthetic legs. Able-bodied high-performance athletes rely on technology in their day-to-day training; yet when these athletes perform in sports like athletics, the technology that

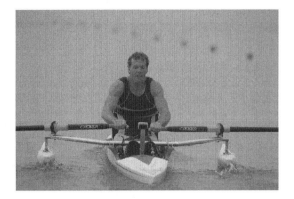

Figure 6.5 Athletes rely on the synergy between their bodies and the competitive technologies. Reproduced courtesy of Lieven Coudenys.

has enabled them to reach the sporting arena may be completely absent from view. An able-bodied athlete takes technology with him/her to the start of an Olympic final as their clothing and footwear are products of advanced technology. However, specialist clothing and shoes appear less like advanced technology in comparison to racing wheelchairs and space age prosthetic limbs as they are not explicitly the aids for mobility. Shogun (1998) has suggested:

> "When persons with disabilities use technologies to adjust the participation in 'normal' physical activity, the use of these technologies constructs this person as unnatural in contrast to a natural, nondisabled participant, even though both nondisabled participants and those with disabilities utilize technologies to participate" (Shogun, 1998, p. 272).

While the debate about naturalness highlighted in the quote above is still ongoing in discussions within the field of the philosophy of sport, sociologically, the greatest importance is that mobility technologies crafted for Paralympic athletes make the public more aware of Paralympic performances. The technology and the incredible things that athletes can do with it has to a limited extent captured the imagination of the general public. Technology, such as racing wheelchairs and flex-feet (artificial legs biomechanically designed for running), has enhanced the performances of athletes whose impairments benefit from their use and are central to the identity of the Paralympic Movement. Bodies that are able to successfully adapt to technology that wherever possible normalizes their movements within society generally and on the field of play.

These technologies should be celebrated, but within limits. Not all Paralympians are able to take advantage of this technology and may be in danger of being marginalized as a result of the fact that they do not engage in the use of mobility technologies. Seymour (1998) suggests that we need to avoid the pitfalls of assuming involvement in high-performance sport impacts on all in a similar fashion.

> "It is undeniable that sport and physical activities provide a context for enjoyment, self-identity and competence, but unless the conditions and ideology of sport are challenged, women, and indeed many men, will continue to operate in a context that compounds their disadvantage" (Seymour, 1998, p. 126).

Summary

This chapter has attempted to highlight how social scientific researchers can explore issues that are central to Paralympic sport, using integration, classification, severity of disability, gender, and technology as exemplars. Structural issues, such as classification, are central to Paralympic sport, but are also inextricably linked to individuals or agents within the movement, the most important of which are the athletes. Athletes' bodies may vary with regards to degree of impairment and gender. Over 15 years ago, criticism was leveled at the IPC which suggests that in the past athletes were not of central concern to the movement:

> "... the Paralympic Movement lurks the danger of becoming top-heavy, of concentrating ever more energies and financial resources on fewer rather than on the equally deserving majority. The sensible chord of overall social responsibility and accountability should thus continue to be the guiding light of the Paralympic Movement. This does not always appear to be the case as concerns the ever-resource-hungry-elite-high-performance-sporting-system" (Landry, 1995, p. 14).

One way by which the IPC has addressed these concerns is to have committees targeted at potentially marginal groups. The IPC women's committee and the ASDC have had a positive impact on assuring continued development of these important areas of the IPC.

From reading this chapter, it should be self-evident that high-quality sociological research could also be usefully combined with historical and philosophical research in order to better understand the culture of the Paralympic Movement. Perhaps just as important could be to actively encourage the use of sociological methods as part of multidisciplinary Paralympic research projects. Such projects might use sociological methods to capture the collective voices of athletes, administrators, and coaches. These data could be used in conjunction with data collected by sport scientists to further the various missions of the IPC. For example, by adopting a multidisciplinary approach on projects related to large substantive issues like—but not limited to—classification that are important to future progress of the IPC, we can possibly gain a more complete understanding of important issues facing the Paralympic Movement than we have to date.

References

Bowen, J. (2002). The Americans with a disabilities act and its application to sport. *Journal of the Philosophy of Sport*, **29**, 66–74.

Brittain, I. (2010). *The Paralympic Games Explained*, pp. 106–121. Routledge, London.

Charles, J.M. (1998). Technology and the body of knowledge. *Quest*, **50**, 379–388.

Cole, B.A. (2005). Good faith and effort? Perspectives on educational inclusion. *Disability & Society*, **20**, 331–344.

Connell, R. (1995). *Masculinities*, p. 54. Polity Press, Cambridge.

Davis, R. & Cooper, R. (1999). Technology for disabilities. *British Medical Journal*, **319**, 1–4.

Deal, M. (2007). Aversive disablism: subtle prejudice toward disabled people. *Disability & Society*, **22(1)**, 93–107.

DePauw, K. (1997). The (in)visibility of disability: cultural contexts and "sporting bodies". *Quest*, **49**, 416–430.

Dijkers, M. (1999). Community integration: conceptual issues and measurement approaches in rehabilitation research. *Journal of Rehabilitation Outcome Measurements*, **3(1)**, 39–49.

Goffman, E. (1963). *Stigma: Notes on the Management of Spoiled Identity*. Penguin, London.

Hall, S. (1996). Introduction: who needs identity. In: S. Hall & P. du Gay (eds.) *Questions of Cultural Identity?* p. 2. Sage, London.

Hargreaves, J. (2000). *Heroines of Sport: The Politics of Difference and Identity*, pp. 187, 195, 199. Routledge, London.

IPC (2004). *The Paralympian: Official Newsletter of the International Paralympic Committee*. No.1: p. 1.

IPC (2005). Annual Report. Bonn. http://www.paralympic.org/export/sites/default/IPC/Reference_Documents/2005_Annual_Report_web.pdf at p. 10.

Landry, F. (1995). Paralympic games and social integration. In: M. De Moragas Spá & M. Botella (eds.) *The Key of Success: The Social, Sporting, Economic and Communications Impact of Barcelona '92*, pp. 1–17. Servei de Publicacions de la Universitat Autónoma de Barcelona, Bellaterra.

Morris, J. (1996). *Encounters with Strangers: Feminism and Disability*, p. 10. Women's Press, London.

Northway, R. (1997). Integration and inclusion: illusion or progress in services for disabled people. *Social Policy and Administration*, **31(2)**, 157–172.

Oliver, M. & Barnes, C. (1998). *Social Policy and Disabled People: From Exclusion to Inclusion*, p. 102. Longman, London.

Ravaud, J.-F. & Stiker, H.-J. (2001). Inclusion/exclusion: an analysis of historical and cultural meaning. In: G.L. Albrecht, K.D. Seelman & M. Bury (eds.) *Handbook of Disability Studies*, pp. 490–512. Sage, London.

Seymour, W. (1989). *Body Alterations*, p. 114. Unwin Hyman, London.

Seymour, W. (1998). *Remaking the Body: Rehabilitation and Change*, pp. 4, 126. Routledge, London.

Sherrill, C. (1999). Disability sport and classification theory: a new era. *Adapted Physical Activity Quarterly*, **16**, 206–215.

Sherrill, C. & Williams, T. (1996). Disability and sport: psychosocial perspectives on inclusion, integration and participation. *Sport Science Review*, **5(1)**, 42–64.

Shogun, D. (1998). The social construction of disability: the impact of statistics and technology. *Adapted Physical Activity Quarterly*, **15**, 269–277.

Sørensen, M. & Kahrs, N. (2006). Integration of disability sport in the Norwegian Sport Organizations: lessons learned. *Adapted Physical Activity Quarterly*, **23**, 184–203.

Steadward, R.D. (1996). Integration and sport in the Paralympic Movement. *Sport Science Review*, **5(1)**, 26–41.

van de Ven, L., Post, M., de Witte, L. & van den Heuvel, W. (2005). It takes two to tango: the integration of people with disabilities into society. *Disability and Society*, **20(3)**, 311–329.

Vanlandewijck, Y.C. & Chappel, R.J. (1996). Integration and classification issues in competitive sports for athletes with disabilities. *Sport Science Review*, **5(1)**, 65–88.

Wu, S.K. & Williams, T. (1999). Paralympic swimming performance, impairment, and the functional classification system. *Adapted Physical Activity Quarterly*, **16(3)**, 251–270.

Recommended readings

Barnes, C. & Mercer, G. (2003). *Disability*. Polity Press, Oxford.

Bourdieu, P. (1977). *Outline of a Theory of Practice*. Cambridge University Press, Cambridge.

Douglas, M. (1966). *Purity and Danger*. Routledge, London.

Giddens, A. (1979). *Central Problems in Social Theory: Action, Structure and Contradiction in Social Analysis*. University of California Press, London.

Howe, P.D. (2008). *The Cultural Politics of the Paralympic Movement: Through the Anthropological Lens*. Routledge, London.

Oliver, M. (1990). *The Politics of Disablement*. Macmillan, London.

Sherrill, C. (1997). Paralympic Games 1996: feminist and other concerns: what's your excuse? *Palaestra*, **13(1)**, 32–38.

Wright-Mill, C. (1959). *The Sociological Imagination*. Oxford University Press, Oxford.

Chapter 7
Psychology

Jeffrey J. Martin[1] and Garry Wheeler[2,3,4]

[1]Department of Kinesiology, Health and Sport Studies, Wayne State University, Detroit, MI, USA
[2]Edmonton Chapter and Alberta Division, MS Society of Canada, Edmonton, AB, Canada
[3]Glenrose Rehabilitation Hospital, Edmonton, AB, Canada
[4]Faculty of Physical Education and Recreation, University of Alberta, Edmonton, AB, Canada

Introduction

Although the history of sport psychology can be dated back to the early 1900s, the most significant growth has occurred in the last 50 years. During this time, the number of journals and textbooks devoted to sport psychology has increased tremendously. Unfortunately, sport psychology research involving athletes with disabilities has lagged behind this historical trend, although a number of sport psychology and adapted physical activity scholars in the 21st century have started to examine common sport psychology theories and research questions with athletes with disabilities. Hence, in the last 10–20 years, a small but rapidly growing body of knowledge has developed.

The purpose of this chapter is to examine the rapidly expanding body of research on the psychology of disability sport. More specifically, reviewing the research to date will help a broad array of individuals to more fully understand and support athletes with disabilities. Sport psychologists, academic researchers, coaches, athletic trainers, administrators, parents, spouses, teammates, and friends of athletes with disabilities should all find value somewhere in this comprehensive overview of the disability sport psychology literature. A holistic human development model is utilized because both sport considerations

The Paralympic Athlete, 1st edition. Edited by Yves C. Vanlandewijck and Walter R. Thompson. Published 2011 by Blackwell Publishing Ltd.

(e.g., sport anxiety) and nonsport considerations (e.g., relationship issues) influence an athlete's ability to train effectively and to perform at optimal levels when it counts most (i.e., Paralympics).

Disability issues

The disability paradox

The disability paradox represents what seems to be a contradiction, i.e., people who have a disability can also simultaneously report enjoying a high quality of life. Dunn (2000), for instance, has reported that people without disabilities regularly believe that the impact of a disability on life quality is much greater than that reported by persons with a disability. However, contrary to this view, many (i.e., >50%) people with disabilities indicate that they have a good to excellent quality of life. Another version of the paradox is that many people with disabilities report feeling discriminated against and having significant limitations in activities of daily living (ADL), but still, nevertheless, report having a good to excellent quality of life (Albrecht & Devlieger, 1999).

To understand this paradox, Albrecht and Devlieger (1999) explored the experiences of people with serious levels of disability and the factors that distinguished the good to excellent quality of life participants from the individuals reporting a poor to fair quality of life. High quality of life participants expressed a balanced view of the value of the mind, body, and spirit. Stated differently, subjects appreciated and valued the importance of the mind and the spirit. Participants also felt supported and integrated with their family, their community, and larger society. Participants with poor-quality lives often reported that the mind, body, spirit, and feelings of connectedness to the larger world were regularly interrupted by pain and fatigue.

Albrecht and Devlieger (1999) speculated that able-bodied people overemphasize the value of the body and marginalize the value of the mind, spirit, and social worlds. In turn, these beliefs contributed to the opinion that all people with disabilities must have an unsatisfying quality of life. The disability paradox is also consistent with a larger phenomenon referred to as "affective forecasting." Affective forecasting occurs when people overestimate how good/bad they will feel in the future as the result of experiencing a happy/sad event. In brief, future events, such as a disabling accident, do not turn out as bad as most people anticipate. The important point for sport personnel interacting with and supporting athletes with disabilities is to avoid assuming that athletes with disabilities have a low quality of life simply because of their disability.

The disability world

People with disabilities share much in common with people without disabilities (Figure 7.1). However, they still move through a world that is different from the able-bodied world and from a holistic systems view of sport involvement, athlete's life experiences directly and indirectly influence their athletic lives. Disability is related to most major life dimensions such as self-esteem, work, school, travel, relationships, and well-being. Children with disabilities, for example, are viewed as less attractive than able-bodied children and often receive looks of pity or "poor you" stares (Goodwin et al., 2004b). Individuals with disabilities also experience negative evaluations of their appearance from others, making it hard to maintain a positive body image.

People with disabilities live in homes with less income compared to people without disabilities. Similarly, a bigger percentage of individuals with disabilities live alone and in poverty relative to people without disabilities. Many more people, percentage-wise, without disabilities also graduate from high school and college compared to individuals with disabilities. Individuals with disabilities are

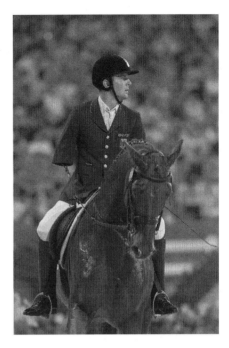

Figure 7.1 Athletes with a disability share much in common with people who have no physical impairment. Reproduced courtesy of Lieven Coudenys.

more likely to be the victims of crime. Women with disabilities, for example, have a 40% greater chance of being assaulted compared to women without disabilities. Even simple tasks such as getting in a car to go to practice or competition take more time for wheelchair athletes compared to the able-bodied. In short, athletes with disabilities work and live in a world that is often profoundly different from the one in which an able-bodied person lives. Recognition of that reality can enhance the quality of support offered to athletes with a disability.

Coping with a disability

About 15% of athletes have a congenital disability (i.e., since birth) and have not experienced life without a disability. However, most athletes with disabilities (i.e., 85%) have had a serious traumatic injury (i.e., acquired disability). A major ramification of such a sudden and permanent injury is a significant disruption of psychological well-being.

Significant psychological and physical adjustment demands are placed on individuals when they go from jumping, running, and skating one day to being permanently unable to move their arms or legs a day later. One example of how severe some individuals react can be found in the words of this former rugby player who stated, "Now I am nothing. Life moves on, without me. That is how it is. How it will always be. I just survive. No ambitions. Nothing . . . Sometimes I don't think I can go on" (Smith & Sparkes, 2005, p. 1101).

As discussed earlier, many people over time will eventually adjust to an acquired disability and enjoy a high quality of life. However, the previous quote illustrates that some people are devastated and may consider suicide due to the life-changing nature of their injury. A loss of function is an obvious and far-reaching ramification of a severe disability and often becomes the most dominating feature of the disability experience. In brief, a primary characteristic of experiencing a significant and permanent injury is a loss of function, and people often become defined by others as their disabilities.

Relationships are also placed under severe challenges. Lyons et al. (1995) interviewed a 43-year-old woman with a spinal cord injury (SCI) who noted, "Your friendships are greatly affected by your disability. I don't have any friends except maybe two from the pre-disability days" (p. 38). Lyons et al. found that people with disabilities see their friends less, have more difficulty relating to old friends, and often experience rejection by old friends. Marriages are often severely disrupted and disability is a risk factor for divorce. For adult athletes with disabilities who are parents, parent–child relationships are also affected.

A disabled person ("Donald") once stated "another thing that makes it hard is the fact that I can't run with them [his children]" (Kleiber et al., 1995, p. 293). Young children who are still cognitively developing cannot understand the nature of a disability, and this exacerbates the frustration that parents feel when managing the change in the parent–child relationship. For example, "Donald" reported on his daughter and noted that "She's not accepting the fact, I don't think, that I can't walk, she'll tell me to put on my shoes, and I can walk. So, see that makes it hard on me" (p. 293).

Sparkes and Smith (2002) and Smith and Sparkes (2005) described men's SCI-related experiences. Able-bodied male athletes who had strong masculine athletic identities and who derived substantial self-esteem from sport had both of these critical aspects of their identities damaged when they became disabled. One participant indicated, "Your masculinity is gone, broken, you just struggle to live up to it [being a man]" (Sparkes & Smith, 2002, p. 269). In fact, some athletes will dismiss disability sport as a choice. One man, for example, stated, "How can you play sports like that? I mean I can understand people using sport for rehabilitation and everything. For me though, they aren't real sports, not really" (Sparkes & Smith, 2002, p. 270). A related sentiment was expressed by a former able-bodied basketball player who noted, "No way would I settle for less with a sport I had excelled in on my feet. So in the hospital I set my mind on the triathlon" (Hutchinson & Kleiber, 2000, p. 50).

Experiencing an acquired disability is world changing. Able-bodied athletes, who acquire a disability and were heavily invested in their sport, will likely struggle with disruptions to their self-schema and will face particularly difficult challenges. It is not unusual for athletes to start participating in disability sport shortly after their acquired injuries and then have short careers (e.g., <2 years). This time line suggests that some athletes may be adjusting to a major trauma, becoming immersed in disability sport, and even preparing for a major competition. An understanding of how athlete's lives are altered by a disability, particularly a recent disability, can help significant others provide a better quality of social support to the athletes in their lives.

Sport psychology considerations

Self-esteem

Self-esteem refers to the favorable or unfavorable judgments people have of themselves. Self-esteem is thought to be based on success experiences that promote feelings of mastery and favorable judgments of value from significant others (i.e., reflected appraisals). Hence, one reason why individuals with disabilities may experience low self-esteem is that their disability directly and indirectly limits their ability to experience success. For instance, Smyth and Anderson (2000) reported that children with movement difficulties, compared to children without movement difficulties, fail more in sport and physical activity. Poorly coordinated children may also withdraw, watch, and be less active at play, thereby limiting their opportunities for success.

Favorable appraisals from significant others may be lacking and, conversely, increased negative feedback may be present. Adults with developmental coordination disorder (DCD), for instance, report experiencing humiliation and anxiety as a result of other's reactions to their condition. However, Cacciapaglia et al. (2004) found that nondisabled people were more willing to talk to a person with a visible disability (i.e., amputee) than the same person who "hid" their disability.

In sport, positive and negative appraisals may be based on ability perceptions. Parents of children with disabilities, for example, believe that peers are more accepting of their children with physical disabilities in physical activity and sport settings if they were viewed as being physically capable. This finding is consistent with previous research examining able-bodied children. Some individuals with disabilities note that their participation in sport and physical activity is trivialized and their physical abilities often doubted.

Even well-intended offers of aid can go awry. For example, Goodwin (2001) interviewed 12 early to later elementary-aged children in order to understand their perceptions of help from peers in physical education classes. She reported that children's self-esteem was threatened when they perceived that help was offered based on a negative assessment of their ability (e.g., "he thinks that I don't have muscles", p. 297). In contrast, Rees et al. (2003) reported on the experiences of six men with SCIs who became disabled as a result of a rugby accident. One of the themes emerging from a discussion of social support was how others (e.g., father, therapist) bolstered their self-esteem and perceptions of ability.

Martin (1999) examined varied self-referent cognitions of adolescent swimmers with varied physical disabilities (e.g., cerebral palsy, CP) and found self-esteem scores comparable to elite adolescent soccer players, gymnasts, and figure skaters. Campbell and Jones (1994) found no self-esteem differences between wheelchair athletes and nonathletes, but still suggested that sport participation has

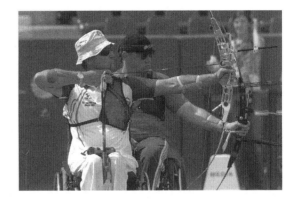

Figure 7.2 International-level athletes report higher self-esteem when compared to other athletes not competing at that level. Reproduced courtesy of Lieven Coudenys.

self-esteem boosting qualities. Additional analyses indicated that the international-level athletes reported higher self-esteem compared to national-, regional-, and recreational-level athletes, supporting the notion that a high level of sport involvement (and presumably success) may be necessary to generalize to increases in global self-esteem (Figure 7.2). Using Harter's (1988) multidimensional self-concept scale, Sherrill et al. (1990) surveyed 158 youth athletes (mean age = 14) with disabilities to determine if their self-esteem scores paralleled those of nondisabled youth based on established norms. The pattern of scores across the global self-worth scale and eight subscales indicated no differences. However, the close friends and job competence subscale scores were 0.10 below the range of normative scores. The investigators suggested that these results were emblematic of youth's unmet needs in these areas as people with disabilities are often socially isolated and underemployed.

In one of the few sport intervention studies assessing self-esteem, Hedrick (1985) examined the effects of a 4-week wheelchair tennis program on children's (N = 36) general perceived competence (i.e., self-worth) and, as he anticipated, found no evidence to support this hypothesis. As Hedrick noted, increases in self-esteem likely require increases in mastery behavior over a significant range of behaviors (i.e., not just sport) over a period of time longer than 4 weeks. Goodwin et al. (2004a) reported that both children (N = 5, aged 6–14 years) and their parents saw wheelchair dance as instrumental in promoting a stronger sense of self. Finally, Valliant et al. (1985) compared athletes with disabilities to nonathletes with disabilities. They found athletes with disabilities had higher global self-esteem compared to nonathletes with disabilities. It should be noted, however, that the disability group was quite heterogeneous (i.e., wheelchair, amputee, blind, CP) and was significantly ($N = 139$) larger than the comparison group ($N = 22$).

In conclusion, the limited research examining the self-esteem scores of individuals with disabilities does not support the notion that they have lower self-esteem compared to nondisabled individuals. Furthermore, it is not likely that intervention programs of short duration focused only on sport skill mastery are likely to have a significant impact on global self-esteem unless program participants have low self-esteem and their athletic identity constitutes a significant aspect of their self-worth. Sport and physical-activity-based interventions have the potential to enhance multidimensional self-esteem, if the specific component of self-esteem targeted (i.e., social self-esteem, friendships) is an area where participants have had limited opportunities to interact with peers and particularly peers with similar disabilities and life experiences.

Efficacy and confidence

Athletes with a disability, particularly elite Paralympians, must feel confident in their capabilities in order to perform consistently and to enjoy superior sport performances at major important competitions (e.g., Paralympics). Fortunately, self-confidence and self-efficacy have assumed a prominent position in disability sport psychology research. Self-confidence represents athlete's beliefs that they can be successful in sport (Figure 7.3). In contrast, self-efficacy is more specific and reflects athlete's beliefs in their abilities to execute a skill (e.g., shooting a basketball) to obtain a particular outcome (e.g., scoring a basket). For instance, Lowther et al. (2002) examined self-efficacy, psychological skills, and performance for 15 elite amputee male soccer players over a six-game Amputee World Cup tournament. Athletes with the strongest self-efficacy performed better relative to soccer players with weaker efficacy. Higher self-efficacy was also associated with stronger psychological

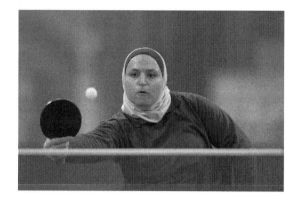

Figure 7.3 Self-confidence represents athletes' belief that they can be successful in sport. Reproduced courtesy of Lieven Coudenys.

skills. In a study of Greek athletes participating in the National Wheelchair Basketball Championships, self-efficacy (along with past performance) predicted passing performance (Katartzi et al., 2007). Schliermann and Stoll (2007) also examined self-efficacy with 45 elite female German basketball players. Contrary to their expectations, basketball self-efficacy was unrelated to somatic anxiety, worry, and concentration disruption. In their study, they employed a sport, but nonbasketball-specific measure of anxiety and a basketball-specific measure of self-efficacy. The lack of congruence between the measures may have been substantial enough, combined with a small sample, to result in the nonsignificant findings.

Training self-efficacy, performance self-efficacy, efficacy for overcoming barriers to successful racing, and positive affect have all been shown to be positively linked with wheelchair road-racing performance. Athletes with stronger multidimensional efficacy and positive affect raced faster compared to "wheelers" who were less efficacious and reported lower positive affect. In a similar study with wheelchair basketball players, Martin (2008) also found positive relationships among training efficacy, performance self-efficacy, thought control self-efficacy, and resiliency self-efficacy. Wheelchair basketball players who could control distressing thoughts and maintain an upbeat attitude also had greater efficacy in their ability to play basketball and train well, despite barriers relative to players who had fewer efficacies in their ability to manage their negative thoughts.

Swimmers with disabilities, who had strong training self-efficacy, also reported receiving high levels of emotional and technical challenge support from their coaches and parents. This finding affirms the value of a strong support system. In a study of 42 national- and international-level athletes with disabilities, Ferreira et al. (2007) reported on their confidence leading up to competition. They found that athlete's confidence decreased just prior to competition. Although effect sizes were not reported, in absolute terms, the decrease from 2 h prior (27.7 to 27.3 and from 28.7 to 28.4) to 20 min before seems insubstantial.

As might be expected, quad rugby athletes had much stronger quad rugby skill self-efficacy (e.g., sprint right, cut left, catch ball from feeder) compared to nonquad rugby players (Adnan et al., 2001). Of additional importance, however, athlete's sport self-efficacy likely transferred to feelings of efficacy for ADL. In particular, athletes expressed much stronger self-efficacy for transferring from wheelchair to bed and seat (and vice versa) compared to nonathletes. Adnan et al.'s (2001) findings supported earlier research on wheelchair tennis players. Greenwood zet al. (1990) found that wheelchair tennis self-efficacy was correlated with wheelchair mobility self-efficacy. They suggested that participation in wheelchair tennis led to enhanced efficacy for nonsport efficacy such as wheeling up ramps and going down curbs. Cumulatively, the above findings support the relevance and important role of efficacy and confidence in sport performance.

These findings also suggest that sport-specific support personnel such as coaches, teammates, and sport psychologists should help athletes build efficacious sport cognitions by focusing on controllable personal performance goals and by employing positive, helpful, self-talk while minimizing negative efficacy destroying self-talk. Finally, the research by Adnan et al. (2001) and Greenwood et al. (1990) suggests that sport participation has nonsport-specific benefits in the area of ADL.

Coping, stress, and anxiety

Research on stress and coping have been prominent in disability sport. Campbell and Jones (1994, 1997, 2002a,b) examined stress and anxiety in elite wheelchair athletes in a series of published research studies. In their 1997 study, they found that somatic anxiety increased as competition approached. Somatic anxiety was high compared to relevant norms and intensity varied greatly indicating heightened individual variability. Campbell and Jones (1997) suggested that the relatively low levels of somatic anxiety may have been reported because athletes simulated physiological "arousal" via imagery to prepare for competition.

Campbell and Jones (2002a) also examined sources of stress in elite male wheelchair basketball players. Athlete's stressors were as follows:
- precompetition issues (e.g., team selection);
- negative competition readiness (e.g., concerned about faulty equipment);
- performance worries (e.g., playing time);
- postmatch performance concerns (e.g., playing badly);
- downside of participating in major events (e.g., being away from home);
- low group cohesiveness (e.g., conflict with teammates);
- negative coaching (e.g., not enough encouragement);
- relationship worries (e.g., concern about partner's well-being);
- sport demands (e.g., limited funds for expensive equipment);
- poor disability awareness (e.g., inaccessible toilets).

From the above list of concerns, it is clear that athletes' worries ranged from unique disability sport stressors (e.g., equipment concerns) to disability-specific worries (e.g., concern about pressure sores) and, finally, to common sources of sport anxiety (e.g., a lack of fitness).

In a follow-up study with the same athletes, Campbell and Jones (2002b) asked participants to appraise the previous sources of stress. Athletes who viewed stressors as challenges also viewed the same stressors as being in their control. This finding suggests (as many sport psychologists have noted) that framing stressful events as challenges to overcome, instead of uncontrollable problems, is helpful. Athletes who viewed stressors as severe were also likely to rate them as threatening and harmful. The most severe stressors were negative coaching behaviors, relationship issues, and the financial costs of

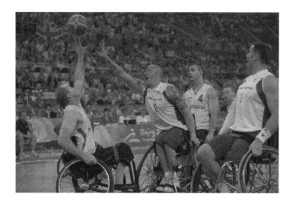

Figure 7.4 In one study, basketball players had low to moderate levels of anxiety prior to competition. Reproduced courtesy of Lieven Coudenys.

wheelchair basketball. The demands of wheelchair basketball were the most frequent stressors.

Perreault and Marisi (1997) found that wheelchair basketball players had low to moderate levels of anxiety prior to competition (Figure 7.4). Ferreira et al. (2007) examined the temporal pattern of anxiety for 42 athletes with disabilities and found that over the week prior to competition, anxiety increased in athletes. Cognitive anxiety remained relatively stable over a 1-week period. Although the pattern of somatic anxiety was similar for all athletes, international-level athletes and more experienced athletes reported lower somatic and cognitive anxiety when compared to national-level athletes and less experienced athletes, respectively. Similarly, Schliermann and Stoll (2007) found that the mean scores for somatic anxiety, worry, and concentration disruption of elite female wheelchair athletes were slightly lower on all three measures compared to a sample ($N \approx 1000$) of German able-bodied female athletes.

Pensgaard et al. (1999) examined Norwegian Paralympians and found that they reported moderate use of functional coping skills such as planning and redefining stress as an opportunity for growth. Scores for more ineffective coping skills such as behavioral disengagement and denying stress were substantially lower. In general, Paralympians and Olympians reported similar levels of coping.

Overton et al. (1995) examined 197 adult athletes, most with CP, to assess if they used sport to cope with their disability and if their coping skills were adequate. Social competence and life quality were proxies for coping skills. Athletes reported being moderately high on coping ability for managing social relationships and they reported a satisfying quality of life. Overton et al. also found differences between athletes planning to continue sport (i.e., "persisters") and those who were thinking of quitting (i.e., "nonpersisters"). First, persisters tended to find positive aspects in stressful situations, whereas nonpersisters were more likely to deny or avoid stress. Second, persisters had plans for managing their stress. Finally, nonpersisters were more likely to respond to anger with stress. They concluded that sport helped athletes cope with their disability, promoted coping skills, and that these skills transferred to other life domains.

In short, athletes with disabilities experience both sport-specific and disability-specific anxiety. In addition, limited evidence suggests that elite-level athletes with disabilities develop skills for effectively coping with sport stress. Sport may also contribute to the development of coping skills, particularly in committed athletes, that can extend to stressful nonsport situations. The above information has implications for sport personnel such as coaches and sport psychologists in regard to anxiety management. At the same time, the finding that athletes traveling abroad worry about their partner's well-being has ramifications for problem solving how athletes and their partners can best manage their separation so that athletes can focus on performing to the best of their ability.

Mood and emotion

Athletes with disability mood states have been researched extensively with the profile of mood states (POMS). Most researchers have sought to determine if athletes report an "iceberg profile," indicative of positive mental health. The iceberg profile is supported when athletes have scores below the norm for anger, confusion, depression, fatigue, and tension with vigor, the only positive mood state, above the norm.

Campbell and Jones (1994) found that wheelchair athletes reported lower anger, confusion, depression, and tension scores and higher vigor scores compared to wheelchair users who were inactive. Additionally, athletes exhibited iceberg profiles, indicative of mental health. The most accomplished athletes reported the strongest feelings of vigor. Similar findings have been found with wheelchair tennis players and nontennis players with disabilities. Tennis participants reported higher than the norm on vigor scores and lower than the norm on tension, anger, confusion, fatigue, and depression, indicative of the iceberg profile of mental health. Tennis players also scored higher on vigor and lower on the negative states compared to nontennis players. Fung and Fu (1995) compared 150 Chinese wheelchair athletes—who were finalists in the National Games—to 150 nonfinalists, and found that, collectively, mood scores for vigor, confusion, tension, and sport commitment distinguished finalists from nonfinalists in 78% of the cases. Finalists were less tensed and confused, and expressed having more vigor and commitment than nonfinalists.

Jacobs et al. (1990) compared wheelchair athletes and nonathletes to able-bodied athletes. Both groups of athletes reported greater feelings of vigor, whereas nonathletes reported higher scores for depressed mood. Jacobs et al. speculated that sport participation provides physiological benefits leading to increased feelings of vigor. Horvat et al. (1989) compared able-bodied athletes with athletes with disabilities, who were similar in years of sport experience and in training habits. Again, athletes with disabilities exhibited iceberg profiles, and the authors concluded that sport helps athletes with disabilities learn to cope with their disability.

Campbell (1995) compared mood states among wheelchair athletes with congenital versus acquired disabilities. Both groups reported iceberg profiles, but athletes with acquired disabilities reported lower scores for anger, confusion, fatigue, and depressed mood and higher scores for vigor, compared to those with congenital disabilities. Athletes did not differ on tension. Campbell suggested that athletes with an acquired disability, relative to athletes with congenital disabilities, may learn coping skills in order to manage their affect.

Although many researchers have focused on wheelchair basketball athletes, Mastro et al. (1987) examined 49 visually impaired, national-level athletes and found that male athletes reported iceberg profiles. Female athletes tended to report profiles similar to nonathletic populations. Also, Masters et al. (1995) examined mood responses among elite athletes with CP, or comparable levels of brain trauma. Athletes reported reduced tension and anger from the beginning to the end of the 6-day camp, followed by an increase in tension and anger 1 month later at the Paralympic trials. Further, Mastro et al. (1988) compared 75 visually impaired and 46 sighted male beep baseball players competing in the World Series of beep baseball. Unsighted athletes were higher in depressed mood and tension. Visually impaired athletes may have experienced more tension because of limited time to adjust to an unfamiliar competition site.

In summary, athletes with disabilities have usually reported iceberg mood profiles, suggesting that athletic participation might be associated with positive moods and buffer against negative mood states. One path of influence is that sport participation provides physiological benefits leading to increased feelings of energy and vigor. Mastery experiences from sport and increased social support are two other plausible mechanisms acting to reduce negative mood states. Of course, individuals with positive mood states may simply be drawn to sport. Given that individuals with disabilities are prone to higher levels of depression relative to individuals without disabilities, the potential mood enhancement abilities of sport should not be underestimated.

Disability sport considerations

The purpose of this section is to provide information that does not "fit cleanly" within disability or sport psychology, but is nevertheless relevant to the world of disability sport. The following information can inform and guide sport (e.g., coaches) and nonsport personnel (e.g., spouses) in their interactions with athletes. For example, in the next section, information is presented that readers can use to help them avoid glorifying or minimizing athletes with disabilities when they interact with them. Other information is unique to disability sport performance (e.g., classification) and training (e.g., training barriers) and can help the athlete's sport support system.

Athletes, supercrips, or pseudo-athletes?

Research on athletic identity has demonstrated that although many athletes with disabilities view themselves as committed and serious athletes, they typically feel that the public does not view them as legitimate athletes. One reason for this is that individuals with disabilities are often equated with their disabilities and their athletic capabilities go unrecognized. Being an athlete is thought to counteract the stereotype of a helpless disabled person (and as a result make them somewhat immune from negative attitudes and prejudice). Unfortunately, researchers have shown that even athletes with disabilities face strong negative biases when "implicit" attitude measures are used.

Contrary to the above view is the "supercrip" stereotype, whereby athletes with disabilities are viewed as heroes simply because they play a sport. However, most athletes with disabilities do not view themselves as heroes or that their achievements represent a personal victory over their disabilities. Athletes perceive the supercrip and hero label as inaccurate because they view their sport successes as normal athletic achievements.

Most elite-level athletes with disabilities do not want to be reduced to a "supercrip" stereotype or be viewed as a pseudo-athlete. They simply want their legitimate athletic accomplishments to be recognized as such. There are two important messages for individuals working with athletes with disabilities. First, recognize that even elite athletes with disabilities, who may have medaled at the Paralympics, may face a public that diminishes their accomplishments. Second, coaches, trainers, and sport psychologists should interact with athletes with disabilities as individuals who play sport and focus on their athletic goals and not on their disabilities. At the same time, these same individuals should not act as if athlete's disabilities are irrelevant.

Training

Social support

Many athletes with disabilities have to train by themselves. This can be particularly problematic for team sport athletes where the ability to practice together is critical. For instance, the 2009 US National Wheelchair Rugby Team came from 11 different states and can only work together at national training camps. Many sport psychologists have found that athletes receive social support as a result of team sport involvement, and sport friendship is one reason to continue playing sport. Clearly, the sport-related support obtained from training partners and teammates can be critical in helping athletes adhere to demanding training schedules. Martin (2002, 2008) suggested that one reason athletes training self-efficacy for overcoming common training barriers was less than optimal was because they faced many social (e.g., lack of training partners) and environmental (e.g., inaccessible exercise facilities) barriers to training.

Fitness facilities

Rimmer et al.'s (2005) line of research examining fitness and health clubs suggest that athletes who wish to train for their sport in such locations would have difficulty in doing so. They examined 35 health clubs across the United States in urban and suburban settings. They found that most facilities were likely (>50%) to have helpful assistive devices such as shower grab bars. In contrast, most facilities were not likely (<50%) to have curb cuts for easy access or paths to lockers that were not blocked. Many facilities did not allow adequate room for wheelchair to exercise equipment transfers, although they had adequate access to the exercise area in general. Many of the exercise facility shortcomings had no adaptive exercise equipment. They concluded that people with mobility disabilities and visual impairments would "have difficulty accessing various areas of fitness facilities and health clubs" (p. 2022). This conclusion can clearly be extended to include athletes with disabilities.

Neighborhood

While able-bodied runners, for example, take for granted the ability to step out their door and go running in the surrounding urban area or park, persons with disabilities are not afforded this luxury. Even outdoor areas often designed to facilitate and support play and sport can present barriers to individuals with disabilities. Poorly lit walking paths or wooded walking trails with rocks or fallen branches can be barriers to individuals with vision loss. Without audible signals at traffic lights and curb cuts that do not have high-color contrast markings that make them distinctly visible, individuals with vision loss cannot train outside without a partner.

Spivock et al. (2007) surveyed 112 neighborhoods in Montreal, Canada, for their activity friendliness for people with disabilities. They examined walking surfaces (e.g., paths wide enough for a wheelchair), signs (e.g., auditory signals on the crosswalks), and surrounding areas (e.g., access ramps, parking). Mean scores were low in absolute terms (i.e., under the scale midpoint) and in relative terms, they were significantly lower than reference items for nondisabled individuals.

Even if wheelchair athletes living in the northern climates used creativity to avoid inclement weather by using shopping malls to train/wheel, for example, they would likely be frustrated. McClain (2000), for example, studied three large shopping malls by examining various features such as the parking lots, elevators, ramps, and restrooms to see if they met the *Americans with a Disability Act* requirements. She obtained mixed results and found that although the malls had ramps for wheelchairs, two of the three malls had slopes too steep for wheelchair users. Finally, even when athletes are members of disabled sport teams and can train in sport facilities, they still rate difficulties with accessing and using toilet and changing facilities as their number one complaint. Few ramps and a lack of room to accommodate a wheelchair are also common barriers in sport facilities. In summary, athletes with disabilities, relative to able-bodied athletes, face more training barriers in the form of reduced social support and increased built environment obstacles.

Pain

Athletes with and without disabilities will at times have to deal with physical pain in training and competition. Most of the research examining pain in individuals with disabilities has not focused specifically on physical activity or athletes. However, the role of pain in the sporting lives of athletes with disabilities is significant and may play a larger role compared to nondisabled athletes (Figure 7.5).

The premise for the above idea is based on research conducted with active individuals involved in exercise and some sport-based research. This small body of research indicates that pain may interfere with

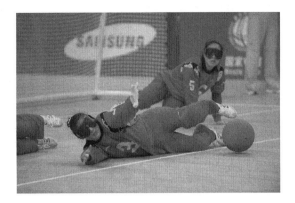

Figure 7.5 Injury and pain are a part of an athlete's life. Reproduced courtesy of Lieven Coudenys.

training for people with SCI as up to 94% of them indicate that they have pain. Other researchers have reported that pain limits physical activity, and in some cases individuals have indicated that their pain is more limiting of their physical activity than their disability. Even physical activity itself can be painful. Finally, athletes with disabilities report more sport-related muscle pain (SRMP) as their training volume increases (Bernardi et al., 2003). Furthermore, 18% reported that SRMP interrupted their training from 1 to 4 weeks. Sport personnel should be particularly sensitive that athletes do not try and train through pain that might exacerbate an injury or their disability.

Injury and illness

Training is also disrupted by injury and illness. Relative to their able-bodied counterparts, athletes with disabilities lose more training time due to injury. Researchers examining athletes at the 1996 Atlanta Paralympic Games found that visually impaired runners experienced lower-leg overuse injuries that were similar in nature to nonvisually impaired athletes (Nyland et al., 2000). Athletes with unilateral amputations (i.e., one leg) suffered more injuries in the ankle area of the nonamputated foot/leg. For other athletes, their disability, sport-specific stressors, and adaptive or guidance aids (e.g., prosthetic device) often interact, leading to the development of an injury. Nyland et al. found that shoulder injuries were the most common among wheelchair athletes. Bernardi et al. (2003) speculated that the everyday demands of wheeling, combined with wheeling for sport, did not allow enough time for rest and adaptation to occur. Athletes with disabilities may also be at risk of upper respiratory tract infections (URTIs). For instance, wheelchair marathon racers experienced more (19%) URTIs than did the able-bodied control subjects (15.4%) in the 2 weeks after a race. Wheelers who trained hard postmarathon also experienced more URTI episodes compared to marathoners training less, suggesting that they were overtraining when they should be recovering (Furusawa et al., 2007). Finally, it is important to understand the increased risk of heat exhaustion and related outcomes (e.g., heat stroke) for athletes with SCI, because they have difficulty regulating body temperature, particularly when competing in high temperatures. In brief, athlete's support personnel should be aware of overtraining and other practices that might heighten athlete's risk of injury and illness.

Coaching

Some high-level athletes (e.g., Paralympians) from wealthy countries (e.g., United States, United Kingdom, and Canada) are increasingly able to benefit from excellent coaching. For instance, Canadian Paralympic swimmers have access to the same high-level coaches as nondisabled swimmers. However, most athletes with disabilities do not have a coach or their coaches do not have the appropriate sport science education. Even elite athletes (e.g., Kenyans competing in the Paralympic Games) from poorer countries may have no coaches, and being from a wealthy country (e.g., United States) is no guarantee of adequate coaching. For example, as of 1996, only 58% of 319 elite adult athletes from the United States (Ferrara & Buckley, 1996) and 33% of a diverse group of international athletes (e.g., Australian, Dutch, and Japanese) reported having coaches. Britain, a country with a proud history of supporting disability sport, has athletes who report having limited access to coaches.

Many athletes overtrain, train inconsistently in nonsport-specific ways, fail to taper for major competitions, and fail to rest after major performance efforts. For athletes who self-coach, appropriate disability sport-specific information is often hard to find. The ramifications of an inadequate coaching support system are that athletes may need extra support and encouragement when pursuing their athletic dreams.

Classification

Most able-bodied athletes who are classified (e.g., according to weight) usually know their classifications and, thus, can reasonably predict or control them. However, athletes with disabilities are functionally classified, which means they are graded based on their abilities to perform physical tests. As a result, athletes with different disabilities may compete against each other. Hence, a swimmer with CP may race against a swimmer missing a limb. Being classified, which occurs prior to competition, can be stressful for a few reasons. First, the process can be stressful if athletes fear being reclassified at a different level than they have been previously. Second, if athletes are reclassified, they may have to compete against athletes whose impairment has less impact on performance and can perform better than their previous competitors who were at a lower level. It is certainly plausible that competing under such circumstances may reduce confidence and increase anxiety at a critical time (e.g., 48 h before competition). Functional classification is clearly a potential stressor. Hence, coaches and sport psychologists should consider helping their athletes prepare for any anxiety about the classification process.

Leaving sport

The foregoing has addressed factors that impact on athletes' performance during their careers. However, at some point, an elite sports career must come to an end and the athlete is faced with a transition out of sports. In the context of transition theory, a transition involves an adjustment to personal identity and requires new adaptive behaviors. An athlete may face the question of *if not athlete who am I now?* and face a life in which he/she is no longer required to engage in intense daily training. How do athletes with disabilities cope with transition out of sports? In the previous sections, a number of factors were raised, which provide some clues as to how athletes may cope and the difficulties they may face. For example, intense commitment to sport and training, the lack of coaching and qualified coaches, and issues of overtraining raises questions as to how the quality of life may be affected in athletes with chronic pain due to overuse injuries. In this section, the concept of transition from elite disability sport is explored. Suggestions are made with regard to helping athletes manage what can be a difficult period in their lives.

A highly sophisticated and complex elite sports system, with its elaborate and often excessive reward systems, places extreme demands on athletes and requires extremely high levels of commitment early in their lives and throughout their careers. It has been suggested that this level of commitment coupled with an institutional focus on creating an "athletic person" may leave an athlete poorly prepared for coping with life after making the transition to retirement from sports. This has been described in able-bodied sport in a classic article by Thomas and Ermler (1988) and serves as an important introduction to this section.

> ". . . what we see happening with the gifted athlete is not a caring for the whole person but all too often caring for the athletic person. We allow the individual to define the self in terms of athletic talent and to lose touch with the truer self. We allow the athlete to narrow his or her personal development and self concept and become identified only in terms of athletic achievement" (Thomas & Ermler, 1988, p. 138).

Furthermore, they suggest that the holistic development of the athlete is subjugated to the assumed benefits of elite sports participation, and that athletes are engaged in a power-dependency relationship with coaches, which leave them with little control over or autonomy in their careers. As a result, athletes may be ill prepared to manage life after sports.

> "The pampered treatment he has long received may have left him without basic skills for coping with life; skills like reading and writing, looking for a sale or balancing a checkbook and now he suddenly confronts a mystifying world that is normal to most" (Myslenski, 1986, in Thomas & Ermler, 1988, p. 139).

Research in the area of how able-bodied athletes transition appears to corroborate the concerns and observations mentioned earlier. Transition to retirement has been described as a traumatic event, an identity crisis, role loss, an inevitable metathesis, and social or career death. Others have described athletes as passing through similar stages as to the grieving process. It has been suggested that on leaving sport, athletes lack personal resources to cope. Factors contributing to emotional problems after sports include commitment to sport, ego involvement, development of an athletic identity, loss of autonomy, and control of personal development during the athletic career.

Conversely, others suggest that in spite of emotional difficulties, most athletes make the transition out of sport successfully and perceive transition to the postsport world as a time to explore new opportunities. The postsport period may be characterized by relief at no longer having to manage the stress of training. Although methodological differences and difficulties have contributed to conflicting findings in this area, it is safe to say that the transition from elite sports can be an emotionally difficult or even traumatic event to which athletes must cope with and adapt.

Therefore, a number of questions arise with regard to elite athletes in disability sports. Do athletes with disabilities have similar transition experiences to able-bodied athletes? What is the nature of these experiences? Do they experience emotional difficulties in making the transition to retirement? What action should (if any) the institution of disability sport take to ameliorate the impact of transition to retirement in this population?

If it is assumed that athletes with disabilities are "athletes first," then perhaps one might conclude that this is a redundant area of study and that recommendations for able-bodied athletes are simply transferable. However, there are a number of good reasons for considering this area as worthy of study and for considering interventions for athletes with disabilities making the transition out of sports to retirement. A number of sequels of the sport career and the transition process occur. Some athletes report long-standing emotional issues associated with not having "worked through" their exit from sport and what that meant in their lives. Interviews with such athletes have been characterized by a significant expression of emotional distress. Athletes may acquire a "secondary disability" (e.g., overuse injuries in the shoulder) as a function of overcommitment and overtraining. Such a situation may have significant consequences for coping with the postsport world and functional aspects such as mobility. A number of authors have also suggested that athletes with disabilities may face the issue of coping with their disability for the first time as well as with transition-related emotional issues. This may be a function of a rapid transition to sport and "promotion" to elite sports after an acquired disability combined with a short athletic career. Asken (1989), for example, has suggested that in some circumstances sport can act as a way for disabled athletes to avoid dealing with disability, and hence after retirement, they may have to cope more overtly with their disability.

Consistent with Thomas and Ermler's (1988) thinking, it could also be argued that the institution of disability sports has a moral obligation to help athletes in transition. The institution of elite disability sport cannot exist without its athletes and, hence, there is a reciprocal obligation on the part of the institution to support its athletes in the transition of their careers. It is important for athletic personnel (coaches, administrators, etc.) to understand the experiences of the athlete with a disability, the importance of sport in their lives, and their experiences in making the transition from sports. This will assist in providing targeted programs and interventions for the athlete in transition. Finally, the world of elite disability sports is growing in sophistication and complexity, and performance demands of athletes are increasing. It is not yet known how this will translate into difficulties in making a transition from sport to retirement. Helping athletes as they make the transition from their sports career is as important as helping athletes with psychological issues of performance during their careers.

Perhaps the assumption that athletes with a disability have similar transition and retirement experiences as able-bodied athletes explains why relatively little work has been conducted in the area of retirement from disability sport. As noted earlier, previous research in able-bodied sports suggests that intense levels of commitment to sport and developing an athletic identity may lead to exclusion of other life interests and may leave an athlete ill prepared to cope with retirement. Research on athletes with a disability has demonstrated a similar level

of intense commitment, with many athletes stating that sport is the dominant feature in their lives, a means of demonstrating personal competency and an essential element of personal identity. An athlete in the Wheeler et al. (1996, p. 388) investigation reported:

> "When we are on the track, I think we don't look at ourselves as disabled. When we're in our racing chair it is like putting on a uniform; it's like you are out of it now; you are out of the disability. It gives you that. It's like putting a Superman vest on."

Consistent with Thomas and Ermler's (1988) predictions, the downside to this commitment was the neglect of other aspects of life, including important relationships, and even self-injurious training practices. An athlete in the Wheeler et al. (1996, p. 388) investigation noted,

> "I didn't have a balance in my life. That's where all the injuries were, that's where all the emotional and mental turmoil was as well. Because I never allowed myself to do other things, because I had my whole identity wrapped up in athletics".

Another athlete noted:

> "I never listened or respected my body and what it was doing. I saw through them (injuries). . . . I just had incredible pain . . . It was winning or nothing. I was going to die trying; that was what I was going to do" (Wheeler et al., 1996, p. 389).

Theory would also suggest that neglecting social relationships would predict difficulties with career transition. Researchers have shown that athletes with disabilities do perceive a lack of support from others, including athletes and sports organizations, after they retire.

Clearly, athletes with disabilities often totally commit themselves to their sports to the exclusion of other interests and relationships; may train to the point of creating chronic injury, and develop an athletic identity. The question, then, is whether this is associated with emotional difficulties upon leaving the sports arena? Again, there are a few research studies upon which our response to this question is based. However, the data are convincing.

A number of authors in the able-bodied sports arena have identified athletes experiencing a huge void or a death-like experience upon retirement. Research in disability sport has identified similar emotional issues including shock, grief, hollowness/ emptiness, anger, sadness, and mourning.

For example, an athlete in the Wheeler et al. (1999, p. 228) study noted.

> ". . . it's like somebody in your family died. It's like a death in your family and that thing that was this person or whatever that was so important to you just disappeared. I think you go through all the grieving things you do when somebody dies".

Symptoms of depression meeting the criteria for a major depressive episode have also been reported, albeit this is inferred retrospectively from self-report data. Perhaps the most remarkable, if not disconcerting, example of the emotional impact of leaving sport was stated by an athlete in the Wheeler et al. (1996) study who said the following on arriving home from competition and (essentially) at the end of her career:

> "I honestly believe it is very closely related . . . as if you were to lose a baby. Just like a miscarriage. It is just the sorrow inside and it is something that you have looked forward to and planned for and boom it is taken away . . . all of a sudden you get back and that focus is gone and guess what . . . so are you basically. If you are not involved in sports anymore you are really nobody—that is exactly how you are treated when you get back" (Wheeler et al., 1996, p. 389).

In a review of transition-related work, Martin (1999b) conceptualized the transition experiences of athletes with disabilities in a loss framework. He suggests that athletes with disabilities experience a range of losses including psychological, social, and physiological losses. Psychological losses are associated with a strong athletic identity, resulting in potential for a negative effect upon leaving sport.

Social losses include loss of athlete friends and lack of opportunity to remain engaged in disability sport. Physiological losses refer to the loss of the health and fitness benefits associated with athletic training. However, consistent with able-bodied research in the area, disability sport transition research has shown that athletes may also be either ambivalent or relieved to be leaving the stresses and strains of the competitive sport environment and having the opportunity for and taking time for other important aspects of life. For example, an athlete in the Wheeler et al. (1996, p. 391) study noted:

> "It was just knowing, that there were other things out there for me to explore. I was 'into' (getting) a career and I wanted to pursue things differently in my career. . . . I just wanted to explore ordinary life. I wanted to finish school and establish a career. I was ready to move on".

It would appear that like able-bodied sports, athletes with disabilities are intensely committed, often develop an athletic identity, disregard other important aspects of life, experience a range of negative emotions on leaving sport, but also see the opportunities in life after sport. Leaving sport may represent a period of grieving for psychological, social, and physiological losses. Athletes may report symptoms consistent with unresolved grieving and clinical depression long after they have retired. While the majority of athletes interviewed in the Wheeler et al. (1996, 1999) studies were coping well with their daily lives, for many the memories of the transition out of sport were poignant and many were angry at sports organizations for simply allowing them to drift away from sports.

Finally, it is worthwhile to consider the factors that can help athletes with a disability to cope with the exit from sports. A number of factors are likely important in the athlete's ability to cope with the transition from sport and include level of commitment (maintaining a balanced approach to sport and other life interests), avoiding overtraining and managing sports injuries (e.g., resting an injured shoulder), identity (identifying self with diverse aspects or roles in life), coping style (emotional or problem solving), support structures (family, sports organizations), and remaining involved in sports (e.g., coaching, sports ambassador).

Given that athletes may experience difficulties, what are the (moral, ethical) obligations of the institution of disability sport toward the athlete? Thomas and Ermler (1988) suggest that sport has a number of moral obligations to its athletes in their careers and during transition based on the concepts of autonomy (control over personal career), beneficence (positive gains from sports), and nonmalfeasance (ensuring no harm to athletes). This statement is based on the data available, and it is reasonable to suggest that athletes with a disability should have access to transition/retirement services/programs and would likely benefit from the services recommended for able-bodied athletes during their careers and transition. This would include counseling services (e.g., preparation for exit from sports; exit interviews and follow-up), ongoing communication with athletes, and recognition of athletes (during and after career). Failure to provide athletes with various levels of support during their careers and in transition, and, in particular, helping athletes maintain a balanced life, may have (and has been demonstrated to have) serious negative consequences for the athlete as he/she makes the transition out of sport and into a "new life." The observation of Wheeler et al. (1996, 1999) demonstrated that for some athletes, life after sports became an ongoing reflection on how the athlete had failed to manage other aspects of their lives and now were facing a life with a chronic injury or secondary disability. Furthermore, many expressed significant anger at a sports institution which simply seemed not to care about them.

Given the findings of early research in this area in both able-bodied and disability sport, it is perhaps surprising that more has not been written or done at the level of the athletic institution to help athletes prepare for and cope with the transition from disability sport. However, it is positive to note that the International Paralympic Committee (IPC) has taken steps to provide access to career transition programs for its athletes. This was initiated in 2007 when IPC President Sir Phil Craven signed an agreement with Adecco to ensure that Paralympic athletes had access to the Adecco Athlete Career Program—which had previously been successfully implemented with the International Olympic Committee (IOC) and its athletes. To quote Sir Phil Craven, "The program is an excellent opportunity for Paralympians to manage the difficult transition from their sporting career

to be successful in their new professional lives" (IPC news release, August 12, 2007). In July 2009, the IPC and Adecco Group have extended their cooperation agreement to deliver the Adecco Athlete Career Program to Paralympic athletes during and at the end of their athletic careers (IPC news release, July 22, 2009). This is an extremely important step for the IPC and for disability sport in general, and in concert with other initiatives will do much to ease the transition of athletes into retirement.

Recommendations

In addition to career-focused initiatives such as that mentioned earlier, how else can sport organizers help athletes with a disability to make a smooth transition from sport? Fisher and Wrisberg (2007) suggest that athletes most often use three strategies for coping with retirement: (a) coping strategies, (b) social support, and (c) preretirement planning. Coping strategies may include maintaining a regular workout schedule, talking with someone who is supportive, and staying in touch with athlete friends. Maintaining or reconnecting to social support mechanisms, which may have become "diluted" during the sport career, is an important component. Preretirement planning strategies including career consulting have significant value. In addition, given that intense commitment to sport to the exclusion of other interests and relationships and the development of an identity based on sports participation and performance, it would make sense that the preretirement interventions should focus on ensuring athletes maintain a diverse social network and engage in activities outside of sports. Coaches should speak with their athletes early in their careers about such matters. Coaches should also monitor athlete training regimens closely and minor injuries should be taken care of quickly and appropriate recovery periods employed. This may help avoid chronic overuse injuries which, as alluded to earlier, can impact quality of life for the athlete in retirement. Another important strategy is recognition by their sports bodies and also opportunities to remain engaged in sports in some capacity. Mentoring or sports ambassador roles have been suggested as a means of keeping athletes involved.

Finally, it is important to note that whereas most athletes will experience some degree of loss upon leaving sports, not everyone will have significant emotional difficulties; nor will every athlete wish to take part in a career transition intervention program. However, some athletes do experience intense feelings of loss (including depression) and do require help in making the transition from sports. Coaches and sports organizations should consider developing such programs so that athletes who are experiencing anxiety can be identified prior to or during their transition and help them in this regard.

Summary

Individuals in the world of disability sport such as coaches, sport psychologists, teammates, and even spouses can best support an athlete's efforts to train and reach their potential, if they understand the disability world, sport psychology, and how disability sport is different from able-bodied sport. Knowledge of the disability paradox, coping with a disability, disability stereotypes, and disability culture are just a few salient considerations of value. Researchers investigating self-esteem, confidence and efficacy, coping, stress, and anxiety, and mood states have reported results that mostly parallel research with able-bodied athletes. A few findings specific to the disability sport or disability condition illuminate the subtle differences between disability and nondisability sport. Finally, disability sport challenges also span the areas of identity, training, pain, injury and illness, coaching, classification, and leaving sport.

References

Adnan, Y., McKenzie, A. & Miyahara, M. (2001). Self-efficacy for quad rugby skills and activities of daily living. *Adapted Physical Activity Quarterly*, **18**, 90–101.

Albrecht, G.G.L. & Devlieger, P.J. (1999). The disability paradox: high quality of life against all odds. *Social Science & Medicine*, **48**, 977–988.

Asken, M.J. (1989). Sport psychology and the physically disabled athlete: interview with Michael D. Goodling, OTR/L. *The Sport Psychologist*, **3**, 166–176.

Bernardi, M., Castellano, V., Ferrara, M.S., Sbriccoli, P., Sera, F. & Marchetti, M. (2003). Muscle pain in athletes with locomotor disability. *Medicine and Science in Sports and Exercise*, **35**, 199–206.

Cacciapaglia, H.M., Beauchamp, K.L. & Howells, G.N. (2004). Visibility of disability: effect on willingness to interact. *Rehabilitation Psychology*, **49**, 180–182.

Campbell, E. (1995). Psychological well-being of participants in wheelchair sports: comparison of individuals with congenital and acquired disabilities. *Perceptual and Motor Skills*, **81**, 563–568.

Campbell, E. & Jones, G. (1994). Psychological well-being in wheelchair sport participants and nonparticipants. *Adapted Physical Activity Quarterly*, **11**, 404–415.

Campbell, E. & Jones, G. (1997). Precompetition anxiety and self-confidence in wheelchair sport participants. *Adapted Physical Activity Quarterly*, **14**, 95–107.

Campbell, E. & Jones, G. (2002a). Sources of stress experienced by elite male wheelchair basketball players. *Adapted Physical Activity Quarterly*, **19**, 82–99.

Campbell, E. & Jones, G. (2002b). Cognitive appraisal of sources of stress experienced by elite male wheelchair basketball players. *Adapted Physical Activity Quarterly*, **19**, 100–108.

Dunn, D.S. (2000). Social psychological issues in disability. In: R. Frank & T.R. Elliott (eds.) *Handbook of Rehabilitation Psychology*, pp. 564–584. American Psychological Association, Washington, DC.

Ferrara, M.S. & Buckley, W.E. (1996). Athletes with disabilities injury registry. *Adapted Physical Activity Quarterly*, **13**, 50–60.

Ferreira, J.P.L., Chatzisarantis, N., Gaspar, P.M. & Campos, M.J. (2007). Precompetitive anxiety and self-confidence in athletes with disability. *Perceptual and Motor Skills*, **105**, 339–346.

Fisher, L.A. & Wrisberg, C.A. (2007). How to handle athletes transitions out of sport. *Athletic Therapy Today*, **12**(2), 49–50.

Fung, L. & Fu, F.H. (1995). Psychological determinants between wheelchair sport finalists and non-finalists. *International Journal of Sport Psychology*, **26**, 568–579.

Furusawa, K., Tajima, F., Okawa, H., Takahashi, M. & Ogata, H. (2007). The incident of post-race symptoms of upper respiratory tract infection in wheelchair marathon racers. *Spinal Cord*, **45**, 513–517.

Goodwin, D.L. (2001). The meaning of help in PE: perceptions of students with physical disabilities. *Adapted Physical Activity Quarterly*, **18**, 289–303.

Goodwin, D.L., Krohn, J. & Kuhnle, A. (2004a). Beyond the wheelchair: the experience of dance. *Adapted Physical Activity Quarterly*, **21**, 229–247.

Goodwin, D.L., Thurmeier, R. & Gustafson, P. (2004b). Reactions to the metaphors of disability: the mediating effects of physical activity. *Adapted Physical Activity Quarterly*, **21**, 379–398.

Greenwood, C.M., Dzewaltowski, D.A. & French, R. (1990). Self-efficacy and psychological well-being of wheelchair tennis participants and wheelchair non-tennis participants. *Adapted Physical Activity Quarterly*, **7**, 12–21.

Harter, S. (1988). *Manual for the Self-perception Profile for Adolescents*. University of Denver, Denver.

Hedrick, B.N. (1985). The effect of wheelchair tennis participation and mainstreaming upon the perceptions of competence of physically disabled adolescents. *Therapeutic Recreation Journal*, **19**(2), 34–46.

Horvat, M., Roswal, G., Jacobs, D. & Gaunt, S. (1989). Selected psychological comparisons of able-bodied and disabled athletes. *Physical Educator*, **5**, 202–207.

Hutchinson, S.L. & Kleiber, D.A. (2000). Heroic masculinity following spinal cord injury: implications for therapeutic recreation practice and research. *Therapeutic Recreation Journal*, **34**(1), 42–54.

Jacobs, D.P., Roswal, G.M., Horvat, M.A. & Gorman, D.R. (1990). A comparison between the psychological profiles of wheelchair athletes, wheelchair nonathletes, and able bodied athletes. In: G. Doll-Tepper, C. Dahms, B. Doll & H. von Selzam (eds.) *Adapted Physical Activity: An Interdisciplinary Approach*, pp. 75–79. Springer-Verlag, New York.

Katartzi, E., Theodorakis, Y., Tzetzis, G. & Vlachopoulos, S.P. (2007). Effects of goal setting and self-efficacy on wheelchair basketball performance. *Japanese Journal of Adapted Sport Science*, **5**, 50–62.

Kleiber, D., Brock, S., Lee, Y., Dattilo, J. & Caldwell, L. (1995). The relevance of leisure in an illness experience: realities of spinal cord injury. *Journal of Leisure Research*, **27**, 283–299.

Lowther, J., Lane, A. & Lane, H. (2002). Self-efficacy and psychological skills during the amputee soccer world cup. *Athletic Insight: The Online Journal of Sport Psychology*, **4**, 23–34.

Lyons, R.F., Ritvo, P.G. & Sullivan, M.J.L. (1995). *Relationships in Chronic Illness and Disability*. Sage, Thousand Oaks, CA.

Martin, J.J. (1999). Predictors of social physique anxiety in adolescent swimmers with physical disabilities. *Adapted Physical Activity Quarterly*, **16**, 75–85.

Martin, J.J. (2002). Training and performance self-efficacy, affect, and performance in wheelchair road racers. *The Sport Psychologist*, **16**, 384–395.

Martin, J.J. (2008). Multidimensional self-efficacy and affect in wheelchair basketball players. *Adapted Physical Activity Quarterly*, **25**(3), 1–15.

Masters, K.S., Wittig, A.F., Cox, R.H., Scallen, S.F. & Schurr, K.T. (1995). Effects of training and competition on mood state and anxiety among elite athletes with cerebral palsy. *Palaestra*, **11**, 47–52.

Mastro, J.V., Sherrill, C., Gench, B. & French, R. (1987). Psychological characteristics of elite visually impaired athletes: the iceberg profile. *Journal of Sport Behavior*, **10**, 39–46.

Mastro, J.V., Canabal, M.Y. & French, R. (1988). Psychological mood profiles of sighted and unsighted beep baseball players. *Research Quarterly for Exercise and Sport*, **59**, 262–264.

McClain, L. (2000). Shopping center wheelchair accessibility: ongoing advocacy to implement the Americans with Disabilities Act of 1990. *Public Health Nursing*, **17**(3), 178–186.

Nyland, J., Snouse, S.L., Anderson, M., Kelly, T. & Sterling, J.C. (2000). Soft tissue injuries to USA Paralympians at the 1996 summer games. *Archives of Physical Medicine and Rehabilitation*, **81**, 368–373.

Overton, S., Habeck, R., Ewing, M. & Dummer, G. (1995). Sports, disability, and coping. In: F.M. Robinson, D. West & D. Woodworth (eds.) *Coping Plus: Dimensions of Disability*, pp. 219–223. Praeger Publishers, Westport, CT.

Pensgaard, A.M., Roberts, C.G. & Ursin, H. (1999). Motivational factors and coping strategies of Norwegian Paralympic and Olympic winter sport athletes. *Adapted Physical Activity Quarterly*, **16**, 238–250.

Perreault, S. & Marisi, D.Q. (1997). A test of multidimensional anxiety theory with male wheelchair basketball players. *Adapted Physical Activity Quarterly*, **14**, 108–118.

Rees, T., Smith, B. & Sparkes, A.C. (2003). The influence of social support on the lived experiences of spinal cord injured sportsmen. *The Sport Psychologist*, **17**, 135–156.

Rimmer, J.H., Riley, B., Wang, E. & Rauworth, A. (2005). Accessibility of health clubs for people with mobility disabilities and visual impairments. *American Journal of Public Health*, **95**(11), 2022–2028.

Schliermann, R. & Stoll, O. (2007). Self-efficacy and sport anxiety in German elite female wheelchair basketball players. *Journal of the Brazilian Society of Adapted Motor Activity*, **12**, 135–139.

Sherrill, C., Hinson, M., Gench, B., Kennedy, S.O. & Low, L. (1990). Self-concepts of disabled youth athletes. *Perceptual and Motor Skills*, **70**, 1093–1098.

Smith, B. & Sparkes, A.C. (2005). Men, sport, spinal cord injury, and narratives of hope. *Social Science & Medicine*, **61**, 1095–1105.

Smyth, M.M. & Anderson, H.I. (2000). Coping with clumsiness in the school playground: social and physical play in children with coordination impairments. *The British Journal of Developmental Psychology*, **18**, 389–413.

Sparkes, A.C. & Smith, B. (2002). Sport, spinal cord injury, embodied masculinities, and the dilemmas of narrative identity. *Men and Masculinities*, **4**, 258–285.

Spivock, M., Gauvin, L. & Brodeur, J.J. (2007). Neighborhood-level active living buoys for individuals with physical disabilities. *American Journal of Preventive Medicine*, **32**(3), 224–230.

Thomas, C.E. & Ermler, K.L. (1988). Institutional obligations in the athletic retirement process. *Quest*, **40**, 137–150.

Valliant, P.M., Bezzubyk, I., Daley, L. & Asu, M.E. (1985). Psychological impact of sport on disabled athletes. *Psychological Reports*, **56**, 923–929.

Wheeler, G., Malone, L.A., VanVlack, S., Nelson, E.R. & Steadward, R. (1996). Retirement from disability sport: a pilot study. *Adapted Physical Activity Quarterly*, **13**, 382–399.

Wheeler, G.D., Steadward, R.D., Legg, D., Hutzler, Y., Campbell, E. & Johnson, A. (1999). Personal investment in disability sport careers: an international study. *Adapted Physical Activity Quarterly*, **16**, 219–237.

Recommended readings

Association of Applied Sport Psychology (2009). Becoming a certified consultant. Available at: http://appliedsportpsych.org/consultants/become-certified (accessed September 1, 2009).

Baillie, P. (1993). Understanding retirement from sports: therapeutic ideas for helping athletes in transition. *The Counseling Psychologist*, **21(3)**, 399–410.

Berger, R.J. (2008). Disability and the dedicated wheelchair athlete: beyond the "supercrip" critique. *Journal of Contemporary Ethnography*, **37**, 647–678.

Blinde, E.M. & Greendorfer, S.L. (1985). A reconceptualization of the process of leaving the role of competitive athlete. *International Review for the Sociology of Sport*, **20**, 87–94.

Blinde, E.M. & Stratta, T.M. (1992). The sport career death of college athletes: involuntary and unanticipated sports exits. *Journal of Sport Behavior*, **15**, 3–20.

Coakley, J.J. (1983). Leaving competitive sport: retirement or rebirth. *Quest*, **35**, 1–11.

Cox, R. & Davis, R. (1992). Psychological skills of elite wheelchair athletes. *Palaestra*, **8**, 16–21.

Cregan, K., Bloom, G.A. & Reid, G. (2007). Career evolution and knowledge of elite coaches of swimmers with a physical disability. *Research Quarterly for Exercise and Sport*, **78**, 339–350.

Davis, R.W. & Ferrara, M.S. (1995). Sports medicine and athletes with disabilities. In: K.P. DePauw & S.J. Gavron (eds.) *Disability and Sport*, pp.133–149. Human Kinetics, Champaign, IL.

Deci, E.L. & Ryan, R.M. (1985). *Intrinsic Motivation and Self-determination in a Human Behavior*. Plenum, New York.

Gill, D. (1997). Sport and exercise psychology. In: J.D. Massengale & R.A. Swanson (eds.) *The History of Exercise and Sport Science*, pp. 293–320. Human Kinetics, Champaign, IL.

Goodwin, D.L. & Compton, S.G. (2004). Physical activity experiences of women aging with disabilities. *Adapted Physical Activity Quarterly*, **21**, 122–138.

Greendorfer, S.L. & Blinde, E.M. (1985). Retirement from intercollegiate sport: theoretical and empirical considerations. *Sociology of Sport Journal*, **2**, 101–110.

Hanrahan, S. (1995a). Sport psychology for athletes with disabilities. In: T. Morris & J. Summers (eds.) *Sport Psychology: Theory, Applications and Issues*, pp. 502–513. John Wiley & Sons, New York.

Hanrahan, S.J. (1995b). Psychological skills training for competitive wheelchair and amputee athletes. *Australian Psychologist*, **30**, 96–101.

Hanrahan, S.J., Grove, J.R. & Lockwood, R.J. (1990). Psychological skills training for the blind athlete: a pilot program. *Adapted Physical Activity Quarterly*, **7**, 143–155.

Harbalis, T., Hatzigeorgiadis, A. & Theodorakis, Y. (2008). Self-talk in wheelchair basketball: the effects of an intervention program on dribbling and passing performance. *International Journal of Special Education*, **23**, 62–69.

Hardin, M. & Hardin, B. (2004). The "supercrip" in the sport media: wheelchair athletes discuss hegemony's disabled hero. *Sociology of Sport Online*, **7**, 1–10.

Henderson, K.A. & Bedini, L.A. (1995). "I have a soul that dances like Tina Turner but my body can't": physical activity and women with mobility impairments. *Research Quarterly for Exercise and Sport*, **66(2)**, 151–161.

Henschen, K., Horvat, M. & Roswal, G. (1992). Psychological profiles of the United States wheelchair basketball team. *International Journal of Sport Psychology*, **23**, 128–137.

Hill, P. & Lowe, B. (1974). The inevitable metathesis of the retiring athlete. *The International Review of Sport Sociology*, **9**, 5–29.

James, W. (1890). *The Principles of Psychology*, Vol. 1. Holt, New York.

Kirkby, R.J. (1995). Wheelchair netball: motives and attitudes of competitors with and without disabilities. *Australian Psychologist*, **30**, 109–112.

Martin, J.J. (1996). Transitions out of competitive sport for athletes with disabilities. *Therapeutic Recreation Journal*, **30**, 128–136.

Martin, J.J. (1999a). A personal development model of sport psychology for athletes with disabilities. *Journal of Applied Sport Psychology*, **11**, 181–193.

Martin, J.J. (1999b). Loss experiences in disability in sport. *Journal of Personal and Interpersonal Loss*, **4**, 225–230.

Martin, J.J. (2000). Sport transitions among athletes with disabilities. In: D. Lavallee & P. Wylleman (eds.) *Career Transitions in Sport: International Perspectives*, pp. 161–168. Fitness Information Technology, Morgantown, WV.

Martin, J.J. (2005). Sport psychology consulting with athletes with disabilities. *Sport and Exercise Psychology Review*, **1**, 33–39.

Martin, J.J. (2006). The self in disability sport and physical activity. In: F. Columbus (ed.) *The Concept of Self in Education, Family and Sports*, pp. 75–90. Nova Science, London, England.

Martin, J.J. & Choi, Y. (2009). Parent's physical activity related perceptions of their children with disabilities. *Disability and Health Journal*, 2, 9–14.

Martin, J.J. & McCaughtry, N. (2004). Coping and emotion in disability sport. In: D. Lavallee, J. Thatcher & M. Jones (eds.) *Coping and Emotion in Sport*, pp. 225–238. Nova Science, London, England.

Martin, J.J. & Mushett-Adams, C. (1996). Social support mechanisms among athletes with disabilities. *Adapted Physical Activity Quarterly*, 13, 74–83.

Martin, J.J. & Smith, K. (2002). Friendship quality in youth disability sport: perceptions of a best friend. *Adapted Physical Activity Quarterly*, 19, 472–482.

Martin, J.J., Mushett, C.A. & Eklund, R.C. (1994). Factor structure of the athletic identity measurement scale with adolescent swimmers with disabilities. *Brazilian International Journal of Adapted Physical Education Research*, 1, 87–99.

Martin, J.J., Mushett, C.A. & Smith, K.L. (1995). Athletic identity and sport orientation of adolescent swimmers with disabilities. *Adapted Physical Activity Quarterly*, 12, 113–123.

Martin, J.J., Eklund, R.C. & Adams Mushett, C. (1997a). Factor structure of the athletic identity measurement scale with athletes with disabilities. *Adapted Physical Activity Quarterly*, 14, 74–82.

Martin, J.J., Engels, H.J., Wirth, J.C. & Smith, K. (1997b). Predictors of social physique anxiety in elite female youth athletes. *Women in Sport and Physical Activity Journal*, 6, 29–48.

Martin Ginis, K.A., Latimer, A.E., Francoeur, C., et al. (2002). Sustaining exercise motivation and participation among people with spinal cord injuries: lessons learned from a 9 month intervention. *Palaestra*, 18(1), 38–50, 51.

Martin Ginis, K.A., Latimer, A.E., McKenzie, K., et al. (2003). Using exercise to enhance subjective well-being among people with spinal cord injury: the mediating influences of stress and pain. *Rehabilitation Psychology*, 48, 157–164.

Ogilvie, B.C. & Howe, M.A. (1982). Career crisis in sport. In: T. Orlick, J.T. Partington & J.H. Salmela (eds.) *Mental Training for Coaches and Athletes*, pp. 176–183. Sport in Perspective and Coaching Association of Canada, Ottawa.

Page, S.J. & Wayda, V.K. (2001). Modifying sport psychology services for athletes with cerebral palsy. *Palaestra*, 17, 10–14.

Page, S.J., Martin, S.B. & Wayda, V.K. (2001). Attitudes toward seeking sport psychology consultation among wheelchair basketball athletes. *Adapted Physical Activity Quarterly*, 18, 183–192.

Perreault, S. & Vallerand, R.J. (2007). A test of self-determination theory with wheelchair basketball players with and without disability. *Adapted Physical Activity Quarterly*, 24, 305–316.

Rimmer, J.H. (2006). Building inclusive physical activity communities for people with vision loss. *Journal of Visual Impairment & Blindness*, 100, 863–865.

Rollins, R. & Nichols, D. (1994). Leisure constraints, attitudes and behavior of people with activity restricting physical disabilities. In: I. Henry (ed.) *Leisure: Modernity, Postmodernity and Lifestyles*, pp. 277–290. Leisure Studies Association, Great Britain.

Schifflet, B., Cator, C. & Megginson, N. (1994). Active lifestyle adherence among individuals with and without disabilities. *Adapted Physical Activity Quarterly*, 11, 359–367.

Schlossberg, N.K. (1981). A model of analyzing human adaptation to transition. *The Counseling Psychologist*, 9, 2–18.

Sinclair, D. & Orlick, T. (1993). Positive transitions from high performance sport. *The Sport Psychologist*, 7, 138–150.

Smith, R.E., Schutz, R.W., Smoll, F.L. & Ptacek, J.T. (1995). Development and validation of a multidimensional measure of sport-specific psychological skills: the athletic coping skills inventory-28. *Journal of Sport & Exercise Psychology*, 17, 379–398.

Taub, D.E., Blinde, E.M. & Greer, K.R. (1999). Stigma management through participation in sport and physical activity: experiences of male college students with physical disabilities. *Human Relations*, 52(11), 1469–1483.

Thomas, P.R., Murphy, S.M. & Hardy, L. (1999). Test of performance strategies: development and preliminary validation of a comprehensive measure of athletes' psychological skills. *Journal of Sports Sciences*, 17, 697–711.

Trieschmann, R.B. (1988). *Spinal Cord Injuries: Psychological, Social and Vocational Rehabilitation*, 2nd edition. Demos, New York.

Uchida, W., Hashimoto, K., Takenaka, K., Arai, H. & Oka, K. (2003). The correlates with psychological–competitive ability for male wheelchair athletes. *Japanese Journal of Adapted Sport Science*, 1, 49–56.

Uchida, W., Hiraki, T., Hashimoto, K., Tokunaga, M. & Yamazaki, M. (2007). A study on the effect of mental training in enhancing the psychological competitive ability of a wheelchair athlete. *Japanese Journal of Adapted Sport Science*, 5, 41–49.

Wakaki, U., Takako, H., Kimio, H., Mikio, T. & Masayuki, Y. (2007). A study on the effect of mental training in enhancing the psychological competitive ability of a wheelchair athlete. *Japanese Journal of Adapted Sport Science*, 5, 41–49.

Werthner, P. & Orlick, T. (1986). Retirement experiences of successful Olympic athletes. *International Journal of Sport Psychology*, 17, 337–363.

White, M.J., Gordon, P. & Jackson, V. (2006). Implicit and explicit attitudes towards athletes with disabilities. *Journal of Rehabilitation*, 72, 33–40.

PART 3
EXERCISE TESTING AND PRESCRIPTION

Chapter 8
Aerobic and anaerobic power

Yeshayahu "Shayke" Hutzler[1,2], Yoav Meckel[1] and Judith Berzen[2]

[1]Zinman College of Physical Education and Sport Science, Netanya, Israel
[2]Israel Sport Center for the Disabled, Ramat-Gan, Israel

Introduction

As with all athletes, the incorporation of training both the aerobic and anaerobic aspects of total fitness is vital to success at elite levels of sports. While for many disability conditions training can be done similarly to other athletes, certain groups of disability conditions do have different physiological responses to exercise to be considered when developing a training program. Also, athletes with some disability conditions use unique sport equipment such as prostheses and sport wheelchairs that may influence their mechanical efficiency. Therefore, it is necessary to adapt training processes to these variations in physiology and equipment. This can be done by a basic understanding of the athletes' physical condition and an adjustment to the individual needs of each athlete. In addition, the assessment and evaluation of the impact of training on energy systems is important for coaches and athletes to determine if improvement is occurring. Consequently, some testing methods of able-bodied athletes are not suitable for some groups of disability conditions. Therefore, a variety of adaptations to these methodologies are discussed in this chapter and throughout this book. Due to the number of disability conditions, and the number of sport disciplines at the elite level, this chapter will

concentrate on some specific disabilities in sport including spinal cord injuries (SCIs), cerebral palsy (CP), and amputations that require basic adaptations to programs of training, as well as fitness and skill assessment. Other disability groups may also require some changes to both training and assessment processes, and by in-depth study of particular groups, it is possible for both coaches and athletes to overcome these barriers to participation simply and safely.

Important exercise-related concerns by disability condition

There are certain concerns that coaches and athletes need to keep in mind when designing training and assessment programs for individuals with disabilities. A complete list of these concerns and how to overcome them can be found in the American College of Sports Medicine's *ACSM's Guidelines for Exercise Testing and Prescription* (2010). This manual is an invaluable resource for those working with individuals with disabilities in sport and exercise.

Spinal cord injuries

In reference to the level and completeness of the lesion in the spinal cord, athletes with this condition have a reduced ability to voluntarily perform large muscle group exercises; therefore, the amount of active muscle has an effect on both testing and training programs. Autonomic dysreflexia (AD) can

The Paralympic Athlete, 1st edition. Edited by Yves C. Vanlandewijck and Walter R. Thompson. Published 2011 by Blackwell Publishing Ltd.

occur in SCIs above the T6 level. It is generally indicated by a sharp rise in blood pressure due to an overreaction by the body to various stimuli. Among other things, AD can be induced by exercise at high intensities. The symptoms include flushing above the lesion, sweating, a rise in blood pressure, shivering, headache, nausea, blurred vision, and a reduced heart rate (HR). This can also be caused by other problems including bladder infections, bowel nonfunction, pressure sores, and illness. Coaches and athletes need to be aware of this life-threatening condition, and be vigilant for its onset (see Chapter 4).

For SCI lesions above the T6 level, either training must take place in thermally neutral environments or precautions against the effects of both heat (see Chapter 12) and cold (see Chapter 13) must be taken into account. Some suggestions include that in hot environments, individuals make use of cold water spray bottles to cool body temperature at regular intervals and drink plenty of fluids (allow time for this during training and testing sessions), and in very cold climates, allow ample time for warm-ups (longer and slower than usual) and dress appropriately for the environment, remembering these individuals may not be able to control and or sense their body temperature.

Training and testing should not take place if the individual has a bladder infection, is not adhering to a proper bowel program, has a pressure wound, or has an illness such as influenza. Training or testing on these symptoms can create a life-threatening situation, or skew the results required. Training and testing should be developed with precautions, reducing the risk of creating pressure wounds and/or skin abrasions, and in cases wherein the reduced blood return might deteriorate the recovery process. Similarly, precautions need to be taken to reduce hypo- and hyperthermia risks, which are increased in SCI compared to nondisabled individuals.

In all cases, always acquire medical permission before beginning either a training or testing program.

Cerebral palsy

Individuals with CP present with a wide variety of disability levels, from mild to moderate and severe. The international body governing sport competition in CP (CP-ISRA) adopted an eight-level system to gradually classify between conditions in reference to sport performance. The medical world utilizes a five-level classification system (Gross Motor Function Classification System, GMFCS) in reference to daily living activities. Across levels of impairment, musculature is typically increased in tone. The range of motion in affected joints of those affected by CP is reduced, patterns of joint alignment (e.g., hip internal rotation and adduction) are abnormal, and reactions of limb musculature while stationary or in movement may occur (e.g., excessive flexion of nonthrowing arm while throwing a ball, or backward kicking while cycling).

Always ensure that both exercise and testing programs are done in combination with proper stretching programs (both active and passive). The stiffer the muscle in an individual with CP, the harder it is for them to move and the harder it is to train. So stretch the muscles with increased tone! Remember that muscles have limited mobility and do not overstretch. Stretching is critical to the success of athletes with CP. This practice should be part of both the pre- and postpractice routine as well as before and after competition.

Individuals with CP have initially higher levels of lactic acid in the musculature than do ordinary athletes; this is thought to be due to the contracture nature of the musculature, causing an elevated energy cost of locomotion averaging three times higher than normal for walking and up to seven times higher than normal for stair-climbing. However, latest research shows that recovery as represented in lactic acid clearance follows a similar, if higher, path than able-bodied athletes. The coach is encouraged to make adjustments for this, especially as it concerns fatigue levels, but also that these athletes may also have a higher tolerance for lactic acid.

Finally, research has confirmed that heat transfer and regulation in persons with CP is impaired, a factor that requires careful attention while designing training volume and intensity and the use of cooling methods as described later in this chapter.

Amputations

Athletes with amputations present with a variety of anatomic distributions and sizes of remaining stumps. The number of affected limbs and joints typically determines the level of impairment. For individuals with single-arm or below-knee amputations, little difference from regular exercise or practice programming needs to be made. However, even in these cases, the coach needs to take into account balance, if joints are involved, and pressure on the stumps caused by prosthetic devices if they are worn by the athlete.

For athletes with more than one limb amputation, it is important to consider the amount of working musculature. Decreases in the amount of working muscle has an effect on the impact of aerobic exercise, and may change the limiting factor of performance to peripheral rather than central processes (e.g., arm muscle fatigue may restrict the wheelchair locomotion of a less-trained bilateral amputee before the cardiovascular system is fully exhausted).

Prostheses are generally expensive and difficult to replace and repair. Some of the new brands are highly sophisticated and require proper adjustment. Excessive pressure on the prosthesis or on the stump itself should be avoided. Breakdown of the surrounding tissue may result in skin injury leading to the inability to adhere to a training program. Malfunction of the prosthesis is time consuming and costly to athletes. In the event of a malfunctioning or improperly fitting prosthesis, cross-training programs that may or may not require the use of the prosthesis of an individual is appropriate. Pressure on the stump of an amputation may preclude the athlete from training for large amounts of time, and should be avoided. Personal medical care providers of the athlete will often have ideas for what can be done regarding the stability of the skin of an amputation. However, there are a number of training methods that can be done without the prosthesis or without applying pressure to the stump. Training of the limb remnants, whether used for the activity or not, is of particular importance. In this regard, (a) stability and symmetry of the shoulder, trunk, and hips should be supported via stretching and specific strength exercises; (b) motor learning of the proprioceptive stimuli in the joints and muscles manipulating the prosthetic devices is necessary to control balance and coordination while performing movements; and (c) relaxation of the overstressed muscles in the remaining limbs is warranted.

Energetic background for training aerobic and anaerobic power

Depending on the intensity and duration of exercise, the relative contribution of the body's various means for energy is divided into two main systems: anaerobic and aerobic.

The anaerobic ATP–CP system provides energy in an immediate and rapid way from the high-energy phosphates, ATP and CP, stored within the activated muscles. This system will be the major energy contributor for short-duration, high-intensity sport events such as the 100-m sprint or weight lifting. The rate at which energy is generated from the breakdown of ATP and CP determines the anaerobic power of the individual and the ability to succeed in such sport events. However, there is sufficient stored phosphate energy in the muscle for an all-out exercise of about 6–8 s only. For an intense exercise that lasts more than a few seconds, the energy to phosphorylate ADP comes mainly from glucose and stored glycogen during the anaerobic process of glycolysis, with the resulting formation of lactic acid. This second anaerobic pathway allows for the rapid formation of ATP by substance phosphorylation, even though the oxygen supply to the muscles is inadequate. This system serves as the major energy supplier during intense and relatively long sport events, such as the 400- and 800-m run or the 100- and 200-m swim, that last between 50 and 120 s. The increase in lactic acid becomes greater as exercise becomes more intense, and the level of muscle lactic acid that the individual can tolerate will determine the anaerobic capacity and the ability to succeed in such sport events. The threshold for lactic acid buildup (termed "anaerobic threshold") is determined by the endurance athlete's genetic endowment or specific adaptations with training.

If exercise proceeds beyond 2 or 3 min, oxygen consumption reactions become the major energy supplier via the aerobic system. In order to continue the exercise for a long time, a balance should be maintained between the energy requirements of the working muscles and the rate of ATP production by aerobic metabolism—a condition termed "steady rate." However, if exercise intensity exceeds the anaerobic threshold, the balance cannot be maintained and lactic acid level in the muscles will increase until exhaustion. The higher the anaerobic threshold level, the higher is the aerobic endurance and the individual ability to succeed in continuous sport events such as marathon. If exercise intensity is increased gradually, oxygen consumption is increased as well until reaching the individual maximal oxygen consumption or maximal aerobic power (VO_2 max). The VO_2 max provides quantitative data of an individual's capacity for aerobic energy transfer and his/her ability to succeed in high to moderate intensity level sport events, such as the 1500- and 3000-m runs that last 5–10 min.

Methods to improve anaerobic performance

Generally, anaerobic training is characterized by maximal or high intensity level of exercise. As a result, this type of training is performed in an intermittent manner termed "interval" or "repetition" training. The length, intensity level, and number of intervals are determined according to the specific fitness components that should be trained. Anaerobic training methods are designed to improve three basic fitness components that are related to the anaerobic energy system: power, speed, and endurance. The following sections describe the main training methods and variables for the development of these components.

Plyometrics

This unique method, mostly performed as explosive jump training, is considered the most effective and popular way to develop anaerobic power. Plyometric exercise consists of various jumps in place or rebound jumping (drop jumping from a height) to mobilize the inherent stretch–recoil characteristics of muscles through the stretch reflex. This exercise overloads a muscle to provide forcible and rapid stretch (eccentric or stretch phase) immediately before the concentric or shortening phase of action. As in many sports situations, the rapid lengthening phase in the stretch-shortening cycle produces a more powerful subsequent movement. The extra power produced in this movement is the result of a greater potential energy and the

evoking of segmental reflexes that potentiate subsequent muscle activation. A plyometric drill uses body mass and force of gravity to provide the rapid prestretch phase to activate the muscle's natural elastic recoil elements. Lower-body plyometric drills include a standing jump, multiple jumps, repetitive jumping in place, depth jumps, or drop jumping from a height of 100–200 cm, single- and double-leg jump, and many other various modifications. Similar exercise can be performed for the upper body, using the arms and the shoulder muscles for various appropriate drills according to the athletes' needs. Although the benefit of plyometric exercise is crucial for power athletes, it should be noted that these jumps generate external skeletal loads and may cause acute or chronic injuries to athletes. Therefore, a plyometric training program should be carefully planned with a gradual and controlled increase in training loads. A typical single plyometric training session for a trained athlete consists of about 80–100 jumps (divided into six to eight sets with 10–15 jumps in each set and 2 min rest between sets) where jumping height is as low as up to 40 cm. If jumping height is higher (60–100 cm), then the number of jumps should be reduced to about 40–50 (divided into six to eight sets with six to eight jumps in each set and 5 min rest between sets).

Speed training

The classic and most common training method for speed development is the "repetition" method that consists of short, all-out, series (8–12) of running in each training session. The short running distance prevents the elimination of the high-energy phosphates, ATP and CP, used as an energy source; thus, maintaining top work rate for each repetition preventing the buildup of lactic acid in the activated muscle and avoiding the appearance of any fatigue symptoms during the runs. The distance in each repetition should be long enough to allow completion of the acceleration phase and reaching top speed. According to these steps, the typical distance for each running repetition in this training method should be between 30 and 70 m. In addition, 2–4 and 8–10 min of rest should be given between repetitions and sets, respectively, in order to

Table 8.1 Various models of repetition training for speed development.

Sets	Model A (m)	Model B (m)	Model C (m)	Model D (m)
1	3 × 30	3 × 70	30, 50, 70	5 × 50
2	3 × 50	3 × 50	30, 50, 70	5 × 50
3	3 × 70	3 × 70	30, 50, 70	–

Table 8.2 Various models of anaerobic interval training for anaerobic endurance development.

Model	Distance (m)	Speed (% of max)	Intervals	Rest (min)
1	200	85–90	8–10	4–6
2	300	80–85	8–6	6–8
3	400	75–80	5–7	8–10
4	500	70–75	4–6	10–12

allow the complete replenishment of the ATP and CP in the working muscles before the beginning of the next repetition. Table 8.1 presents the various models of repetition training for speed development. It is noticeable that although the order of distances is different between the models, they all stay within the limits of the repetition method.

These top speed repetitions are believed to train the muscles and the nervous system to more efficient, forceful, and fast movements, leading to a faster and more efficient running. However, it should be noted that the level of improvement for this fitness component is only minor at best, mainly because of the limited improvement potential in the rate of the ATP–CP breakdown.

Anaerobic endurance training

Anaerobic endurance is improved via anaerobic, high intensity, and relatively long-duration intervals that are separated from each other by relatively long rest periods. These intervals bring a high level of lactic acid to the activated muscles and the blood, causing a significant level of fatigue and eventually an inability to continue exercise. The rest periods between intervals should be long enough to allow partial, but not a complete, recovery before beginning the next interval. The specific intensity level, number of intervals, and duration of intervals and recovery periods can be varied largely as presented in Table 8.2, and depend on the specific needs of the individual. Although the interval length and speed are fixed in each model in the table, they can also be manipulated and changed to be gradually increasing or decreasing for each model. These changes can be implemented by the coach according to the desired physiological load and the athlete's specific needs. This training method enables the participants, in time, to work and reach higher

levels of lactic acid and higher level of performance during high-intensity and relatively long-duration sport activities such as a 400- and 800-m run or 100- to 200-m swim. This is believed to be accomplished by the adjustment of key enzymes in the anaerobic glycolysis system to higher level of lactic acid in the blood and muscles.

Methods to improve aerobic performance

Aerobic training is usually characterized by long-term activity that is performed in a continuous or intermittent manner. These training programs are designed to attain two major goals: improved capacity of the cardiovascular system to deliver oxygen and enhanced capacity of the muscle cells to process oxygen. Proper aerobic training will improve the maximal aerobic power (VO_2 max) and/or aerobic endurance. While an improved VO_2 max can enhance the performance mainly in moderate to high intensity level activities that last 5–15 min, an improved aerobic endurance (determined by the anaerobic threshold level) enhances the performance in a long and low to moderate intensity level activities lasting over 30 min. The following sections describe the main training methods that improve these aerobic capabilities.

Aerobic interval training

As in anaerobic intervals, the aerobic intervals training method consists of alternated periods of activity and rest. This training method enables the performance of an extraordinary amount of relatively high-intensity exercise, normally not possible if the exercise progressed continuously. However, due to the relative high intensity level, the overall duration of activity in this training is shorter than the duration time that characterizes the typical continuous aerobic training (which will be described later in this chapter). The aerobic interval training is especially effective for improving the VO_2 max of the participant. Therefore, this training method is very popular among middle- and long-distance runners (800–10,000 m) or swimmers (200–800 m) who attain a high level of VO_2 during their sport. In contrast, this training is not popular among the general population, especially older age groups, due to its high intensity and the possible risks put on the performer. It should be noted that due to its high intensity level, this training method is also used by anaerobic athletes as it may improve their anaerobic endurance. Still, the specific variables that characterize the aerobic interval training are somewhat different than the variables that characterize the anaerobic interval training. The distance that is customary for aerobic intervals range between 600 and 1500 m. The level of intensity for these intervals can be monitored by HR (but can also be determined by a preplanned pace for a given distance). For younger athletes (20–25 years old), individuals with a maximal predicted HR of 200 beats per minute (bpm), the typical HR values during the intervals should range between 170 and 195 bpm. These values are above the anaerobic threshold level of the individual, indicating the involvement of the anaerobic energy system and the appearance of relatively high levels of lactic acid in the blood in this training. The number of intervals should be accumulated and lead to a total of 5000–8000 m for a single training session. These distances enable the appropriate exposure time for the necessary cardiovascular improvement during the training session. Table 8.3 summarizes the typical variables that characterize aerobic interval training.

For a better recovery between the intervals, it is recommended that the performer will stay active and keep on walking or jogging. This light activity may speed up the removal of the accumulated intramuscular lactic acid and fatigue symptoms from the active muscle, enabling the maintenance of the required intensity throughout the entire session. This procedure is also recommended for anaerobic interval training sessions.

Continuous training

Continuous training usually involves steady-paced prolonged exercise at low or moderate intensity, usually 55–75% of the participant's VO_2 max. The exact pace can vary, but it must at least meet a threshold intensity to ensure aerobic physiological adaptations. The continuous training is especially effective for the improvement of the individual's aerobic endurance as represented by the level of the anaerobic threshold. This increase in the anaerobic threshold allows the individual to exercise at a higher intensity level without getting fatigued for a long time. Because of its submaximal nature, continuous exercise training progress in relative comfort. This contrasts with the potential hazards of high-intensity interval training for unfit individuals and the high level of motivation required for such strenuous exercise. Continuous training suits those beginning an exercise program or wishing to accumulate a large caloric expenditure for weight loss. When applied in athletic training, continuous training actually represents "over-distance" training, with most athletes training two to five times the actual distances of competitive events. Since continuous training can be useful for endurance athletes as well as for the general population, two different models (Tables 8.4 and 8.5) can be established to characterize the specific variables of a typical continuous training session. The variables in Table 8.4 suit those individuals of the general population who wish to exercise in order to improve health-related physiological components such as body weight and blood pressure. The variables in Table 8.5 better suit endurance athletes who wish to improve their aerobic endurance and performance in continuous sport events such as the 10,000-m run.

Table 8.3 The typical variables (for running) for aerobic interval training.

Variables	Values
Interval time (min)	1–5
Running distance (m)	600–1500
Interval intensity (% of max HR)	85–95
Rest time between intervals (min)	1–6
Number of intervals	6–12

Table 8.4 Variables that characterize continuous training for recreationally active nonathletes.

Variables	Nonathletes
Type of activity	Running, walking
Time (min)	30–60
Distance (km)	5–7
Intensity (% of max HR)	55–65
Frequency (sessions per week)	3–6

Table 8.5 Variables that characterize continuous training for endurance athletes.

Variables	Endurance athletes
Type of activity	Running
Time (min)	45–90
Distance (km)	10–20
Intensity (% of max HR)	70–80
Frequency (sessions per week)	2–4

Another special version of the aerobic training is the blending of interval and continuous training. In this unique form of training, the performer can run in a slow pace and then pick up speed before slowing down again and picking up again. In contrast to the precise exercise interval training prescription, this type of training does not require systematic manipulation of exercise and relief intervals. Instead, the performer determines the training regimen based on the athlete's personal perception, sports specialization, and current physical condition. This training method can overload one or all of the energy systems according to the athlete's needs. It is therefore hard to establish an accurate set of values that will best describe the appropriate variables for this type of training. Although lacking the systematic and quantified approach of interval and continuous training, this training provides an ideal means of general conditioning and off-season training for different types of athletes. It also adds freedom and variety in the workouts.

Training Anaerobic power in athletes with disability

For many disability conditions, anaerobic training is similar to that of able-bodied athletes described earlier. Adaptations may be needed in time and in intensity progression level, and these should be made according to initial fitness levels of individual athletes. Due to the unique physical and physiological aspects of some disability conditions and task requirements, specific adaptations to training methods are imperative.

Spinal cord injuries

Due to the primary mode of locomotor activity using wheelchair propulsion or walking with crutches, athletes with SCI are prone to have an imbalanced muscular strength distribution around their principal joints. For example, the shoulders may be adducted and internally rotated due to overproportionate function of the pectoralis major. Training guidelines should take this aspect into consideration. Generally, for lesions below the T6 level, the adaptation to training is simply one that requires the training to incorporate only the use of the upper body and the physiological impact of this type of exercise. However, due to the limited muscle mass involved in exercise, local muscle fatigue may become a limiting factor to performance, particularly at the early stages of training. As a result, wheelchair basketball players may not reach the basket after rolling a few laps of the court, and swimmers become exhausted after relative short durations. Therefore, training needs to focus on muscle strength and endurance rather than cardiovascular endurance, as is often the case in able-bodied athletes. However, above the T6 level, changes to the actual function of cardiovascular and muscle function capabilities require more drastic changes to the approach to training. While even below T6, athletes with SCI are often seriously restricted by the amount of working musculature, decreasing the amount of active muscle required for storage of energy and for clearance of lactic acid levels, due to sympathetic dis-innervations, a lesion above T6 limits the ability of the cardiovascular system to increase HR, with most individuals only able to raise maximum HR levels to between 120 and 130 bpm. Thus, the intensity of exercise cannot be increased above this level. The implications for interval/sprint training are that the training intensity is decreased, and the lactate concentrations in the blood plasma and HR increase, which is slower than usual. Thus, short-duration (sprint) exercise seems not to accumulate high lactate levels and increase HR as much as in able-bodied athletes. Therefore, doing longer-duration, high-intensity exercises is more effective, and combining this with shorter duration, high intensity to follow is even better. In other words, do longer sprints first, then decrease sprint distance, rather than the other way round. The longer interval at the beginning of a session raises lactic acid levels in the muscles, while not giving time for total recovery; shorter-duration sprints will theoretically maintain these levels for a longer period of time, causing the anaerobic system to be stressed and thus adapt to the overload, thereby resulting in a training effect.

Interval/sprint training can also be enhanced by the utilization of a variety of additional drag-type equipments—from parachutes to sleds—increasing the amount of work being done and, therefore, escalating training intensity. The balance of the wheelchair and the angle of drag created must be considered. Without improving anaerobic threshold, there can be little improvement in aerobic ability. This type of training is vital to success in all sport disciplines. Some sports, such as marathons, require mostly endurance or aerobic activity; some require mostly sprint or anaerobic activity, but most sports require a basic combination of both. Improving aerobic abilities requires improving the lactic acid tolerance levels, which is an anaerobic ability.

Plyometric training with a medicine ball, to build power, can easily and creatively be designed for all individuals with SCI. Coaches should study the required sport to extract major power areas and develop programs that enhance power in movements used during the activity. Certain guidelines can be followed to institute a positive outcome program. Always ensure that athletes are properly warmed up before starting plyometric training. Plyometrics places an incredible load on the skeleton, and precautions should be taken when deciding the weight of the ball to be used. The success of a plyometric program requires the athlete to complete activity with maximum effort and at high speeds of movement; so again the

correct program for a particular athlete is important. The program should be done at least two to three times per week, best on days where athletes do not lift heavy weights. The duration of the session depends on the individual's structure and fitness level of the athlete. A basic guide is that beginners should do about 80–100 throws, intermediate between 100 and 120 throws, and advanced 120–140 throws during a session. These are broken into sets of repetitions to suit the athletes' requirements and fitness level. Examples of plyometric exercises include overhead throws using both hands, single-arm throws, chest passes, and side throws. In addition, athletes are instructed to hold the ball with two hands for non-throwing activities. Athletes extend the ball in front and anterior to the body, perform a figure of 8, or lift the ball from mid-right wheel overhead to mid-left wheel, or even Russian Twists entailing turning the body while bringing the ball from over and outside of one wheel to over and outside of the other (Figure 8.1). Using various forms of additional equipment, coaches help to tailor mimic movements. For instance, using a mini trampoline for ball return will include downward-angled actions and speed ball return, and sitting at a tilted incline and pushing the ball up the slope provides push power activity (Figure 8.2). Caution should always be taken while using plyometric training, with slow progression, to allow time for the system to properly adapt to the stress. This activity is contraindicated in prepubescent athletes.

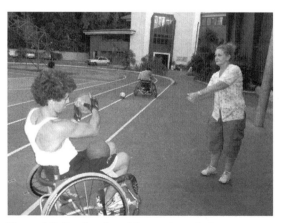

Figure 8.1 Quad rugby athlete and coach demonstrate an anaerobic performance drill.

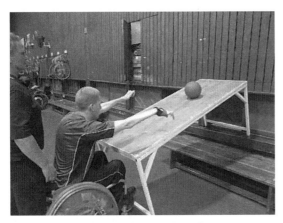

Figure 8.2 Quad rugby athlete and coach demonstrate a plyometric drill.

Ballistic weight training is another useful form of power training. Ballistic training proposes to train power as a combination of both strength and speed. Exercises to develop the combination are started between 30% and 35% of a one repetition maximum for 15–20 repetitions, and develop to a maximum of 50% and 55% of a one repetition maximum for 25–30 repetitions. Sets are a minimum of two and a maximum of three. The idea is to complete the movements at a fast but controlled steady rate. Keep rest periods between the sets to a minimum of 2–4 min, and rest periods between the sets to a maximum of 6–8 min. Again, the gradual progression of the program is important, and should follow the route of increasing repetition to maximum allowed then slowly increasing the weight and reducing the repetition number.

Cerebral palsy

Without training, the anaerobic performance of persons with CP is typically more than two standard deviations below the average of typically developing age and gender compared individuals. It is assumed that the reasons for their reduced anaerobic performance are: (a) impaired coordination, reducing the outcome of fast and powerful movements and (b) a possibility of selectively diminished fast-twitch fibers. However, short-term efforts relying on anaerobic fitness are common in most sport activities available for persons with CP as well as in daily living activities. Therefore, training of anaerobic metabolism is vital for all athletes, including those with CP; yet very little actual scientific research has been done on the effects of anaerobic training in persons with this condition. Based on practice experiences, all the types of anaerobic training suggested in the previous section relating to SCI seem applicable to athletes with CP. However, certain considerations need to be kept in mind, and these are listed in the section regarding important exercise-related issues by disability types.

Increased muscle tone of individuals with CP is a common impairment. This may require that athletes with CP stretch more vigorously and more often than other athletes. Time should be allowed for this, especially between sets, with active-type recovery periods rather than inactive-type recovery periods. Even during recovery periods, muscles should be kept moving. Also, athletes with CP tend to have some degree of internal rotation of the limbs. Movements that require internal rotation mechanisms in these athletes are generally stronger than those that require external rotation. Therefore, it is recommended to include activities that better balance the major joints such as strengthening shoulder and hip abductors and external rotators. The athlete should work on external rotation movements more or away from the body midline to strengthen the opposing muscles. High levels of initial lactic acid have been found in these individuals. Also, higher lactate concentrations have been found after completing an aerobic swimming test. Although evidence is extremely weak, this may have an effect on training intensity and on training duration. Due to the higher lactate levels, athletes with CP may, especially in early training, reach points of localized muscle fatigue at a faster rate than other athletes. Sets and repetitions can be adjusted accordingly to accommodate individual athletes. However, the level of tolerance to lactic acid levels may also be much higher in these individuals and so make it possible for them to train at higher rates. Due to the lack of research in this particular aspect, each athlete should be assessed as an individual and training designed to target the area most required for their particular sport choice.

Amputations

For the most part, individuals with amputations can train their anaerobic mechanisms with similar programs designed for nondisabled athletes. For examples of these programs, see the section on anaerobic training for SCI, but remember that the sets and repetitions, especially regarding interval/speed training, should follow the rules of the able-bodied athletes and not those of the athletes with SCI. However, for individuals with more than one amputation, certain considerations for anaerobic training need to be applied, particularly with regard to prosthetic and stump pressure.

The use of task-specific routines in an aquatic environment called "water-based training," with or without the use of aquatic prostheses and/or buoyancy equipment, may have unique benefits. The weightless aspect of water decreases the probability of pressure on either the prosthesis or the residual limb, but has been proven to be highly effective in anaerobic training of a variety of able-bodied athletes. Water-based programs consist of running in deep water with the aid of flotation devices. No contact is made with the bottom of the pool, and studies have shown that this is a great way to decrease the impact on limbs, which is beneficial to anaerobic training and performance. It can also be used to increase the aerobic capacity. Due to the increased density of water compared with air, the resistance during the running action is increased, resulting in improved performance on land. A typical program protocol is depicted in Table 8.6.

The benefit for amputees (both upper and lower limbs) is that both sides of the body are active at all times, no prosthesis is required, and training is balanced at all times. The decreased active muscle mass in athletes of more than one amputation needs to be taken into consideration. As with other athletes with decreased active muscle, localized fatigue may present in active muscles. With gradual progressive training, this can be overcome. Balance of the body for individuals with amputations is vital to overall health and wellness, and to the athletic participation. Therefore, it is important to work both sides of the body, with and without amputations, at similar rates and intensities so as to prevent muscular imbalance. That is to say, if

Table 8.6 A typical anaerobic training program protocol.

Phase	Warm-up 8–10 min	Main 30 min	Cooldown 5 min
	Running at jogging pace from shallow to deep water and back	(a) A 3-min overload phase: jogging in deep water	Slow pace back swimming, or any other comfortable swimming stroke
		(b) Interval pyramid training phase with sprint effort for 10 s, rest period for 10 s, then sprint effort for 20 s and rest for 20 s, all the way up to 60 s, sprint 60 s rest and back down the pyramid	
		(c) Relay sprints of 10 m with 2 min recovery between sessions, starting with 3 in week 1 and progressing to 6 by week 4	

the good leg is training a particular movement, so should the missing leg, and so on. Without the ability to balance the body properly, the efficient use of prosthetic devices becomes nearly impossible. Consequently, the work and training of core musculature has a greater performance impact on individuals with amputations.

Training aerobic power in athletes with disabilities

Athletes with disabilities require aerobic training for success in all kinds of sports. Aerobic training provides athletes with a base for sports fitness regardless of the energy system demands of the sport. Although the benefit for long- and middle-distance athletes is obvious, coaches and athletes often miss the importance of aerobic training for sprint distance athletes and for those who participate in games such as wheelchair basketball and wheelchair rugby. In the case of a sprinter, proper training for aerobic capacity will allow the athlete to recover better, and race more easily in subsequent events. It also enables an athlete to provide peak performances more than once at a competition. For athletes who participate in intermediate energy source performance such as ball games (wheelchair basketball, wheelchair rugby, seven-a-side soccer, sitting volleyball), aerobic training enhances a quicker recovery, and helps athletes sustain high-energy outputs over the length of a match. Athletes and coaches often mistake aerobic training as long, boring pushes or runs that have to be done. To the contrary, these are vital to the overall fitness of the athlete and can be both enjoyable and challenging. Although general steady-state activity is required at the beginning of the training program, creativity and cross-training methodologies will help to reduce the boredom factor. More than one form of training (e.g., marathoners could handcycle or row), and games players could do any of the above activities, should be considered on all or different days. For the most part, steady-state training takes place in out of season and low season times.

By the middle of low season training, athletes should begin to do threshold training, and once again creativity and variety is the key to keeping athletes motivated and in adherence with the program. This type of training is time consuming, and if done properly will take up at least 3–6 h of time per week for short-duration and multisprint athletes, and more for endurance athletes. The most successful endurance athletes in the world are considered to be the Kenyans who train for 5 months at threshold, including hill training, interval workouts, and tempo sessions two to three times per day, over-rugged terrain at high elevations, only to attend what has been termed a "fire and brimstone" camp for 3 weeks prior to elite-level competitions. At this camp they train 6 days per week, three times per day at HR levels of up to 90% of maximum. These programs take a great deal of dedication and motivation, and athletes should be encouraged to adhere to training by the results that are achieved in participation. Due to the unique physical and physiological aspects of certain disability conditions, some suggestions for improving, starting, and maintaining aerobic capacity in athletes have

been included in this chapter. However, coaches should be creative with an aim to target skills that will improve performance in the athlete's sport of choice.

Spinal cord injuries

The effects of an SCI lesion from a thoracic level are a decrease in the capacity of the cardiorespiratory system to function at full capacity. For individuals with SCI at T6 or above, there is a marked decrease in the function of both the heart and the lungs. Lung capacity is further decreased by a sitting position, and the inability of intercostal muscles to function properly; in quadriplegics, this is further exacerbated by the total loss of intercostal muscle innervations. Therefore, in both training and testing of aerobic function, it is important to keep in mind that the use of HR measures is not always appropriate, and that the VO_2 max values are not the same as are seen in able-bodied athletes. Most individuals with SCI have VO_2 max values that do not exceed 2–3 l/min or 40 ml/kg/min. Some normative data do exist for wheelchair athletes such as basketball players, track athletes, and tennis players, but in general, athletes' results should be compared to previous data.

Steady-state training as with all athletes should be done year-round, but given focus in out of season times. Coaches should be creative to prevent athletes from missing training sessions, by doing different activities on different days; e.g., push for 30–40 min on one day outside on the road, push a different route the next day, or cycle the same route and compare the times. Athletes can also try new activities such as kayaking or rowing. Coaches need to find what works for the athlete by asking what they like to do, and then incorporate it into training. Athletes in colder climates may like to ski or skate on sledges, while in warmer climates they may prefer to swim. It should be noted, however, that while these activities provide full body training, often they incorporate nonspecific activities (such as for wheelchair sports) and, therefore, should be maintained mostly during off-season training.

Once a good base has been achieved, the athlete can do the distances required in the time without too much effort. Aerobic threshold training can then start, due to the lower HR and VO_2 max values in participants with SCI. It is more appropriate to use rating of perceived exertion (RPE) (see section on testing of anaerobic function for SCI) tables to give value to training intensities. Nonetheless, this training is important so that athletes who do long-distance racing do not tire in the second half of the race, and so that both sprinters and ball game players recover well and have sustained energy for the duration of a match.

A variety of methods exist for training of the aerobic systems, including interval aerobic training, or doing high-intensity sections during aerobic training sessions followed by recovery periods at lower intensity levels. Or, in more simple terms, doing sprints during aerobic training followed by recovery periods at lower speeds. To do this training, athletes in wheelchair sports such as wheelchair basketball and rugby should start by incorporating 2×10 min periods at anaerobic threshold level, then progress to 5×5 min periods, then 3×10 min periods, working up to 20 min plus 10 min, and finally a 30-min period of threshold level training. Research shows that this amount of threshold training is ample for proper development of the aerobic system. Another good training program for anaerobic threshold training is continuous hill training that has been adapted from the successful Kenyan long-distance running program. Athletes/coaches should find a hill of between $15°$ and $30°$, depending on the athlete's level of lesion and physical capabilities, incline that runs for approximately 40–45 m in length. Athletes should use the hill to do sets of continuous training taking between 60 and 90 s for an athlete to go up and back down the hill. Start with two sets of 10, developing all the way up to a continuous 30 min of hill training. It is very important to keep in mind that many participants with SCI, especially those with lesions above T6, have temperature regulation difficulties, and aerobic training requires that athletes do increase body temperature. Athletes with these problems must remain hydrated throughout training sessions, with fluid intake at 15-min intervals of approximately 200 ml. Athletes should use spray bottles to cool at least every half hour. To prevent interruptions to training, it is a good idea to have these bottles available on hand for each athlete, or attached to the chair or bike (see Chapters 4 and 12).

Cerebral palsy

Athletes with CP have already raised levels of lactic acid concentrations prior to beginning training, which should be kept in mind when starting a training program for aerobic metabolism. Progressions need to be more gradual than able-bodied athletes, and training may take longer to achieve expected goals. Coaches should be patient, but also demanding of the athlete to adhere to the program. Since their movement economy is reduced (e.g., requiring three times more energy for walking at a comfortable pace than able-bodied persons), HR values of athletes with CP are expected to be higher than those of able-bodied athletes for the same power output. However, there is some thought that this is often due to a lack of conditioning rather than only a physiological problem; therefore, training aerobic systems should vastly improve aerobic capabilities in these athletes. A good base training of long steady-state work will help before threshold training takes place. Coaches should be creative and allow cross-training alternatives to relieve athlete boredom with this type of training and incorporate as many types of steady-state training as possible. Closed-chain exercises such as kayaking, rowing, handcycling, and leg cycling are particularly recommended for these athletes. Swimming, running, and wheelchair pushing are further options. For athletes who are water safety-trained, both pool and open water swims are a great option for aerobic training, but coaches should be aware that colder water temperatures will increase the tone in the musculature of athletes with CP and decrease their ability to reach time requirements for training.

Temperature regulation is a problem for athletes with CP and care should be taken to provide either a temperature-controlled environment or ample water, both to drink and to spray. Each athlete should have these available on hand so as not to interrupt training sessions. In cold climates, coaches should ensure that athletes are appropriately dressed for any outdoor activity.

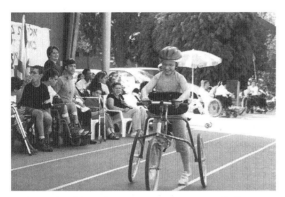

Figure 8.3 Athlete demonstrates running with the "Petra" device.

Cold temperature will increase muscle tone and limit the range of motion.

For those athletes with CP who participate on foot (in sports such as seven-a-side soccer or track and field) as much as possible of the aerobic training should take place in this state in order to improve the aerobic metabolism as well as to enhance skill efficiency. Coaches should use running, stair-climbing, cross-trainer exercising, cycling, and tricycling as the first options for aerobic training. Closed kinetics chain devices such as cycles are encouraged due to their better economy. Applying gear systems with the cycles allow better regulation of resistance and cadence. Three-wheel devices to partially support the body weight and posture while running ("PETRA" running cycles) is another option for more severely impaired participants who could neither run or walk without support, nor propel the pedals of a bike (Figure 8.3). Also, a water aerobic training program in a temperature-regulated pool should be considered, as it improves the range of motion in movement, and has the effect of decreasing muscle tone.

Amputations

For most athletes with amputation, training of aerobic systems follows a similar route to that of able-bodied athletes. Both VO_2 max and HR values are similar to those of athletes without disabilities, and thus training programs should follow similar progressions. Athletes with bilateral lower-limb amputations can utilize wheelchairs, but train at similar HR levels as able-bodied athletes.

Some persons with amputations, who participate in wheelchair sports, may find the reduced weight of the legs a beneficial factor since it decreases person–wheelchair systems' mass and therefore reduces deceleration after each arm stroke. Some athletes with a predominantly anaerobic fiber distribution may find it more effective to use an intermediate stroke pattern for long-distance wheelchair events rather than using a continuous muscle activation pattern. Using this technique may enable such athletes to successfully participate in endurance events.

Athletes with amputations should be encouraged to do at least some of the aerobic steady-state training without their prosthesis in order to protect both the skin integrity of the stump and the prosthesis itself. In this regard, cross-training is vital, and as much variety as possible should be used. Coaches should consider water-based programs such as swimming, both in a pool and in open water and water aerobic programs, as these have the advantage of training residual limb strength at the same time as not using the prosthesis. Training programs of rowing and kayaking, as well as cycling, are other options.

For single lower-limb amputations, a tried and tested program of hopping on one leg that is used by some of the most successful Kenyan athletes is a fun idea to try. The athlete hops rapidly on one foot (2.5–3 hops per second), while standing relaxed with hips level and heel slightly raised, minimizing vertical displacement. The idea is to strike the ground with the mid-foot and spring upward fast. Athletes generally do at least 2×40 s on each leg, or in this case on one leg, and rest for 1 min, working up to doing six to eight sets of 40 s.

Evaluating anaerobic and aerobic function in athletes with disabilities

Changes in both anaerobic and aerobic metabolism in athletes with disabilities should be tracked for a number of important reasons, including the following:
• to evaluate the effectiveness of training programs and to better match programs to individual athletes,
• to predict future performances,

- to measure real improvements achieved,
- to better understand weaknesses and strengths.

Participation of athletes in testing (the actual process or activity) and evaluation (the analysis of the results attained) procedures also provides a motivational benefit to athletes and coaches, by numerically giving evidence of results being achieved during training while satisfying the competitive urge in athletes throughout the season. There are numerous test protocols available to test all aspects of fitness and skill of athletes; however, not all are disability appropriate, and not all are disability specific. Coaches and athletes need to make informed choices about the testing protocols that they choose and stick with what they know. Testing can be either laboratory-based or field-based, or a combination of both. Laboratory-based testing is more accurate and precise; it is also more expensive and results may require some explanation from exercise physiologists in order to apply results to training implementation. Field tests are easier, cheaper, and can be creatively designed by coaches to test what they consider to be important sport-specific aspects. A number of disability- and sport-specific skills tests exist for sports like wheelchair basketball (Figure 8.4) and wheelchair rugby; however, these are skills tests, and testing of aerobic and anaerobic indicators is usually limited at best. The physiological assessment of both aerobic and anaerobic systems in athletes is an important process for the characterization of all athletes and for monitoring progress and effectiveness of training program design.

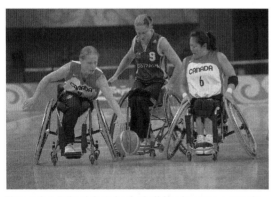

Figure 8.4 Wheelchair basketball has become a popular Paralympic sport. Reproduced courtesy of Lieven Coudenys.

As some athletes with disabilities have atypical physiological responses to certain forms of training, it is important to test and ensure that the best possible evaluation protocols are used for a particular athlete. New research is constantly becoming available to the wider public, and all coaches and athletes are encouraged to stay up to date on new findings and information that are provided in scientific, coaching, and training journals available worldwide. A good way of checking how an athlete is responding to training programs is through the use of anthropometry or body composition (for more detailed description, refer to Chapter 10). Measures can include body mass index (BMI) by simply measuring body mass (BM) and height (i.e., BMI = BM in kg/height in m^2), and/or a measure of body fat compared to lean body weight using at least four skinfold measurements. However, for individuals with disabilities, this formula may not be applicable due to abnormal body density, for example, as a result of atrophy. Also, no normative data exist and the appropriate way to evaluate their progress is against their own previous results.

Anaerobic performance evaluation for persons with disabilities

Before beginning any test procedure on any athlete, it is highly recommended to first get medical clearance for the test. In addition, coaches and athletes should follow and adhere to the section at the beginning of this chapter regarding "important exercise-related concerns by disability condition," as results of any test may vary if these are not taken into account. Also, coaches should try to do subsequent testing on athletes at similar times of the day as results can be diurnal. Testing should also be done under similar environmental conditions as previous tests.

Anaerobic evaluation protocols for athletes with SCI

The American College of Sports Medicine (ACSM, 2010) has a thorough manual with full descriptions of test protocols and how to evaluate the results. However, with the ongoing research into sport and exercise for individuals with disabilities, coaches should be aware of new ideas that may be available for those with the inclination to stay ahead of the game. Goosey-Tolfrey and Tolfrey (2008) have studied safe and effective testing protocols for individuals with SCI. This research found that in a laboratory assessment of propulsion speed, HR and lactate levels could be efficiently done through a submaximal incremental wheelchair test, allowing pushing economy to be calculated. In addition, if this test is done on a wheelchair treadmill or wheelchair ergometer (WERG), the outcomes may be compared with reference values that now exist for wheelchair racers, basketball players, and tennis players with SCI.

Many laboratory tests for persons with SCI are using arm crank ergometry (ACE). While using such equipment, it should be taken into account that some of the upper arm energy may be spent for stabilization rather than only for propelling the ergometer. This may be one reason for differences found between levels of disability. In the assessment of maximal exercise intensity with a Wingate Anaerobic Test (WAnT) protocol, peak power, mean power, and a fatigue index can be calculated. However, the use of this testing protocol is limited by the fact that peak power output (PPO) seems inversely related to level of the lesion (i.e., the lower the lesion, the greater the PPO). In another study (Knechtle et al., 2003), testing the anaerobic threshold via measurement of VO_2 max and lactate levels in a series of sprints with increasing distance, a protocol commonly used with able-bodied athletes, results have shown that these tests may not be appropriate for wheelchair athletes. Both lactate concentrations and HR increased with the length of the exercise duration, and not the other way round (opposite to what is expected in able-bodied athletes).

A good way to assess anaerobic ability in the field is through sprint testing. However, research shows that testing of speed over the generally prescribed distance (in skills tests) of 20 m is often irrelevant. A better protocol is to set timing gates along a court or track at desired intervals (15–25 m apart), marked clearly with cones. Athletes are then required to sprint a minimum of six times, at maximum effort between the cones and are given 10 s for the turnaround. This eradicates the time taken for an athlete to start, and gives a better idea of actual sprint times.

Through the use of this test, and the incorporation of body mass figures, maximum, minimum, and average power output can be calculated. Coaches can also design their own speed and sprint tests, but should be careful when recording the details or protocol, so that the test can be run again in exactly the same manner as previously. The test results are then compared to each other to measure improvement, so testing procedures should not vary.

Research shows that to monitor the training intensity of an athlete with complete SCI above the T6 level, it is not appropriate to use HR as an indicator, so HR monitors do not give an indication of training intensity due to minimized cardiac output function. Most athletes with SCI with lesions above T6 have difficulties in raising their HR above 140 bpm. Therefore, it is best to use an RPE, acquired from the athlete during training to assess the intensity of a program. RPE scales are available from a number of sources, or coaches can detail their own. It is important that all the details of the scale are known by the athletes in order to get a true reflection on this scale. The standard RPE most used is a Borg Scale (Borg, 1998) that ranges between 6 and 20, with 6 being no exertion at all and 20 being maximum exertion. Borg also developed a shorter version of a similar scale known as the CR10 Scale that may be easier for athletes to follow. Coaches should keep clear records of the responses obtained from athletes at various stages of training and adjust the intensity and duration of sessions accordingly. Examples of both these scales are given in Table 8.7.

Anaerobic evaluation protocols for athletes with CP

In all testing of athletes with CP, it is important to remember that the concentrations of lactic acid are higher and vary from one athlete to other, when compared with standard values of other athletes (Figure 8.5). However, test protocols that are used on able-bodied athletes have been found to be appropriate for athletes with CP, if considerations for the higher resting or baseline lactate levels and increased time for event completion are given. The increased muscle tone in athletes with more severe CP may also lead to cessation of performance in testing at

Table 8.7 Examples for evaluating levels of exertion with the Borg Scale.

Number	Level of exertion
(a) *Example of RPE Scale 6–20*	
6	No exertion at all
7	Extremely light
8	
9	Very light
10	
11	Light
12	
13	Somewhat hard
14	
15	Hard (heavy)
16	
17	Very hard
18	
19	Extremely hard
20	Maximal exertion
(b) *Example of CR10 Scale*	
0	Nothing at all
0.5	Extremely weak
1	Very weak
2	Weak (light)
3	Moderate
4	Somewhat strong
5	Strong (heavy)
6	
7	Very strong
8	
9	
10	Extremely strong (almost max)
**	Maximum

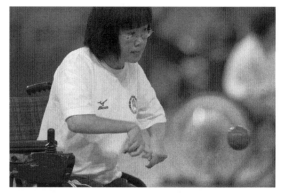

Figure 8.5 The lactic acid accumulation for athletes with CP may be elevated. Reproduced courtesy of Lieven Coudenys.

10 times 5-m running performance were designed for walking individuals with CP (Verschuren et al., 2009). Encouraging moderate correlations have been reported between the anaerobic performance in these tests and gross motor function. However, the sensitivity of these tests in elite athletes training has not yet been established, and, therefore, research into the effects of training for individuals with CP is still an important need.

As with athletes with SCI, a great way to evaluate the intensity of a training session is to use the RPE scales like the ones provided earlier, or the one developed by the coach. Athletes should understand the various levels and what they indicate before implementation in order for the scale to be of some use. For athletes with cognitive/intellectual difficulties, color versions of the RPE scales are available that may ease their ability to understand both visually and without numbers. These scales are affected by the way the athlete is feeling that day, so they also give the coach a good idea of athlete mood swings and health issues that may affect performance. Records should be kept of the responses of athletes to training sessions and adjusted intensity and duration as required.

Anaerobic evaluation protocols for athletes with amputations

Athletes with amputation are generally able to take part in able-bodied protocols, with a few minor considerations to be taken into account.

an earlier stage than is usual. Coaches should use individual results as comparative measures against each other, rather than trying to match these with normative data of able-bodied athletes.

Two types of valid and reliable anaerobic performance field tests based on six times 15-m or

Athletes' weight data will not usually fit the profile for test protocols, especially if the amputations are above knee or above elbow. In addition, for both single and bilateral lower-limb amputations, it is best to use ACE or wheelchair-friendly protocols (e.g., WERG), rather than to try to do bicycle tests with prostheses, as this may put the prosthesis or the athlete in danger. All test protocols should be carried out under conditions of balance and stability for the athlete, as fears of insecurity will skew results and lead to poor performances. For example, harnesses may be a useful aid while performing treadmill tests. Providing the most comfortable environment possible is the best way to ensure clear and precise results. Allowing the athletes to choose from a variety of equipments (e.g., arm crank, cycle, or treadmills) will prevent any balance problems that may arise.

Due to a loss of active muscle mass in higher-level amputees, there may be variations in blood lactate concentrations and clearance. The coach should keep this in mind when reviewing results. No normative data exists for specific levels of amputations, so it is best to compare subsequent results within the athlete with each other. Field sprint tests should be kept to a minimum to prevent injury to both the athlete and the prosthesis. However, it is a good idea to do some testing in the field to get a clearer picture of future performance capabilities of athletes. Standard sprint testing and testing of power are all advised.

Aerobic evaluation protocols for athletes with disabilities

Aerobic evaluation of athletes is traditionally done in a laboratory, and typically refers to values of VO_2 max and HR. Due to the variable amounts of working muscle in some disability conditions, and variable functioning in cardiorespiratory systems, some of the test protocols and normative values for able-bodied athletes are not appropriate for athletes with disabilities. However, it is important for coaches and athletes to keep records of aerobic performance. Aerobic metabolism is the base for all fitness in all sports and should be regarded as vital to achieve success at any level (Figure 8.6).

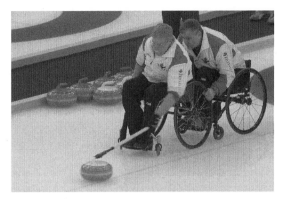

Figure 8.6 Athletes in all sports should engage in regular exercise to improve aerobic capacity. Reproduced courtesy of Lieven Coudenys.

Aerobic evaluation protocols for athletes with SCI

Due to decreases in cardiorespiratory function in most sport participants with SCI, VO_2 max in athletes with lesions of thoracic level and above do not exceed 2–3 l/min or 40 ml/kg/min. This makes the normative values of VO_2 testing for able-bodied athletes inappropriate. However, values for VO_2 max in SCI are available (Bhambhani, 2002; Hutzler et al., 1998), and can also be compared to previous individual levels. For athletes with SCI lesions above the T6 level, HR is mostly limited to between 120 and 140 bpm, thus HR reference values of able-bodied athletes cannot be applied. In addition, laboratory testing is both expensive and limited with regard to availability of wheelchair-friendly equipment. However, these tests are of considerable worth, should these factors not exist.

Field testing of aerobic function has the advantages of not requiring specialized equipment, and larger groups of athletes can be tested in shorter amounts of time. Research shows that at least two tests of aerobic metabolism for field use are both valid and reliable means of evaluating athletes' aerobic function (Goosey-Tolfrey & Tolfrey, 2008). The first is a multistage fitness test (MSFT), which is a 20-m shuttle run test protocol at increasing speed until the athlete can no longer achieve times at markers. However, the skill needed for turning appears to be a factor considerably affecting the performance in this test. Also, variations in floor surface and wheelchair–user interface have been found to compromise the validity of another version of the shuttle run test. The other recommended aerobic field test is the 12-min Cooper Push, which requires athletes to push as far as they can in the given time of 12 min. However, research is still warranted to establish the predictive validity of this test. Due to the limited amount of valid specific sport tests, coaches may need to be creative and design their own tests based on available space and amount of time that athletes are typically required to exert themselves for any given sport, or adapt any of the able-bodied protocols available. With these types of tests, it is once again best to compare the results for each individual athlete with previous results for the same test.

Aerobic evaluation protocols for athletes with CP

Research done on swimmers with CP by Pelayo et al. (1995) found that although swimmers with CP had higher HR values during the test and during recovery, slopes for recovery were the same as those for able-bodied swimmers. This implies that aerobic testing for athletes with CP can be done with able-bodied protocols if consideration is given for higher values at start and for slower times to complete. Valid and reliable multistage 10-m shuttle run test for measuring aerobic performance in young individuals with CP who have a walking ability has been demonstrated by Verschuren et al. (2007). However, the sensitivity of this test for measuring change due to athletic training has yet to be disclosed. A selection of protocols for testing aerobic capacity using WERG and ACE in athletes with CP who use wheelchairs for mobility has been reviewed by Bhambhani (2002).

Aerobic evaluation protocols for athletes with amputations

Aerobic function in athletes with amputations is generally not impaired; therefore, test protocols of able-bodied athletes can be applied if consideration is given to balance and active muscle mass issues. However, coaches should pay attention to the higher-energy cost while walking and running and, thus, it is recommended to use nonweight-bearing measuring devices such as cycle ergometers and particularly ACE, which have proved valid and reliable for aerobic evaluation.

References

American College of Sports Medicine (2010). *ACSM's Guidelines for Exercise Testing and Prescription*, 8th edition. Lippincott Williams & Wilkins, Baltimore, MD.

Bhambhani, Y. (2002). Physiology of wheelchair racing in athletes with spinal cord injury. *Sports Medicine*, 32, 23–51.

Borg, G. (1998). *Borg's Perceived Exertion and Pain Scales*. Human Kinetics, Champaign, IL.

Goosey-Tolfrey, V. & Tolfrey, K. (2008). The multi-stage fitness test as a predictor of endurance fitness in wheelchair athletes. *Journal of Sport Sciences*, 26, 511–517.

Hutzler, Y., Ochana, S., Bolotin, R. & Kalina, E. (1998). Aerobic and anaerobic arm crank power outputs of males with lower limb impairments: relationship with sport participation intensity, age, impairment and functional classification. *Spinal Cord*, 36, 205–212.

Knechtle, B., Hardegger, K., Müller, G., Odermatt, P., Eser, P. & Knecht, P. (2003). Evaluation of sprint exercise testing protocols in wheelchair athletes. *Spinal Cord*, 41, 182–186.

Pelayo, P., Morreto, P., Robin, H., Sidney, M., Gerbeaux, M. & Latour, M.G. (1995). Adaptation of maximal aerobic and anaerobic tests for disabled swimmers. *European Journal of Applied Physiology*, 71, 512–517.

Verschuren, O., Takken, T., Ketelaar, M., Gorter, J.W. & Helders, P.J. (2007). Reliability for running tests for measuring agility and anaerobic muscle power in children and adolescents with cerebral palsy. *Pediatric Physical Therapy*, 19, 108–115.

Verschuren, O., Ketelaar, M., Gorter, J.W., Helders, P.J. & Takken, T. (2009). Relation between physical fitness and gross motor capacity in children and adolescents with cerebral palsy. *Developmental Medicine and Child Neurology*, 51, 866–871.

Recommended readings

Bompa, T.O. (1995). *Power Training for Sport: Plyometrics for Maximum Power Development*. Mosaic Press, Ontario.

Durstine, J.L., Moore, G., Painter, P. & Roberts, S. (2009). *ACSM's Exercise Management for Persons with Chronic Diseases and Disabilities*, 3rd edition. Human Kinetics, Champaign, IL.

Hargereaves, M., McKenna, M.J., Jenkins, D.G., et al. (1998). Muscle metabolites and performance during high-intermittent exercise. *Journal of Applied Physiology*, 5, 1687–1691.

http://www.impactimages.com.au/waterbasedtraining/index.htm.

Hutzler, Y. (1998). Anaerobic fitness testing for wheelchair users. *Sports Medicine*, **25**, 101–113.

Jones, A.M. & Carter, H. (2000). The effect of endurance training on parameters of aerobic fitness. *Sports Medicine*, **29**, 373–386.

Laursen, P.B. & Jenkins, D.G. (2002). The scientific basis for high-intensity interval training. *Sports Medicine*, **32**, 53–73.

Maltais, D., Wilk, B., Unnithan, V. & Bar-Or, O. (2004). Responses of children with cerebral palsy to treadmill walking exercise in the heat. *Medicine and Science in Sports and Exercise*, **36**, 1674–1681.

Morgulec, M., Kosmoi, A., Vanlandewijck, Y. & Hubner-Wozniak, E. (2005). Anaerobic performance of active and sedentary male individuals with quadriplegia. *Adapted Physical Activity Quarterly*, **22**, 253–264.

Neumann, G., Pfutzner, A. & Berbalk, A. (2000). *Successful Endurance Training.* Meyer & Meyer, London.

Pitetti, K.H., Snell, P.G. & Stray-Gundersen, J. (1987). Maximal response of wheelchair-confined subjects to four types of arm exercise. *Archives of Physical Medicine and Rehabilitation*, **68**, 10–13.

Sawka, M.N., Latzka, W.A. & Pandolf, K.B. (1989). Temperature regulation during upper body exercise: able-bodied and spinal cord injured. *Medicine and Science in Sports and Exercise*, **21**, S132–S140.

Van der Woude, L.H., Bouten, C., Veeger, H.T. & Gwinn, T. (2002). Aerobic work capacity in elite wheelchair athletes: a cross-sectional analysis. *American Journal of Physical Medicine & Rehabilitation*, **81**, 261–271.

Vanlandewijck, Y.C., Daly, D.J. & Theisen, D.M. (1999). Field test evaluation of aerobic, anaerobic, and wheelchair basketball skill performances. *International Journal of Sports Medicine*, **20**, 548–554.

Vanlandewijck, Y.C., van de Vliet, P., Verellen, J. & Theisen, D.M. (2006). Determinants of shuttle run performance in the prediction of peak VO_2 in wheelchair users. *Disability and Rehabilitation*, **30**, 1259–1266.

Wilmore, J.H. & Costill, D.L. (1993). *Training for Sport and Activity: The Physiological Basis of the Conditioning Process.* Human Kinetics, Champaign, IL.

Chapter 9
Strength training

Marco Cardinale[1,2] and Lee Romer[3]

[1]British Olympic Medical Institute, Institute of Sport, Exercise and Health, University College London, London, UK
[2]University of Aberdeen, School of Medical Sciences, Aberdeen, UK
[3]Centre for Sports Medicine and Human Performance, Brunel University, London, UK

Introduction

Strength is the ability to produce maximal force. Muscle strength is important not only for physical performance, but also for injury prevention. The basic principles of strength training involve a manipulation of the number of repetitions (reps), sets, tempo, exercises, and intensity to cause desired improvements in strength, endurance, and size by overloading a single muscle or a group of muscles. Strength training has received a lot of attention by the scientific community in the last 20 years due to its effectiveness in enhancing force, power-generating capacity and speed. Historically, the focus of training in Paralympic athletes has been on improving cardiorespiratory capacity. When strength training was introduced into training programs, athletes and coaches were opposed to its use due to the misconception that such training might actually be deleterious to athletic performance. After much research, it is now accepted that strength training (or resistance exercise as it is referred to in the literature) not only can contribute to performance improvement in many sports but also can help in injury prevention. Modern Paralympic athletes have refined their preparation plans and have adapted to lessons learned in able-bodied sports to maximize sporting performance. In many countries, strength and conditioning specialists are

developing *ad hoc* training solutions for disabled athletes and are advancing practical knowledge in this field.

Several studies have examined the dose–response relationship for various strength training paradigms in able-bodied individuals, and various special populations. Few studies, however, have focused on Paralympic athletes. This lack of scientific information makes it difficult to produce clear and effective guidelines for strength training in Paralympic athletes. The aims of this chapter are to review the literature pertaining to strength training of disabled athletes and to provide guidelines to develop not only safe and effective training paradigms but also suggestions for future research efforts in this area.

This chapter has been divided into sections that focus upon the disability groups eligible to compete at the Paralympic Games, namely amputees, visually impaired, cerebral palsy (CP), spinal cord injury (SCI), intellectually disabled (ID), and les autres ("the others" a broad category including various disabilities such as multiple sclerosis (MS) and dwarfism).

Amputees

Amputation in Paralympic athletes is primarily the result of traumatic injuries or congenital abnormalities. Amputation in the general population, however, is due also to vascular, bone, and circulatory pathologies (often induced by metabolic disorders such as diabetes).

The Paralympic Athlete, 1st edition. Edited by Yves C. Vanlandewijck and Walter R. Thompson. Published 2011 by Blackwell Publishing Ltd.

Lower-limb amputees participate in many Summer (Figure 9.1) and Winter (Figure 9.2) Paralympic sports and have recently received a great deal of attention due to the advancements in prosthetics which seem to guarantee similar locomotor capabilities to able-bodied athletes. Lower-limb amputations, independent of the precise site of limb interruption, always elicit an initial significant reduction in the individual's physical abilities, which is due not only to the missing limb or part of the limb but also to subsequent alterations in proprioception and muscle mass. Reduced proprioception and muscle mass have a negative influence on force-generating capacity and movement control, and in this particular group of athletes there is clear evidence that these two aspects represent an area where performance gains can be made with strength training.

Above-knee amputation has been associated with impaired physical performance due to balance disturbance and proprioceptive deficit. Recent advancements in prosthetic design have contributed to enormous improvements in gait patterns of above- and below-knee amputees. However, one of the main causes of impaired gait is the imbalance of the muscles acting on the hip joint following removal of the femoral ends of major muscles such as the hamstrings, adductors, rectus femoris, and sartorius during the surgical procedure. The muscles such as the iliopsoas, gluteus maximus, and gluteus medius, act on the hip joint as agonists only and mostly without the counterpart antagonists. Under such conditions of imbalance,

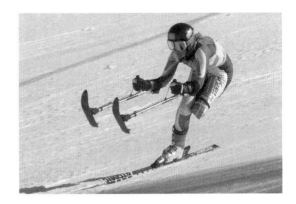

Figure 9.2. Lower-limb amputee participating in winter event. Reproduced courtesy of Lieven Coudenys.

muscle function is reduced and eventually becomes ineffective. Muscle atrophy in the glutei is an obvious consequence and is particularly evident in physically inactive amputees. The muscle atrophy contributes to changes in gait due to altered gluteal control during the contact phases of gait and stair climbing. Therefore, while prosthetics have solved the biomechanical aspects of walking and running gaits, neuromuscular control still requires understanding in terms of assessment and training prescription. Running and sprinting in particular present challenges to amputee athletes independent of the prosthetics used. The main biomechanical deficits of amputee running are insufficient power generation at prosthetic push-off, increased impact forces on the intact limb, and inter-limb asymmetry. Each of these deficits could lead to serious injuries when muscle imbalances are not properly addressed by the strength program.

Few studies have investigated the effects of strength training on gait and running abilities in amputee athletes. Nevertheless, it seems clear that strength training in amputee athletes should be directed to the trunk and hip flexors/ extensors because of the likely occurrence of low back pain in this population. Even for amputees involved more in wheelchair sports than in running activities, training of trunk strength and gluteal activation is important to enable specific rotational movements to be performed safely and repeatedly.

Strength training for below-knee amputees should also be targeted at increasing leg-extensor

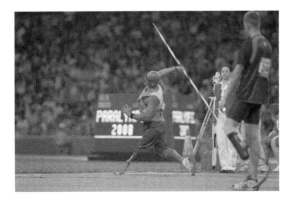

Figure 9.1. Lower-limb amputee participating in summer event. Reproduced courtesy of Lieven Coudenys.

strength. Untrained amputees often have asymmetries in leg-extensor strength, which are not totally attributable to muscle atrophy. Furthermore, imbalances in hip strength have also been observed. However, recent work has shown that physically active transtibial amputees have little strength asymmetry and overdeveloped hip extensor strength, suggesting a potential influence of sporting use of prosthetics (Nolan, 2009). Strengthening the leg extensors can be a challenge due to the limited possibilities offered by conventional equipment. While squats and Olympic lifts can still be used, care should be taken to avoid overloading the stump, and alternative training modalities should be considered in this population. Strength training exercises that require lifting from the floor should also be carefully assessed with video analysis and biofeedback techniques. In the work setting, lower-limb amputees have been shown to use different lifting biomechanics than able-bodied individuals, and incorrect strength training technique can increase the risk of injury when lifting heavy weights. Specific isoinertial devices, hydraulic or robotic devices, and even

rubber bands can be used to train the leg extensors. Particular care needs to be placed on training not only the injured side, but also the noninjured leg, as asymmetrical exercises could exacerbate the already existing asymmetries in muscle strength around the lower back and the hip joint. Balance should also be assessed routinely and improved through specific exercise prescriptions using unstable surfaces of various difficulties with a progressive overload approach. Therefore, progressive overload needs to take into account not only the amount of external loading but also the instability of the surface used. Improvements in balance and in running gait can translate into performance gains and for this reason less conventional training modalities (in combination with resistance exercise) could also be beneficial. Recent work by Lee et al. (2007) suggested the use of low-level electrical stimulation in combination with visual and auditory feedback to improve balance control in sedentary amputees. Similar systems could be adapted for use in Paralympic amputee athletes to improve balance performance (Figure 9.3).

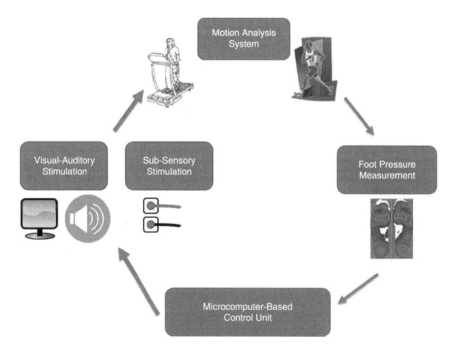

Figure 9.3. Example of a visual and auditory feedback system similar to the one used by Lee et al. (2007). Similar systems could be evolved for use in Paralympic athletes to provide information during strength training exercises.

Vibration training could also be used as an adjunct to improve strength and power in amputee athletes. Studies conducted in able-bodied athletes suggest that whole-body vibrating platforms alone or in combination with conventional resistance exercise has the potential to enhance strength and reduce low back pain. Locally applied vibration has been shown to produce a tonic vibration reflex which might also elicit a training stimulus. Recent evidence suggests the possibility of using vibration directly applied to the neck or the hip to improve postural asymmetry in lower-leg amputees. The combined use of voluntary muscle activation with percutaneous electrical stimulation could also be used as an effective modality to increase strength and to reduce muscle mass deficits. Despite limited information on the effectiveness and safety of vibration or electrical stimulation in amputees, it seems reasonable to presume that these techniques would improve strength in such individuals. However, it would be important to monitor the athletes to ensure neither vibration nor electrical stimulation exacerbates phantom limb pain. Practical advice for strength training this group of athletes includes the following:

• Use prostheses of equal limb length to minimize asymmetries.
• Consider the use of weighted vests or shoulder-mounted systems to perform squat-like strengthening exercises for upper-limb amputees.
• Ensure appropriate spotting techniques to guarantee the safety of the athlete before performance gains are sought.
• Always monitor the stump and how the athletes cope with heavy lifts and/or plyometric activities.
• Make sure exercise prescription takes into account the need to balance agonist and antagonists' muscles around the stump.

Vision impaired

There is limited information regarding the strength and power capabilities and trainability of visually impaired individuals. Logic dictates that strength and power production would not be impaired by an inability to adapt to training, but rather by the coordinative aspects and the ability to transfer strength gains into sporting performance.

Physical fitness of visually impaired adolescent games players is higher than that of more sedentary adolescents. This suggests that individuals with visual impairment are not limited from getting stronger. Visually impaired recreationally active adults have also been shown to be as fit as normal sighted individuals. Visually impaired young sedentary individuals are weaker and less aerobically fit purely because they are not as physically active as an age matched able-bodied group. However, totally blind sedentary individuals are weaker and less aerobically fit than semi-blind and individuals with amblyopia. It is then clear that the main difficulties in improving strength and power in this group are due to the limited ability of these athletes to perform strengthening exercises that require high coordinative demands and/or complex motor skills. Visual deficiency has been shown to impair children's neuro-psychomotor development as demonstrated by the finding that visually impaired children performed worse than an age matched normal sighted group in balance and coordination (Navarro et al., 2004). However, when children with low vision are appropriately trained, they can significantly improve coordination, balance, and strength supporting the concept that improved performance in this population resides in the coach's abilities to impart appropriate instructions. Generally, individuals with visual impairment are more cautious when performing movements and have more difficulty performing tasks when their centre of gravity is outside of their base of support.

The following aspects should be considered when planning a strength training program for visually impaired athletes:

• Choice of exercise progression should take into account the coordinative demands of the exercise as well as the load lifted.
• The visually impaired athlete should be well supervised and provided with enough space so he/she can lift heavy weight and/or perform complex lifting movements safely.
• Individuals who are blind from birth will need additional instruction to perform complex lifting movements.

Cerebral palsy

Impairments in muscle strength and motor control are major causes of performance deficits in individuals with CP. Such impairments, together with adaptive changes at neural and musculoskeletal levels, disturb muscle and bone growth and the learning of motor skills. CP results from damage to part of the brain. For many people the cause is unknown. The outcome of the brain damage is a permanent physical condition that affects movement. Children with CP learn to move stereotypically due to reduced and disordered muscle force generation, increased muscle stiffness, and soft tissue contracture. As a consequence, individuals with CP who enroll in competitive sport late in life might have difficulty learning the complex movements typically used in able-bodied strength training programs. It is necessary to assert that strength is fundamental to guarantee individuals affected by CP a better quality of life. Indeed, a positive relationship between muscle strength and function has been found in children and adults with CP. Therefore, strength training should be an integral part of exercise programs in this population, regardless of the competitive level of the individual. A recent systematic review (Scianni et al., 2009) concluded that strengthening interventions are ineffective and not worthwhile in children and adolescents with CP who are able to walk. However, a more comprehensive review (Verschuren et al., 2008) concluded that children with CP benefit from exercise programs that focus on lower-extremity muscle strength, cardiovascular fitness, or a combination of both. However, the outcome measures used in most of the studies reviewed were not intervention specific, which suggests that additional studies are needed. Based on the available evidence, an appropriately supervised and individually tailored strength training program combined with other interventions (e.g., stretching, massage, and so on) has the potential to improve strength and reduce spasticity in athletes with CP.

Before planning a strength program for athletes with CP it is important to understand which part of the body is affected. Figure 9.4 shows the wide range of impairment in people with CP. It is difficult, therefore, to provide a blanket approach to strength

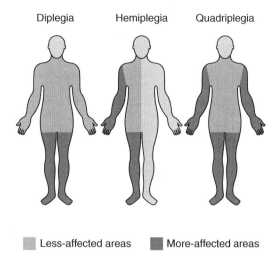

Diplegia   Hemiplegia   Quadriplegia

Less-affected areas   More-affected areas

Figure 9.4. Areas of the body affected by CP. Diplegia affects mainly the lower limbs and partly the upper limbs and the trunk. Hemiplegia affects one side of the body. Quadriplegia affects all four limbs and trunk.

training in athletes with CP. It is necessary to identify the areas of the body affected and the particular movement dysfunctions. Thus, strength training programs for athletes with CP might be either very simple or relatively complicated, depending on the areas of the body affected.

From a neurophysiologic standpoint, excessive muscle co-activation of functional antagonists during voluntary agonist contraction is a common clinical feature associated with spastic, diplegic CP. Thus, an athlete with CP who is required to perform strengthening exercises with heavy loads needs to be monitored closely and heavy loads need to be introduced progressively because voluntary drive to the agonist muscle can result in spasticity and co-contraction thereby altering the joint motion pattern. Leonard et al. (2006) suggested that deficits in long-latency (presynaptic) inhibition appear to be the main determinants of voluntary movement impairment in individuals with CP. The authors used a task for which the subjects had to contract isometrically the tibialis anterior muscle at various percentages of the maximal voluntary contraction force. Neural contributions to reciprocal inhibition of the soleus motor neurons during this task were assessed in either spastic, diplegic CP or able-bodied individuals. The results suggested that neural pathways subserving reciprocal inhibition are not functioning properly in individuals diagnosed with spastic diplegia.

When athletes with CP are required to produce maximal voluntary contractions during strength training, it is necessary to provide appropriate instruction and supervision. However, other aspects such as temperature and emotional state also need to be controlled to ensure the athlete does not become too tense or stiff around the joints used during training. Despite the relatively large amount of literature on exercise and motor control issues in individuals with CP, there is a paucity of information regarding the effectiveness of strength training in athletes with CP. Clearly, there is a need for well-controlled studies to determine the implications of strength training in this population. That people with CP benefit from competitive sport participation in terms of fitness and quality of life, it is advisable to include strength training in the overall training regime.

Additional training modalities such as vibration and electrical stimulation might also benefit individuals with CP. Vibration has been suggested to improve muscle strength and reduce spasticity in this population. Small vibrations applied directly to the arm improved movement patterns of a hemiparetic shoulder (Shirahashi et al., 2007). Whole-body vibration in combination with the Cologne Standing-and-Walking-Trainer improved mobility in children and adolescents with CP (Semler et al., 2007). Direct application of vibratory stimulation to muscles had already been suggested in the 1970s as an effective intervention to improve strength in individuals with CP; however, no further studies have been conducted in well-trained individuals with CP. There is certainly scope for using vibration in athletes with CP, not only as a training aid but also potentially as a "preconditioning" activity before strengthening exercises due to its potential to reduce spasticity and enhance alpha motor neuron activity in agonist muscles. Adult sedentary individuals affected by spastic diplegia have also been shown to benefit from whole-body vibration training to the same extent as conventional resistance exercise modalities, further supporting the need to

investigate whole-body vibration use in an athletic population.

Currently, there is no information on the ability of adult athletes with CP to maximally activate specific muscle groups. Evidence in children with CP suggests that large deficits in voluntary activation are apparent. Hence, using voluntary contractions for strength training in individuals with CP may not produce forces sufficient to induce muscle hypertrophy and/or significant gains in muscle strength. In this light, techniques such as enhanced feedback and neuromuscular electrical stimulation may be helpful for strengthening muscles that cannot be sufficiently recruited with conventional strength training programs that require a voluntary activation of muscle groups. Indeed, isometric strength training with superimposed electrical stimulation has been shown to produce better gains in strength and in the ability to activate the muscle groups treated than a conventional exercise program. The use of vibration and electrical stimulation techniques could solve the problem of the reduced motor drive and the inability to recruit high threshold motor units observed in this population by allowing athletes with CP to reach near maximal levels of muscle activation. The integrated use of conventional strength training modalities with vibration and electrical stimulation could represent an effective way of improving muscle strength and power in athletes with CP. However, more studies are needed to determine the effectiveness of this approach and the safest modalities.

The following aspects need to be considered for the delivery of strength training in this population:
• Training plans need to take into consideration which parts of the body are affected by CP and the demands of the sport.
• An assessment of functional movement should be conducted in a controlled environment and with increasing loads to assess co-contraction and the occurrence of jerky movements.
• Fatigability and co-contraction need to be assessed in order to prescribe the correct training volumes and avoid the athlete performing repetitions with high levels of joint stiffness.
• Warm-up procedures should be incorporated to reduce spasticity before heavy loads are used.

• A safe and emotionally stable environment should be sought, particularly when training with heavy loads.

• Periodized programs and progressive overload need to be tailored to the adaptive abilities of the individual athlete.

• It is important to check not only improvements in strength and power but also how such improvements affect spasticity and hence overall health-related quality of life.

Spinal cord injury

The extent of functional limitation in people with SCI depends on the level (distance from the brain) at which the spinal cord is injured. The impact of SCI is therefore often described using a letter and a number (e.g., T11), indicating the most distal uninvolved segment of the spinal cord. Further details indicate if the lesion is complete or incomplete, indicating the extent of interruption of nerve transmission. Complete indicates an absence of sensory and motor function below the lowest sacral segment, and incomplete indicates a partial preservation of sensory and/or motor function below the neurological level. In this light, having precise information on the level and completeness of the lesion is paramount in order to prescribe appropriate strength training programs. Spasticity and spasm are typical in athletes with SCI and motor control in specific joints is dependent on the characteristics of the lesion.

It is important to assess trunk control when selecting strength training exercises, particularly if the aim is to perform overhead lifts. Patients with thoracic SCI try to compensate for the loss of postural function of the erector spine through the increased use of different nonpostural muscles. Studies have shown differences between individuals with high and low thoracic SCI, with those with high thoracic SCI requiring more complex strategies to maintain and restore sitting balance. Trunk extension strength seems to play only a minor role in sitting stability; however, motor control strategies can be improved by strengthening the trunk not only in flexion and extension but also in various positions with a variety of techniques to facilitate static strength and postural control. The level and the characteristics of the lesion will of course dictate how much trunk stability training can be performed and which exercises can be safely executed. With this in mind, it is advisable to assess sitting stability as well as trunk strength in these athletes to verify the effectiveness of strength programs in the overall ability to control trunk motion. While it is relatively easy to assess isometric strength, the assessment of sitting postural control requires more complex tools such as force platforms and/or specifically designed benches with strain gauges and dedicated software packages to measure the sway path of the center of mass. Strapping and backrest aids should be used to stabilize the trunk during heavy lifts.

Upper extremity strength training is important for athletes with SCI as it insures better independence and quality of life as well as providing a clear performance benefit in wheelchair sports. Assessment of motor control and neuromuscular function should precede training prescription as there is clear evidence that, depending on the level and completeness of the lesion, marked inter-differences exist in muscle activation patterns. The individual demands of the sport also need to be assessed for effective exercise prescription. Heavy resistance training for five sets of 10–12 repetitions has been shown to improve strength as well as wheelchair sprinting performance. Strength training conducted on ergometers has also been shown to produce significant gains in strength. Strength training should also include less conventional forms of resistance exercise. Low cadence functional electrical stimulation-assisted cycling has been shown to produce strength gains in T4–T5 individuals. Other forms of functional electrical stimulation have also been shown to be beneficial, even if its effectiveness in athletes has still to be proved. Vibration exercise by means of vibrating dumbbells has been suggested as an effective modality to improve strength and power of upper limb muscles. Direct application of vibration has also been shown to benefit individuals affected by SCI, but its effectiveness in an athletic population has still to be demonstrated.

Strength training prescriptions in this population have to always consider the consequences not only for performance but also for safety. Wheelchair athletes present overuse injuries of the shoulder; hence, the strength training program should be aimed not only at improving wheelchair propulsion but also at protecting the shoulder, elbow, and wrist joints. Strength training prescriptions should be focused on strengthening muscles of the back (e.g., trapezius and rhomboids) and the posterior deltoid to protect the shoulder from repetitive strain injuries. Safeguarding already stressed joints due to the high demands of normal daily activities should also be taken into account when planning training sessions. Ideally, rest and recovery prescription after heavy sessions should also include a reduction in wheelchair use/training as well as appropriate recovery from intense forms of wheelchair-specific sessions.

Consideration needs to be given to gymnasium safety (including the safety of "spotters") due to the potential for uncontrolled jerky movements. Therefore, it is important to ensure there is enough free space around the athlete while lifting and to practise safe spotting techniques. Gymnasium safety also requires control over ambient temperature, as the impaired thermoregulatory responses of SCI athletes puts them at risk in hot and humid environments. For this reason, appropriate cooling procedures need to be implemented when in hot and humid environments.

Respiratory muscle training in SCI

Respiratory function in people with SCI is impaired due to complete or partial denervation of the respiratory muscles. The extent of respiratory impairment is primarily dependent on the level of injury, completeness of injury, and time since injury. Higher lesions result in progressively more of the respiratory muscles becoming denervated (Figure 9.5). Complete lesion above the phrenic motor neurons (C3–C5) results in paralysis of the major muscles of inspiration and expiration. When injury is to the lower cervical or upper thoracic cord, the diaphragm and sternocleidomastoid muscles may function normally. However, denervation of the other muscles of inspiration (inspiratory intercostals and scalenes) and to the major muscles of expiration (abdominals and expiratory intercostals) causes a reduction in the strength and endurance of these muscles.

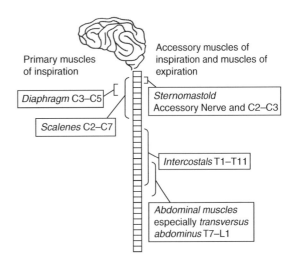

Figure 9.5. Innervation of the respiratory muscles. Reprinted with permission (Sheel et al., 2008).

The effect of profound respiratory muscle weakness is a decrease in vital capacity through reduction in both inspiratory and expiratory reserve volume. Inspiratory volumes are further compromised because the intercostals and other chest wall muscles may not provide the normal expansion of the middle and upper rib cage as the diaphragm descends during inspiration. Denervation of the abdominal muscles and the associated increase in abdominal compliance may also decrease inspiratory volumes by reducing appositional forces during inspiration that act to expand the lower rib cage. A decrease in the force-generating capacity of the respiratory muscles may conspire to limit exercise performance by mechanically constraining ventilation, especially given that some respiratory muscles also partake in nonventilatory tasks during upper-body exercise. Thus, specific respiratory muscle training (RMT) may provide a means of improving the ventilatory capacity, exercise ventilation, and, hence, exercise performance.

Techniques of RMT

The most commonly used methods of RMT include inspiratory flow resistive loading, inspiratory pressure threshold loading, and voluntary hyperpnea. Inspiratory flow resistive loading requires a person to inhale via a variable diameter orifice, whereby,

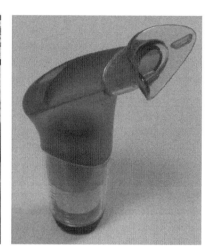

Figure 9.6. A Paralympic athlete with SCI undergoing pressure threshold inspiratory muscle training (left panel); and a close-up view of the training device (right panel).

for a given flow, the smaller the orifice the greater the resistive load. An inherent limitation of resistive loading is that inspiratory pressure, and thus training load, varies with flow and not just to orifice size. It is vitally important, therefore, that flow or pressure is targeted if an effective training stimulus is to be provided. Inspiratory pressure threshold loading requires a person to produce an inspiratory pressure sufficient to overcome a negative pressure load and thereby initiate inspiration (Figure 9.6). An advantage of threshold loading is that it permits variable loading at a quantifiable intensity by providing near-flow independent resistance to inspiration. Voluntary hyperpnea training requires a person to maintain a high target level of ventilation. To ensure that the partial pressure of carbon dioxide does not decrease below resting levels it is necessary to increase the inspired fraction of carbon dioxide, either by partially rebreathing the expired air or by titrating carbon dioxide into the inspired gas.

Influence of RMT on respiratory function

Each of the aforementioned techniques of RMT has been shown to improve respiratory function in healthy able-bodied subjects and in patients' groups with respiratory conditions such as chronic obstructive pulmonary disease. Although there is some evidence for efficacy of RMT in people with SCI, improvements in respiratory function have not been consistently demonstrated in this population. Only two studies used a randomized design with a separate control group. Loveridge et al. (1989) found a significant increase in inspiratory muscle strength and endurance after 8 weeks of inspiratory resistive loading in six patients with chronic cervical SCI. However, similar changes in inspiratory muscle function were noted in a control group such that the improvements were not different between groups. Liaw et al. (2000) found a significant increase in pulmonary function, respiratory muscle endurance, and resting dyspnea after 6 weeks of inspiratory resistive loading in 10 patients with acute cervical SCI. The improvements were greater in the treatment group compared with the control group. While these results do not provide strong support for the efficacy of RMT, it is necessary to assert that poor study design may have concealed the true therapeutic potential of RMT. For example, comparable improvements in respiratory function for control and treatment groups may reflect the influence of learning or recovery from SCI. Furthermore, use of inspiratory resistive loading without targeting flow or pressure may produce an inadequate training stimulus.

Despite insufficient evidence to strongly support inspiratory muscle training as a means to improve respiratory function in people with SCI, there is some evidence to support the efficacy of expiratory muscle training. Many people with high-thoracic or cervical SCI compensate for loss of expiratory muscle function by recruiting their accessory expiratory muscles. The clavicular portion of the pectoralis major, for example, increases its activity during expiration and cough. Repetitive isometric contraction of the pectoralis major for 6 weeks in six subjects with chronic cervical SCI produced marked increases in maximal isometric muscle strength and in expiratory reserve volume, and a decrease in residual volume compared to control subjects (Estenne et al., 1989). The effect persisted when subjects were retested 10 weeks after discontinuing training. An alternative approach to expiratory muscle training in people with SCI has been to magnetically stimulate the thoracic nerve roots using a coil placed over the lower thoracic spine. Using this approach for 4 weeks in nine subjects with chronic cervical SCI resulted in an increase in voluntary expiratory muscle strength, expiratory reserve volume, and peak expiratory flow (Lin et al., 2001). The benefits, however, disappeared within 2 weeks after the cessation of training. Interestingly, neuromuscular stimulation of the expiratory muscles has been shown to improve inspiratory as well as expiratory muscle function. The reason for an increase in inspiratory function with expiratory muscle training is unclear, but could be due to an improvement in diaphragm performance consequent to a training-induced decrease in abdominal compliance.

Influence of RMT on exercise responses

There is clear evidence in healthy able-bodied subjects and in patients with pulmonary disease that RMT can elicit small but significant improvements in exercise performance and related outcomes such as dyspnea. Whether RMT has the potential to improve exercise responses in people with SCI is less clear. Uijl et al. (1999) found a small but statistically significant increase in peak oxygen uptake during arm–crank exercise after 6 weeks of flow-targeted inspiratory resistive loading in nine sedentary subjects with chronic cervical SCI; these changes were greater than those induced by 6 weeks of prior sham training. In contrast, Litchke et al. (2008) found no change in peak oxygen uptake after 10 weeks of flow-resistive inspiratory and expiratory muscle training in three recreational athletes with cervical SCI when comparisons were made with a lesion-matched control group. A concern with both studies, however, is that a separate placebo group was not incorporated into the experimental design, making it difficult to determine whether improvements in exercise performance were the result of the treatment, or merely a learning or placebo effect.

Only a few studies have evaluated the effects of RMT in highly trained athletes with SCI. Mueller et al. (2008) reported an increase in respiratory muscle endurance after 6 weeks of voluntary hyperpnea in six wheelchair-racing athletes with SCI (T4–L3). Despite a strong trend toward an increase in 10-km simulated time-trial performance in the treatment group, the improvement in performance was not different versus that in a lesion-matched control group. Verges et al. (2009) found an increase in both expiratory muscle strength and respiratory muscle endurance after 4 weeks of voluntary hyperpnea in nine national/international level endurance athletes (T4–L1 or post-polio) who served as their own controls. There was a reduction in dyspnea and a trend toward an increase in field-based measures of endurance exercise performance. More recently, Goosey-Tolfrey et al. (2008) reported an increase in inspiratory muscle strength after 6 weeks of inspiratory threshold loading in eight highly trained wheelchair basketball players. However, a similar improvement in inspiratory muscle strength in a sham-training placebo group rendered the changes statistically nonsignificant. Similar changes in the treatment and placebo group were also noted for expiratory muscle strength, which suggests that most of the improvements in respiratory muscle strength were due to a learning effect rather than training. It is perhaps unsurprising, therefore, that the change in total recovery time during a repetitive sprint test was also not different between the treatment and placebo group.

A concern with most of the studies of RMT in highly trained athletes is that they did not use a randomized placebo-controlled experimental design. Where a placebo group was included, the intervention appeared to elicit an improvement in respiratory muscle function of similar magnitude to that observed in the treatment group. In an attempt to address these concerns, West et al. (2009) used a randomized placebo-controlled study design. Twelve Paralympic wheelchair rugby players with cervical SCI were paired by functional classification and randomly assigned to either a treatment or placebo group. The treatment group underwent 6 weeks of inspiratory pressure threshold loading while the placebo group underwent sham bronchodilator treatment. The participants were informed that they were taking part in a study to compare the effects of RMT versus bronchodilator medication, and were therefore blinded to the true purpose of the study and the expected outcomes. Compared to placebo, the treatment group showed a small but significant increase in inspiratory muscle strength. Chronic activity-related dyspnea and pulmonary function were unchanged after RMT. During maximal incremental arm exercise, however, the treatment group demonstrated increases in tidal volume and ventilatory efficiency that exceeded the changes in the placebo group. Moreover, there was a strong trend, with large effect size, toward an increase in peak work rate. These preliminary findings suggest that inspiratory pressure threshold loading provides a useful adjunct to exercise training in athletes with cervical SCI.

Practical recommendations

Optimal protocols for RMT in people with SCI have not been identified. Thus, it is advisable that training recommendations be guided by the current evidence available in people with other respiratory conditions such as chronic obstructive pulmonary disease. For this population, inspiratory pressure threshold loading, targeted flow resistive loading, and voluntary isocapnic hyperpnea have been shown to improve respiratory muscle strength and/or endurance, improve exercise capacity and quality of life, and decrease dyspnea. To elicit an increase in inspiratory muscle strength, it is important that training loads exceed 30% of maximum pressure-generating capacity. Training with a moderate strength bias increases strength and velocity of shortening nearly as much as specifically training for each alone, and

such intermediate loads also elicit improvements in inspiratory muscle endurance. Thus, threshold and resistive loads should be set at about 30–50% of inspiratory muscle strength. Improvements in inspiratory muscle strength are also specific to the lung volume at which training occurs. The range of vital capacity over which strength is increased is greatest when training occurs at low rather than at high lung volumes. Therefore, inspiratory efforts during threshold or resistive RMT should encompass the greatest range of lung volume possible, commencing below relaxation volume. The training should last at least 4–6 weeks, after which the number of sessions per week can be reduced by as much as two-thirds without loss of function.

While the preceding discussion has centered on the practical application of threshold and resistive loading, there is also some evidence that voluntary hyperpnea may benefit athletes with SCI. For healthy able-bodied subjects, respiratory muscle endurance is improved when voluntary hyperpnea is performed for 10–20 min at 60–70% of maximal voluntary ventilation. To achieve similar durations of voluntary hyperpnea in people with SCI, the initial minute ventilation should be set at about 60% of maximal voluntary ventilation for those with thoracic or lumbar lesions, but should be reduced to about 40% for those with cervical SCI. Regardless of the type of loading, RMT has generally been carried out continuously or in intervals, 1–2 times per day, 4–6 days per week, with increases in load of about 5% per week.

Future directions

Clearly, there is a need for large randomized controlled trials of RMT in highly trained athletes with SCI. Studies should use a research design that controls for the influence of learning and recovery on outcome measures. Training techniques should include inspiratory pressure threshold loading, flow- or pressure-targeted resistive loading, or voluntary isocapnic hyperpnea. Specific training of the expiratory muscles using maximal volitional contractions of the pectoralis major or neuromuscular stimulation of the abdominal muscles should also be considered. Outcome measures should include respiratory muscle strength and endurance, exercise performance, and associated responses such as dyspnea. Studies are also needed to compare the effectiveness of RMT relative to or as an adjunct to other interventions such as exercise training.

Future research is needed to determine which activities might derive the greatest benefit from RMT. To date, most studies of RMT have assessed its influence on endurance performance. Because the diaphragm is important for postural control in people with SCI, activities that require forward flexion of the trunk (e.g., wheelchair propulsion) or maintenance of stable posture may also benefit from RMT. Studies are also needed to determine whether there may be value in implementing RMT in athletes with neuromuscular disorders other than SCI. Despite evidence of an improvement in respiratory function in people with post-polio or muscular dystrophy, no study has specifically investigated the effect of RMT on exercise performance in these groups.

Finally, more research is needed to evaluate the extent to which the respiratory system limits exercise performance in people with SCI. The respiratory impairments associated with SCI would be expected to create a mismatch between the demand for respiratory muscle work and the capacity to meet that demand. However, recent findings in highly trained athletes with cervical SCI suggest that such individuals rarely reach mechanical ventilatory constraint during exercise and do not exhibit objective evidence of exercise-induced inspiratory muscle fatigue (Taylor et al., 2010). These findings suggest that any decrease in ventilatory capacity with SCI could be accompanied by a similar decrease in the ventilatory demand consequent to a reduction in the active muscle mass. Clearly, further studies are needed to characterize the complex interactions among exercise responses and the respiratory system in people with SCI.

Intellectual disability

Individuals with ID demonstrate developmental delays in the acquisition of basic motor skills. Their difficulty in obtaining gains from strength training lies primarily from an inability to follow complex instructions. Such language comprehension barriers often deter individuals with ID from exercise. The unfortunate outcome is that inactive individuals with ID tend to exercise less than individuals without disabilities, thereby increasing the risk of sarcopenia and obesity.

Physically active individuals with ID do not present clear fitness impairments. There is some evidence that both male and female Paralympic athletes with ID are similar if not better than age-matched physical education students in many areas of fitness except for strength (van de Vliet et al., 2006). Although no studies have assessed maximal voluntary contraction force, there is evidence that individuals with ID cannot fully activate their skeletal muscles. The physiological reasons why individuals with ID are unable to maximally activate their muscles may reside in the malfunctioning of central and peripheral structures. Indeed, damage of the corpus callosum and the corticospinal tract has been identified in individuals with mental retardation. The corpus callosum and the corticospinal tract are important structures for communication of sensorimotor information and a major pathway in the central nervous system that transmits the neural drive to motor neurons. Corticospinal lesions have been shown to impair the voluntary drive to muscles in several pathological conditions suggesting that the structural alterations observed in individuals with ID could be one of the reasons for the reduced strength in this population. Longer pre-motor times and reduction in nerve conduction velocity have also been suggested as potential mechanisms affecting the ability to produce force in individuals with ID. From a practical standpoint, coaches should aim to motivate athletes with ID to perform lifts and strengthening exercises using maximum effort to ensure high neural drive to the muscles targeted by exercise.

Strength testing in athletes with ID also presents a challenge as the athlete may not only have limited ability to maximally activate the muscle groups tested but also they may be unable to fully understand the requirements of the tests. It is important therefore to familiarize the athletes with the testing procedures to ensure reliable data are obtained. Previous studies have shown that reliable strength data can be obtained in mentally retarded patients with isometric and isokinetic testing modalities (Horvat et al., 1993; Suomi et al., 1993; Surburg et al., 1992). There is, however, a paucity of data on the reliability of strength measurements in athletes with ID. Strength training programs for people with ID should be tailored to the sport's needs and designed to reduce the likelihood of injury. An appropriate loading and difficulty progression should be considered, taking into account the individual's ability to learn complex motor tasks such as Olympic lifts. The safety of the athlete is paramount. Therefore, it is important that heavy loads are only used in movements and exercises that the athlete can master. Appropriate steps should be taken to ensure the intended instructions are understood by the athlete. For this reason, various coaching strategies should be employed that incorporate audiovisual aids and biofeedback systems. Coaches need to be patient and create an environment in which athletes are not surrounded by distraction or noise. Importantly, the athletes need to be reassured and able to experiment with movement patterns. Occam's razor approach (i.e., the simplest explanation is the best) should be used in this population when introducing new strength training exercises.

Les autres

Les autres (French for "the others") is a term used to describe athletes whose disabilities do not fit into the traditional classification systems of the established disability groups. This category includes a wide range of conditions resulting in locomotor disorders, such as dwarfism, MS, muscular dystrophies, and congenital disorders.

As with many of the established disability groups, the scientific literature regarding strength training in les autres athletes is limited. For example, the literature does not provide insight into how to train effectively individuals affected by dwarfism. For this reason it is difficult to understand how this disability affects physical capacity of an individual. Takken et al. (2007) showed that children with achondroplasia had a lower cardiorespiratory capacity and muscle strength than age-matched

subjects. To our knowledge, no intervention study has been conducted in athletes with achondroplasia. Despite the lack of scientific studies, it is important not to overload the spine in athletes with dwarfism. Spinal deformities have been observed in such individuals with achondroplasia (King et al., 2009; Shirley & Ain, 2009) and care is needed when overloading the spine. Furthermore, appropriate screening to assess any alterations in normal spinal curvatures is suggested. Attenuated responsiveness to strength training may occur in athletes with dwarfism due to deficiencies affecting the growth hormone-IGF-1 axis and steroid hormones in this population. Needless to say, more research is needed in this area.

Strength training has been shown to benefit patients with MS by improving gait and mobility (Dalgas et al., 2009; Gutierrez et al., 2005; Taylor et al., 2006). Strength and functional capacity have also been shown to improve with strength training in such individuals. While the evidence suggests that strength training may benefit individuals with MS, care is needed in the setting of training loads as fatigue patterns can be variable in this population.

Generic suggestions for strength training prescription

Strength training prescription for Paralympic athletes is much more challenging than for able-bodied athletes. With the mindset that challenges can be transformed into opportunities, innovative training and coaching solutions can be developed. Strength training is essential in this population, not only to improve athletic performance, but also and probably more importantly to ensure a better quality of life when the athlete's career finishes.

Strength training prescriptions can be developed if an appropriate needs analysis is performed together with a clinical assessment. In Figure 9.7, a framework is suggested to guide the planning of strength training programs for Paralympic athletes. In this population, it important to have a multidisciplinary approach to strength training that involves the strength and conditioning coach, physiotherapist, and doctor. The best results are

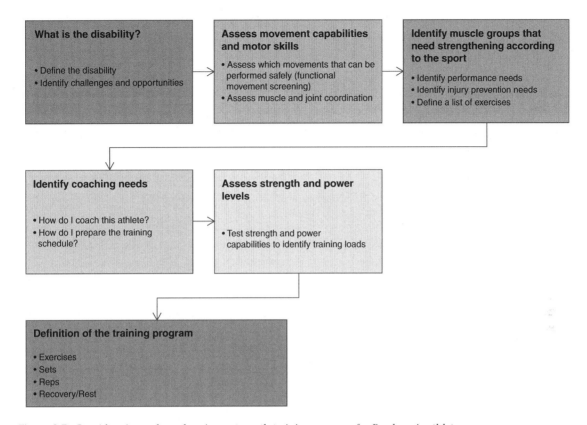

Figure 9.7. Considerations when planning a strength training program for Paralympic athletes.

obtained when clinical and performance aspects are carefully identified and monitored. Information from a variety of sources should be collected to decide not only the best use of specific exercises and loading patterns but also to explore alternative and less conventional ways of improving strength and power in athletes with a disability. Creative ways of presenting the training program should be sought in order to motivate the athletes and facilitate comprehension of prescribed exercise routines. Biofeedback and video analysis should also be used to help and support the Paralympic athlete, particularly when performing complex movements with heavy loads. Modern technology enables the use of multimodal feedback systems based on motion, visual and auditory information, which when combined with effective coaching can provide an enjoyable and productive training environment.

Particular attention should also be paid to the monitoring of training. The ability to measure force and power during key lifts and/or strengthening exercises combined with the measurement of balance and/or movement patterns is becoming easier due to portable technology. Such technology should be implemented in this population. Other simple forms of assessment could include visual-analogue or perceived exertion scales. The use of computerized, interactive and biofeedback data collection and training devices should also be implemented with this population. Providing multimodal feedback and control to maximize force production and appropriate execution of specific strengthening exercises might improve the quality of strength training in this population. The ability of coaches to impart the correct information, stimulate and motivate the athlete, and judge loading and effectiveness of training modalities cannot be substituted by computerized equipment. The key to a successful strength training program still resides in the relationship between the coach and the athlete and the coach's ability to apply scientific knowledge and principles to the design of the training program.

References

Dalgas, U., Stenager, E., Jakobsen, J., et al. (2009). Resistance training improves muscle strength and functional capacity in multiple sclerosis. *Neurology*, **73**, 1478–1484.

Estenne, M., Knoop, C., Vanvaerenbergh, J., Heilporn, A. & De Troyer, A. (1989). The effect of pectoralis muscle training in tetraplegic subjects. *The American Review of Respiratory Disease*, **139**, 1218–1222.

Goosey-Tolfrey, V.L., Foden, E., Perret, C. & Degens, H. (2010). Effects of inspiratory muscle training on respiratory function and repetitive sprint performance in wheelchair basketball players. *British Journal of Sports Medicine*, **44**, 665–668.

Gutierrez, G.M., Chow, J.W., Tillman, M.D., McCoy, S.C., Castellano, V. & White, L.J. (2005). Resistance training improves gait kinematics in persons with multiple sclerosis. *Archives of Physical Medicine and Rehabilitation*, **86**, 1824–1829.

Horvat, M., Croce, R. & Roswal, G. (1993). Magnitude and reliability of measurements of muscle strength across trials for individuals with mental retardation. *Perceptual and Motor Skills*, **77**, 643–649.

Lee, M.Y., Lin, C.F. & Soon, K.S. (2007). Balance control enhancement using sub-sensory stimulation and visual-auditory biofeedback strategies for amputee subjects. *Prosthetics and Orthotics International*, **31**, 342–352.

Leonard, C.T., Sandholdt, D.Y., McMillan, J.A. & Queen, S. (2006). Short- and long-latency contributions to reciprocal inhibition during various levels of muscle contraction of individuals with cerebral palsy. *Journal of Child Neurology*, **21**, 240–246.

Liaw, M.Y., Lin, M.C., Cheng, P.T., Wong, M.K. & Tang, F.T. (2000). Resistive inspiratory muscle training: its effectiveness in patients with acute complete cervical cord injury. *Archives of Physical Medicine and Rehabilitation*, **81**, 752–756.

Lin, V.W., Hsiao, I.N., Zhu, E. & Perkash, I. (2001). Functional magnetic stimulation for conditioning of expiratory muscles in patients with spinal cord injury. *Archives of Physical Medicine and Rehabilitation*, **82**, 162–166.

Litchke, L.G., Russian, C.J., Lloyd, L.K., Schmidt, E.A., Price, L. & Walker, J.L. (2008). Effects of respiratory resistance training with a concurrent flow device on wheelchair athletes. *The Journal of Spinal Cord Medicine*, **31**, 65–71.

Loveridge, B., Badour, M. & Dubo, H. (1989). Ventilatory muscle endurance training in quadriplegia: effects on breathing pattern. *Paraplegia*, **27**, 329–339.

Mueller, G., Perret, C. & Hopman, M.T. (2008). Effects of respiratory muscle endurance training on wheelchair racing performance in athletes with paraplegia: a pilot study. *Clinical Journal of Sports Medicine*, **18**, 85–88.

Navarro, A.S., Fukujima, M.M., Fontes, S.V., Matas, S.L. & Prado, G.F. (2004). Balance and motor coordination are not fully developed in 7-year-old blind children. *Arquivos de Neuro-Psiquiatria*, **62**, 654–657.

Nolan, L. (2009). Lower limb strength in sports-active transtibial amputees. *Prosthetics and Orthotics International*, **33**, 230–241.

Scianni, A., Butler, J.M., Ada, L. & Teixeira-Salmela, L.F. (2009). Muscle strengthening is not effective in children and adolescents with cerebral palsy: a systematic review. *The Australian Journal of Physiotherapy*, **55**, 81–87.

Semler, O., Fricke, O., Vezyroglou, K., Stark, C. & Schoenau, E. (2007). Preliminary results on the mobility after whole body vibration in immobilized children and adolescents. *Journal of Musculoskeletal & Neuronal Interactions*, **7**, 77–81.

Shirahashi, I., Matsumoto, S., Shimodozono, M., Etoh, S. & Kawahira, K. (2007). Functional vibratory stimulation on the hand facilitates voluntary movements of a hemiplegic upper limb in a patient with stroke. *International Journal of Rehabilitation Research*, **30**, 227–230.

Shirley, E.D. & Ain, M.C. (2009). Achondroplasia: manifestations and treatment. *The Journal of the American Academy of Orthopaedic Surgeons*, **17**, 231–241.

Suomi, R., Surburg, P.R. & Lecius, P. (1993). Reliability of isokinetic and isometric measurement of leg strength on men with mental retardation. *Archives of Physical Medicine and Rehabilitation*, **74**, 848–852.

Surburg, P.R., Suomi, R. & Poppy, W.K. (1992). Validity and reliability of a hand-held dynamometer applied to adults with mental retardation. *Archives of Physical Medicine and Rehabilitation*, **73**, 535–539.

Takken, T., van Bergen, M.W., Sakkers, R.J., Helders, P.J. & Engelbert, R.H. (2007). Cardiopulmonary exercise capacity, muscle strength, and physical activity in children and adolescents with achondroplasia. *The Journal of Pediatrics*, **150**, 26–30.

Taylor, N.F., Dodd, K.J., Prasad, D. & Denisenko, S. (2006). Progressive resistance exercise for people with multiple sclerosis. *Disability and Rehabilitation*, **28**, 1119–1126.

Taylor, B.J., West, C.R. & Romer, C.M. (2010). No effect of arm-crank exercise on diaphragmatic fatigue or ventilatory contraint in Paralympic athletes with cervical spinal cord injury. *Journal of Applied Physiology*, **109**, 358–366.

Uijl, S.G., Houtman, S., Folgering, H.T. & Hopman, M.T. (1999). Training of the respiratory muscles in individuals with tetraplegia. *Spinal Cord*, **37**, 575–579.

van de Vliet, P., Rintala, P., Frojd, K., et al. (2006). Physical fitness profile of elite athletes with intellectual disability. *Scandinavian Journal of Medicine & Science in Sports*, **16**, 417–425.

Verges, S., Flore, P., Nantermoz, G., Lafaix, P.A. & Wuyam, B. (2009). Respiratory muscle training in athletes with spinal cord injury. *International Journal of Sports Medicine*, **30**, 526–532.

Verschuren, O., Ketelaar, M., Takken, T., Helders, P.J. & Gorter, J.W. (2008). Exercise programs for children with cerebral palsy: a systematic review of the literature. *American Journal of Physical Medicine & Rehabilitation/ Association of Academic Physiatrists*, **87**, 404–417.

West, C.R., Taylor, B.J., Campbell, I.G. & Romer, L.M. (2009). Effect of inspiratory muscle training in paralympic athletes with cervical spinal cord injury. *Medicine and Science in Sports and Exercise*, **41**, S31–S32.

Recommended reading

King, J.A., Vachhrajani, S., Drake, J.M. & Rutka, J.T. (2009). Neurosurgical implications of achondroplasia. *Journal of Neurosurgery*, **4**, 297–306.

Sheel, A.W., Reid, W.D., Townson, A.F. & Ayas, N. (2008). Respiratory management following spinal cord injury. In: Eng, J.J., Teasell, R.W., Miller, W.C., et al. (eds.) *Spinal Cord Injury Rehabilitation Evidence*, pp. 8.1–8.40. Vancouver.

Chapter 10
Nutrition, body composition and pharmacology

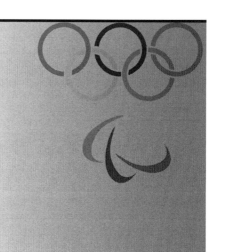

Peter Van de Vliet[1,2], Elizabeth Broad[3] and Matthias Strupler[4]

[1]International Paralympic Committee, Bonn, Germany
[2]Health, Leisure and Human Performance Research Institute, Faculty of Kinesiology and Recreation Management, University of Manitoba, MB, Canada
[3]Clinical Services, AIS Sports Nutrition, Australian Institute of Sport, Canberra, ACT, Australia
[4]Institute of Sports Medicine, Swiss Paraplegic Center, Nottwil, Switzerland

Introduction

Nutritional and pharmacological recommendations for an athlete must be taken into consideration to assist the athlete to prepare for training and competition. This requires an understanding of sport nutrition principles and its interaction with body composition, as well as of medications and pharmacological supplies that adhere with actual standards of doping and drug-free sport. This chapter describes the knowledge available today and the challenges for the future to optimize athletes' sportive careers.

Nutritional strategies for Paralympic athletes

Sports nutrition principles

The knowledge and understanding of sports nutrition principles for elite able-bodied athletes has grown rapidly over the past 30 years. The scope of this text does not allow for complete discussion of all sports nutrition issues. Excellent reviews can be found in the recommended citations at the conclusion of this chapter. Although limited research has been undertaken on sports nutrition principles and applications to Paralympic athletes, the depth and breadth of research in able-bodied athletes provide important insights into the biochemical and physiological working of skeletal muscle and neurological and cardiovascular systems, enabling our knowledge of able-bodied athletes to be extrapolated to the disabled athlete population with some degree of confidence.

The application of sports nutrition strategies to an individual athlete requires careful consideration of the specific characteristics of the athlete (e.g., age, stage of development, training history, gender, body composition), the technical requirements of the sport/event, and the environmental conditions. There is no "one-size-fits-all" approach. For example, athletes and coaches may argue that sports nutrition is not important in skill-based events, yet appropriate hydration strategies and well-managed timing and content of food can ensure optimal concentration while minimizing detrimental issues such as gastrointestinal discomfort, hence potentially can improve performance. The application of these principles to a Paralympic athlete requires the same considerations, with additional factors to consider including the nature of the impairment and its impact on functional capacity, the use of medications, and any coexisting medical conditions. The following is a summary of the core training nutrition principles which can be applied to most sports, specifically highlighting the adaptations critical for the Paralympic athlete.

The Paralympic Athlete, 1st edition. Edited by Yves C. Vanlandewijck and Walter R. Thompson. Published 2011 by Blackwell Publishing Ltd.

Energy expenditure

The area causing the greatest concern among sports nutrition practitioners is how to estimate energy expenditure in many Paralympic athletes. Daily energy expenditure is the sum of four primary sources of energy output:

1. Resting metabolic rate (RMR)—comprising metabolism in a thermoneutral environment during sleep and the early stage of arousal from sleep. Age, gender, and fat-free mass (FFM) predict up to 80% of RMR.
2. Thermic effect of feeding (TEF)—energy expended in the digestion, absorption, transport, metabolism, and storage of food within the body.
3. Adaptive thermogenesis (AT)—temporary shifts in energy expenditure due to cold, heat, fear, stress, and certain medications or drugs (such as caffeine, alcohol, and smoking).
4. Thermic effect of activity (TEA)—otherwise known as energy expenditure of exercise, this is the most variable component of energy expenditure in humans, contributing more than 50% of total daily energy expenditure in athletes. TEA also incorporates:

   a. Nonexercise activity thermogenesis (NEAT)—sometimes known as activities of daily living, this is the energy expended in undertaking normal daily activities, including cooking, shopping, dressing, and watching television.

   b. Spontaneous physical activity (SPA)—such as fidgeting and shivering.

Energy expenditure can be measured directly using metabolic chambers or doubly labeled water. The cost and technical expertise required for these methods limit their use to research or large educational institutes. In a practical setting, RMR can be estimated using one of a number of published equations. Total daily energy expenditure is calculated by applying a multiplication factor according to estimated physical activity levels (PALs) (e.g., 1.4 for sedentary through 2.3 for very heavy exercise); or a multiple is applied to RMR for sedentary/maintenance activity (e.g., 1.4) with the energy expenditure of training estimated from heart rate recordings and additional time spent undertaking specific exercise.

Complexities involved in assessing each of these components of daily energy expenditure in Paralympic athletes include:

1. RMR is usually estimated using equations that include age, body mass, height, and/or lean body mass (LBM). For example, the Harris–Benedict equation estimates RMR from body mass (BM), height (ht), and age in an able-bodied population. It is recognized that the Harris–Benedict equation underestimates energy expenditure in an athlete population; however, it can be useful when LBM is difficult to measure (Table 10.1). The Cunningham equation requires estimating LBM and has been found to be one of the best predictors of RMR in a trained athlete population. Body composition methods used to estimate LBM, as considered later in this chapter, may not be valid for some Paralympic athletes, making the Cunningham equation not applicable to this population. In the case of a spinal-cord-injured (SCI) athlete, lower-limb amputees, and some athletes with cerebral palsy (CP), height may be difficult to measure accurately, and the assumptions as to how much LBM contributes to total body mass may be violated due to significant atrophy of, or lack of, leg musculature. Hence, at this stage, the question remains unresolved as to how to estimate the energy expenditure in a practical setting for many Paralympic athletes.

2. TEF may be reduced in some Paralympic athletes due to lower total energy intake and less feeding frequency over the day.

3. AT may not be different from able-bodied individuals in the majority of Paralympic athletes. However, individuals with SCI may be more prone to greater variations due to an impaired thermoregulatory capacity, and the influence of medications should be investigated on a case-by-case basis. Athletes with CP or amputation may also demonstrate thermoregulation issues.

4. Estimates of TEA are currently based on energy expenditures of different activities measured in an

Table 10.1 Equation estimates for energy expenditure.

Harris–Benedict equation (1919)	
Males	RMR (kJ/day) = [66.47 + (13.75 × BM in kg) + (5 × ht in cm) − (6.76 × age in years)] × 4.2
Females	RMR (kJ/day) = [655.1 + (9.56 × BM in kg) + (1.85 × ht in cm) − (4.68 × age in years)] × 4.2
Cunningham equation (1980)	
	RMR (kJ/day) = [500 + (22 × LBM in kg)] × 4.2

RMR, resting metabolic rate; BM, body mass; LBM, lean body mass.

able-bodied population and presented relative to LBM, but not to absolute body mass. SPA in an athlete with CP could vary considerably depending on whether the athlete has the spastic or athetoid form of CP. NEAT could be increased in some individuals as mobility difficulties will increase energy expenditure of movement, yet decreased in others due to a smaller total muscle mass. For example, amputee athletes have higher energy expenditure in ambulation due to the balancing required of prosthetic limbs, or the lack of an upper limb.

5. Finally, there is almost no data reported on energy expenditure during exercise of Paralympic athletes, other than those with an SCI. Energy expenditure of exercise is lower than in able-bodied individuals (e.g., 17–27 kJ/min at heart rates ranging from 102 to 145 beats per minute), due to the smaller absolute muscle mass used.

The ability to estimate energy expenditure from equations may be less of a concern if reliable data were available in the literature regarding energy expenditure in Paralympic athletes. Energy expenditure of nonexercising individuals with an impairment is unlikely to be useful since active individuals, especially elite athletes, have a greater LBM than their sedentary counterparts and hence will have a higher RMR. However, information on nonathletes can provide an indication of the degree of variation in RMR that could be expected. For example, the typical daily energy expenditure of individuals with CP varies substantially depending on their mode of ambulation. Individuals who are wheelchair (WC) dependent have lower total energy expenditures than those who are ambulating (Figure 10.1). Regardless of ambulatory status, having athetosis (uncontrollable, jerky movements) increases estimated RMR; however, athetosis also reduces the amount of day-to-day activity undertaken. As a result, total energy expenditure does not appear to differ compared to nonathetotic individuals with CP.

Resting metabolic rate in those with an SCI is relative to the level and completeness of the lesion, which can result in substantial variations in RMR even within different members of a Paralympic team with similar impairment (e.g., SCI, up to 25%). Abel et al.'s (2008) report measured RMR (indirect calorimetry) of male paraplegic tennis and basketball players to average 6300–6712 kJ/day while quadriplegic rugby

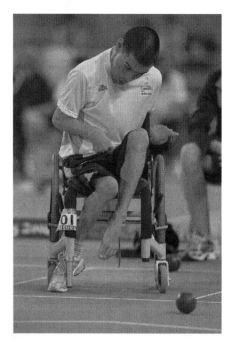

Figure 10.1 Athlete with CP participating in boccia. Reproduced courtesy of Lieven Coudenys.

players averaged 6380 kJ/day. These values are 9–12% lower for paraplegics and 15% lower for quadriplegics than the estimated RMR using the Harris–Benedict equation for these athletes.

Without the ability to estimate energy expenditure, the task of advising athletes on changes to dietary intakes required to alter body composition, or adjust nutrient balance within the same energy profile, becomes more difficult. Self-reported dietary records, however, are not always a reliable alternative with studies in able-bodied populations commonly underreporting total energy intake by 20–50%. Even in the hands of an experienced practitioner, a dietary history has been shown to overestimate nutrient intakes. Sports nutrition practitioners, therefore, should be highly trained in assessment and interpretation of dietary intakes, and have a solid understanding of the specific needs of athletes, in order to provide optimal advice for managing energy intakes.

Muscle fuels

In able-bodied individuals, the predominant muscle fuel at low exercise intensities is fat in the forms of intramuscular triglyceride and blood-borne free fatty acids, reaching a maximal capacity for oxidation at around 65% of maximal oxygen uptake (VO_{2max}). Muscle glycogen and blood glucose become increasingly important fuels as exercise intensity increases, with muscle glycogen being the primary fuel source during "anaerobic" exercise. Since humans have a limited capacity to store muscle and liver glycogen, dietary carbohydrate (CHO) intake recommendations have been proposed for athletes to ensure sufficient fuel to support training (Table 10.2).

In contrast, fat stores are plentiful for training needs in all athletes, so recommendations for dietary fat intake are generally considered as being a balance of remaining energy requirements once CHO and protein needs have been met. One important training adaptation of working muscles is a greater capacity to utilize fat during exercise, therefore reducing reliance on CHO stores at the same power output.

There is no evidence to suggest that the working muscles of Paralympic athletes would respond any differently to a single exercise bout, or adapt differently to training, compared to an able-bodied athlete. Peak fat oxidation rates have been reported to occur at anywhere between 55% and 75% $VO_{2\,peak}$ in trained athletes with SCI depending on the type of ergometry being undertaken (e.g., lower for wheelchair ergometry or handbike cycling than for arm ergometry). Fuel utilization in athletes with CP has not been reported, and it is clear that more studies are required to determine relative fuel utilization during exercise in Paralympic athletes and how this varies with different muscle groups. Consequently, while absolute fat and CHO usage may vary, CHO remains an equally important fuel source in Paralympic athletes as it is for able-bodied athletes.

Current CHO intake recommendations for able-bodied athletes should be considered appropriate for use in Paralympic athletes and applied according to daily training loads. The appropriate application of these guidelines to any athlete relies on an in-depth understanding of training demands (duration, intensity relative to the individual's maximal capacity, frequency) of the athlete, an assessment of the contribution of muscle to total body mass, training status, and the athlete's energy expenditure. For example, consider an 85-kg male wheelchair rugby player who is training once a day for 1–2 h (Figure 10.2). Daily energy expenditure could be estimated to be 10,000–11,000 kJ/day. If CHO intake was recommended to be at 6 g/kg/day (according to Table 10.2), it would account for 8160 kJ or 80% of the total energy intake. Hence, it may be more appropriate to set CHO intake at the lower end of the recommended range (e.g., 5 g/kg/day) to allow room to include protein requirements and some dietary fat. In contrast, the CHO requirements for a wheelchair-bound shooter are not as important, as the training demands from a muscle fuel perspective are much lower. In this case, adequate CHO

Table 10.2 Guidelines for CHO intakes in everyday training.

Activity	CHO intake (g kg BM $^{-1}$ d $^{-1}$)
Immediate recovery after exercise (0–4 h)	1.0–1.2 g kg BM $^{-1}$ h $^{-1}$
Daily recovery: moderate duration/low-intensity training	5–7
Daily recovery: moderate to heavy endurance training	7–12
Daily recovery: extreme exercise program (4–6+ h/day)	10–12+

Adapted from Burke & Deakin (2010). *Clinical Sports Nutrition*, 4th edition. McGraw-Hill.

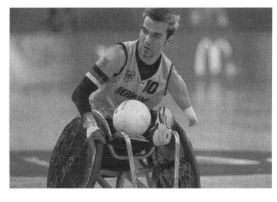

Figure 10.2 The daily energy expenditure for a male wheelchair rugby player could be in excess of 10,000 kJ/day. Reproduced courtesy of Lieven Coudenys.

is more important from the perspective of daily mobilization and maintenance of stable blood glucose concentrations and liver glycogen stores.

Some of the athlete's daily CHO needs may be achieved by consuming CHO during an exercise bout (whether it be training or competition), but this depends on a number of variables. There is no evidence that performance during exercise of less than 1 h duration is improved by consuming CHO unless exercise is commenced in a glycogen-depleted state. In contrast, exercise bouts longer than 90 min have consistently been shown to benefit from the ingestion of CHO during exercise, especially where the exercise includes high-intensity efforts and/or is undertaken in the heat. In these circumstances, recommendations suggest that a CHO ingestion rate averaging 1 g/min is well tolerated in most athletes, although this can be up to 1.5 g/min if a combination of glucose/glucose polymer and fructose is consumed. Some Paralympic athletes may avoid consuming CHO during exercise in fear of exceeding energy requirements or a lack of understanding about the role of CHO in the working muscle. Education of the athlete and coach about how prudent shifting of CHO timing to optimize the training output can enhance long-term training adaptations while simultaneously achieving body composition goals is crucial. Further, the inclusion of some CHO in fluids consumed during exercise can promote increased fluid consumption and may be a useful adjunct to promote optimal blood glucose concentrations for neurological functioning, particularly in an athlete who commences training in a fasted state.

Protein requirements

The dietary protein requirements of able-bodied athletes are recognized as being higher than those of nonexercising individuals, due to the contribution of protein to energy expenditure, increased breakdown of protein (mechanical damage), and the protein requirements of training adaptations (development of mitochondria, enzymes, and muscle tissue). The protein requirements of athletes range from 1.2 to 1.7 g/kg BM/day regardless of whether they are endurance- or strength-trained (Figure 10.3). Dietary surveys of athletes indicate that it is not

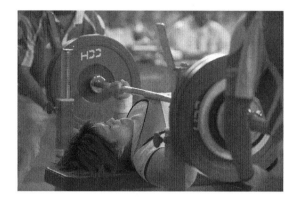

Figure 10.3 The protein requirements of power athletes may increase to 1.7 g/kg body mass per day. Reproduced courtesy of Lieven Coudenys.

difficult to meet these needs, partly due to higher energy intakes of many athletes as well as the wide range of dietary protein sources. There have been no studies published on either the protein needs or the dietary intakes of Paralympic athletes. As with CHO requirements, there is no reason to expect that there would be any difference in a Paralympic athlete's muscle response to exercise and adaptations to a progressive training program. Equally important is the timing of this protein intake relative to an exercise bout (see "Postexercise recovery" section) and its regular distribution throughout the day (together with an adequate energy intake) to support maintenance of muscle mass. Protein intakes above recommendations are unnecessary, and may result in compromised CHO or other nutrient intakes, especially where daily energy expenditure is low due to low total LBM.

Hydration

Hydration status is an important consideration for all athletes. Dehydration increases the physiological strain of exercise and the athlete's perception of effort during exercise. The importance of adequate hydration status is accentuated as environmental temperature increases. Commencing exercise in a dehydrated state, and/or allowing sweat losses to exceed fluid replacement during exercise such that a 2% or greater loss in body mass occurs, will reduce aerobic exercise performance, degrades mental or cognitive performance, and can increase the risk of heat stress. Current fluid intake recommendations to athletes, therefore, are to:

1. commence exercise in a hydrated state;
2. consume fluid during exercise at a rate that prevents excessive dehydration (>2% body mass), yet does not exceed individual athlete's sweat rates.

Sweat rates of individual athletes are known to vary with environmental conditions, gender, and exercise intensities. Sweat rates of various able-bodied athlete populations have been published as examples of the variations within- and between-athlete groups, highlighting the need for individualized fluid intake plans as opposed to generic fluid intake guidelines. It is also recognized that most athletes fail to consume sufficient fluid during exercise, especially when sweat rates are high.

In contrast, sweat rates and fluid requirements of Paralympic athletes have not commonly been reported, despite hydration requirements being similar, if not greater than their able-bodied athletic counterparts. In particular, athletes with SCI and CP are sensitive to hydration problems. Wheelchair-bound athletes tend to reduce their intake of liquids to avoid the complexity associated with toilet hygiene (particularly in the final lead up to a race or game when strapped into the sports chair). Athletes with CP tend to underestimate the amount of fluid loss due to evaporation (e.g., athletes with severe athetosis), or the need of sufficient quantities of fluid to be supplied (e.g., boccia players).

Sweat losses in athletes with SCI have received the most attention within this athlete population since they are commonly lower than able-bodied populations due to a reduced sweating capacity and vasomotor adjustments (Figure 10.4). As ambient temperatures increase, the divergence in sweat rates between able-bodied athletes and athletes with SCI becomes greater. Sweat losses also tend to become smaller as the level of spinal cord lesion goes higher; however, even within similar levels of spinal cord lesion, there remains variability between individuals.

Assessment of an athlete's sweat loss is not difficult to undertake, and can be a useful practical tool to optimize fluid intake recommendations during exercise. The athlete can be weighed immediately prior to, and after, an exercise bout ensuring minimal clothing and the athlete has toweled down. The

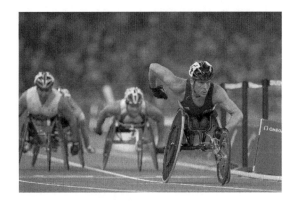

Figure 10.4 Sweat loss in athletes with SCI is a special concern to sport scientists. Reproduced courtesy of Lieven Coudenys.

body mass change, when fluid intake is accounted for, provides an estimate of sweat rate and comparative fluid intake. Urine loss can be estimated by body mass change prior to and after a visit to the bathroom. Sweat loss is calculated as:

Sweat loss (ml/h) = [change in BM (g) + fluid ingested during exercise (ml) − urine loss (g)]/ duration of exercise (h)

When undertaken during different training sessions, environmental conditions, training state, and locations, the athlete can better understand how their fluid requirements change and specific plans can be put in place to minimize the amount of dehydration incurred during exercise. Such planning also minimizes the risk of developing hyponatremia (an electrolyte disturbance in which the sodium concentration in the plasma is lower than normal), which can be a consequence of consuming fluid at a rate that exceeds sweat losses during exercise.

Undertaking assessments of daily hydration status is an important tool, enabling the athlete to monitor fluid needs and the effectiveness of current hydration practices. There are various tools available to do this, with varying degrees of complexity and expenses associated with them. The most convenient and practical tool for most athletes is a visual assessment of urine color, with a variety of color charts available. However, the athlete and/or his support staff need to be aware that the precision of urine color is not always accurate, and can be influenced by various medications. Furthermore, urine color changes over time, so the assessment must be done soon after the collection of the sample.

In contrast, urine specific gravity (USG) can be measured simply through a portable electronic or optical refractometer. USG is a stable, reliable, and valid measure of 24-h hydration status where a first morning, midstream sample is collected. Its validity is reduced if it is used within 2–3 h of consuming a bolus of fluid, hence interpretation must be well considered for samples collected through the day. A USG below 1.020 is considered to indicate euhydration, with recordings higher than 1.025 indicating significant dehydration. USG is a useful tool in educating athletes about their current hydration practices and how effectively they drink fluids over an entire day, rather than just in relation to an exercise bout. This may be particularly important in some Paralympic athlete populations, such as those with CP, who can have higher nonsweat fluid losses than able-bodied populations, even outside training or competition. Feedback regarding USG values and recommendations regarding changes to fluid intake over a day should consider practical issues such as access to toilet facilities and habitual bladder control mechanisms of an athlete, particularly in individuals with SCI. Additionally, prescribed fluid intakes may need to be modified for individuals with an ileostomy or any gastrointestinal tract incompetence to prevent "dumping" of fluid.

One of the other important reasons why attention is paid to hydration status is to support optimal cooling and maintenance of core body temperature. It is important to acknowledge that maintaining adequate hydration status alone may not be sufficient to control the core temperature of some Paralympic athletes. Individuals with an SCI may have a reduced thermoregulatory capacity related to the disruption of neural innervations to the periphery, hence their core body temperature is more difficult to regulate in extremes of environmental conditions (both heat and cold), regardless of whether they are exercising or not. External cooling in the heat, or heating in cool conditions, may become a higher priority than fluid intake for maintenance of core body temperature. However, external cooling in the heat may reduce the drive to drink, and

increase the risk of dehydration, hence monitoring of athletes remains important.

Water remains the fluid of choice on a day-to-day basis, and during most exercise sessions. However, there is good evidence for the inclusion of CHO (as discussed previously) and electrolytes (particularly sodium) under particular circumstances. While sodium losses during exercise has not been studied in a Paralympic population, sweat sodium losses have been shown to vary considerably between able-bodied athletes, and there is evidence that sodium may be important to consider in athletes with high liquid losses. Including sodium in a fluid may also enhance total fluid consumption by maintaining the drive to drink until the body has been adequately hydrated.

Postexercise recovery

The importance of good nutritional recovery practices has become increasingly apparent. While originally this was focused primarily on CHO consumption to optimize glycogen restoration, it has now been expanded to include rehydration and protein intake to promote muscle repair and adaptations to the training stimulus. In practice, however, many Paralympic athletes fail to recognize the importance of eating and drinking soon after exercise. Paralympic performances are constantly improving, and with that many athletes are training at least once a day, if not several times in line with their able-bodied counterparts. Hence, the time available between training sessions is becoming shorter, and the role of recovery is more crucial in sustaining training loads and promoting the positive adaptations to training.

Refueling

Consuming CHO within a 2-h period immediately after exercise has been shown to increase the rate of regeneration of muscle glycogen stores. This is particularly important when a second exercise bout is to be undertaken within 8 h of the first bout, and where muscle glycogen stores are a limiting factor to exercise performance. While high glycemic index CHO may result in faster muscle glycogen restoration in the short term (2 h), the practicality of consuming mixed forms of CHO—which can meet other nutrient goals—still achieves a similar outcome over 6–8 h.

Repair/adaptation

Consuming 10–20 g of protein soon after resistance exercise has been shown to increase muscle protein synthesis compared to waiting several hours before eating. The same is likely to be true for any exercise bout that could cause muscle protein breakdown, including a high-intensity training session or any session involving impact (such as running). Similarly, consuming protein after endurance exercise can enhance the synthesis of proteins involved in the adaptive response to this type of training (such as mitochondrial proteins). It is not necessary for this protein to be in the form of special "protein powders" or amino acids—it can easily be consumed in the form of fluid (such as milk) or food, and can be combined with CHO.

Rehydration

Rapid rehydration following exercise is important, especially when another exercise bout is to be undertaken in a relatively short period of time (<8 h). Sweat losses usually continue following cessation of exercise as the body continues to cool itself, so it is not sufficient to simply replace the fluid lost in the exercise bout itself. Recommendations are to replace 125–150% of the fluid lost during exercise (i.e., 1.25–1.5 l for every kg body mass loss). Fluid retention is also maximized if this volume is consumed over time rather than in one large bolus. If the fluid loss was greater than 2% of the body mass, adding sodium to the fluid may be useful in improving the uptake and distribution of fluid throughout the body. Sports drinks are one useful choice in this instance, but there are many practical ways to achieve this target. Examples include milk-containing fluids or water consumed with foods which can supply sodium (as well as CHO and protein, such as a ham or cheese sandwich).

Nutritional supplementation and ergogenic aids

The plethora of nutrition supplements and ergogenic aids available to athletes increases almost daily.

While many can be useful adjuncts in particular circumstances (such as sports drinks, sports bars, gels), the vast majority of proposed ergogenic aids not only have no scientific evidence to support their use, but also carry the risk of inadvertent doping offences due to poor manufacturing or packaging regulations. It is documented that up to 15% of the packaging ingredient lists fail to report the presence of prohibited substances. Surveys of athletes consistently show their regular use of supplements and/or ergogenic aids without an understanding of the reason for use, the recommended doses, the potential side effect or the risk of inadvertent doping or lack of "active ingredient." Furthermore, athletes often look to supplements to give an "edge" over competitors without full consideration of, and attention to, the factors that result in the majority of performance advantages in sport, such as diet, hydration, recovery practices, training consistency, and sleep. The scope of this chapter does not allow for an exhaustive discussion of this topic. However, three ergogenic aids that have consistently proven benefits in able-bodied athletes will be mentioned briefly. For greater details, readers are referred to other key manuscripts in this area (see recommended reading). It is important to note that no research has been published using any ergogenic aids in Paralympic athletes.

The application of any ergogenic aid to an athlete requires an in-depth understanding of the mechanism of action of the supplement as well as the physiological processes involved in the particular athlete's activity. Since the duration and intensity of some Paralympic sports can differ from their able-bodied counterparts, it remains up to the sport scientist, nutritionist, and coach to determine whether any benefits are likely within this athlete population. There is also potential for different side effects, or more acute sensitivity to side effects, in some Paralympic athletes, hence any use of ergogenic aids must be trialed in a structured manner in training first.

Caffeine

Caffeine is a central nervous system stimulant found in many commonly consumed foods and fluids such as tea, coffee, cola drinks, "energy" drinks, and chocolate. Caffeine was removed from the World Anti-Doping Code (WADC) Prohibited List (see further discussion under "Doping") in 2004 and has been studied in a wide range of sports and activities as a potential ergogenic aid. Caffeine has been found to improve performance in endurance events, intermittent high-intensity sports (e.g., team and racquet sports), and sustained high-intensity efforts, to reduce the rating of perceived exertion, and to increase alertness and reaction times. Less evidence is available on single high-intensity efforts such as throws, jumps, and single sprints. Doses used in research have commonly ranged from 3 to 6 mg/kg body mass, taken around 1 h prior to the start of exercise. In practice, athletes often use lower doses with good effect (down to 1.5 mg/kg body mass), and endurance athletes will often take some during an event. Furthermore, the timing of ingestion may require individualization due to differences in absorption rates. The side effects of caffeine should be carefully considered in Paralympic athletes, particularly neurological stimulation and gastrointestinal irritability. Those competing in the afternoon and evening should also consider the potential impact on sleep, as disturbed sleep will impact on recovery. Athletes considering experimenting with caffeine in competition are advised to trial controlled doses of caffeine in training first to ensure full consideration of potential positive and negative effects. Consideration should also be made of potential interactions with medications.

Creatine

Phosphocreatine is an immediate source of ATP at the initiation of, and first few seconds of, muscle contraction. Phosphocreatine can be rapidly regenerated, but limited amounts are available. Consumption of 20–30 g creatine monohydrate daily in split doses for 5 days (or alternatively 3 g creatine daily for 3–4 weeks) has been shown to increase muscle phosphocreatine stores in approximately 70% of individuals. There appears to be an upper limit of phosphocreatine storage, which makes consuming more creatine than recommended unnecessary. The elevated stores can be maintained by consuming 3 g of creatine monohydrate daily, and it takes several weeks for stores to return to baseline following cessation of supplementation. Creatine loading

has been shown to be beneficial for short-term, high-intensity efforts (6–30 s), especially where little rest (20 s to 5 min) is provided between bouts. Examples include team and racquet sports, and strength or resistance training individuals. Effects on a single sprint event are uncertain; however, it may be useful as a training tool where repeat sprints constitute a training session. Effects on endurance performance are absent. Currently, the main side effect of creatine loading is body mass gain, which is considered to be mostly fluid in the loading phase, and as such athletes are advised to ensure adequate fluid intake if loading with creatine. Athletes with preexisting renal disease should avoid supplementation with creatine.

Buffers

Performance of very high-intensity exercise is limited by the decrease of pH in the muscle, which inhibits muscular contractile and energetic enzymes and processes. Bicarbonate has been studied in high-intensity efforts in an attempt to control the change in pH by buffering it in the blood. More recently, B-alanine supplementation has been studied as it is taken up into the muscle to form carnosine, an intramuscular buffer. Studies using bicarbonate have been shown to consistently benefit performance in near maximal intensity efforts lasting 1–7 min duration. Few studies are currently available using B-alanine; however, the benefits are believed to be for the same type of activities. Bicarbonate loading involves an acute dose of 0.3 g/kg body mass sodium bicarbonate consumed 1–2 h prior to the start of exercise. Doses are best split over a 1-h period and consumed with sufficient water. The side effects are primarily gastrointestinal, including nausea, vomiting, and diarrhea, so supplementation must be trialed in training before use in competition. B-alanine is a chronic loading supplement, requiring at least 4 weeks of continuous daily supplementation (4–5 g/day in split doses) to achieve maximal muscle carnosine stores. As with creatine, there appears to be a prolonged period of washout following cessation of supplementation. Side effects of B-alanine supplementation known to date are acute paresthesia symptoms (tingling, burning sensations in the peripheral limbs), which can be reduced by using smaller single doses repeated periodically over the day or a slow release form.

Practical issues

Not only may an impairment require modification of sports nutrition advice, it may also require modification of some practicalities of eating and drinking. Examples include:

• having someone available to assist a visually impaired athlete in selecting food at a buffet, or purchase and prepare food in an unfamiliar environment;
• adjusting fluid intake in the latter part of the day in an individual with SCI to minimize the disruption overnight in having to go to the toilet;
• providing quick and easy meal ideas to an individual with CP for whom food preparation may take longer and involve greater exertion;
• ensuring suitable cooking facilities and equipment if self-catering for wheelchair-dependent individuals and amputees;
• considering the impact of dietary changes on bowel and bladder function in those with SCIs;
• nutrition education of the support person/caretaker.

Assessment of body composition

There are numerous methods to assess body composition in athletes, varying in expense, portability, and ease of use. All that may be required is body mass and stretch stature (height), although the latter may need to be modified to a seated stretch stature for which there is no reference data available. However, assessing body composition and changes over time in an athlete can provide useful feedback regarding adaptations to training and dietary manipulations. All methods of body composition assessment have underlying assumptions that need to be recognized before applying to Paralympic athletes. It is important from the outset of body composition monitoring to determine the goals of such monitoring as this will assist in choosing the method best suited for the individual athlete. In practice, the method chosen should also be inexpensive, safe, and noninvasive.

Discussion of such methods in this chapter is limited to the most commonly used methods in athletes.

The assessment of body composition in sports science has four fundamental applications:
1. to identify physique characteristics of elite performers,
2. to assess and monitor growth,
3. to monitor responses to training programs,
4. to determine optimal body composition for weight category sports.

Indirect methods (Level 2 methods)

Indirect measures of body composition are derived by measuring parameters that are associated with body composition but do not actually measure body composition directly. Direct body composition measurement can only be achieved by cadaver dissection (Level 1 method). Due to this, all indirect methods of measurement are associated with validity issues and none are absolutely accurate. The expense and lack of portability results in these evaluation techniques having greater use in research settings, and for validation of Level 3 methods of body composition assessment.

Hydrodensitometry (underwater weighing)

Historically considered the "gold standard" method of assessing body composition, hydrodensitometry uses Archimedes principle to determine body density, and uses either the Siri or Brozek equations to convert body density to a percent body fat. This technique divides the body into two compartments—fat and FFM—and assumes each compartment has a constant density. This can be an issue in Paralympic athletes as it is documented, for example, that individuals with SCI have lower whole body bone mineral density (BMD) than control subjects, reducing the potential density of the fat-free compartment. Hydrodensitometry has two other primary sources of error—the inability to measure air trapped in the lungs and in the gastrointestinal tract.

Air displacement plethysmography

More recently, air displacement plethysmography has been implemented as an alternative to underwater weighing, using the BOD POD™ (Life Measurement, Inc., Concord, CA). The principles of air displacement plethysmography are the same as for hydrodensitometry (using air displacement to estimate body volume) and thus are subject to the same assumption errors. Both densitometry techniques require highly standardized testing protocols and present unique challenges for some Paralympic athletes in relation to transfer in and out of the measuring areas. Three-dimensional (3D) body scanning, a relatively new technology, may enable an accurate measure of body surface area, which combined with other body composition assessment tools may provide a means to better estimate body density in Paralympic athletes. However, as of today, no data are available on Paralympic athletes.

Dual X-ray absorptiometry

Dual X-ray absorptiometry (DXA) was originally developed to measure bone mineral content (BMC) and BMD, and is considered the "gold standard" for these measures. The technology has been developed to also include the ability to measure body composition through the use of sealed X-ray tube and dual-energy photons since the relative attenuation of photons in soft tissue changes in proportion to the fat content of the soft tissue, and soft tissue can be clearly distinguished from bone. While DXA now appears in the literature as the standard comparison method for body composition assessment, it is rarely recognized that the use of DXA to measure body composition comes with limitations. Standardization of protocols to control placement of the subject, dietary and hydration status, and limited diurnal variations and inter-machine variations are essential. Although the radiation dose is very low, it is not recommended for routine monitoring of body composition in athletes.

Dual X-ray absorptiometry has been used and has been stated to be a useful and valid technique for assessing body composition changes following SCI. DXA may be useful in the Paralympic population in the monitoring of segmental differences in muscle mass and tracking changes in specific body regions as a result of training. Paralympic athletes with large stretch stature (>190 cm) and large body mass (>120 kg) will have difficulty fitting within the scanning area of most DXA machines, and innovative methods will need to be used to gain accurate complete scans.

Doubly indirect (Level 3) methods

Doubly indirect methods of body composition require validation against Level 2 methods of body composition when determining percentage body fat. Provided assumptions of both Level 2 and Level 3 methods are acknowledged and methods are used in a standardized manner by trained individuals. Level 3 methods of body composition present simple, low-cost, portable methods to monitor change in body composition parameters.

Surface anthropometry

In the hands of a skilled, trained practitioner, surface anthropometry can be a reliable and valid method of assessing body composition. In its most simple form, this involves the measurement of stretch stature, body mass, and skinfold thickness at seven to eight sites across the body (e.g., biceps, triceps, subscapular, iliac crest, supraspinale, abdominal, mid-thigh, and maximal calf). Surface anthropometry can also be expanded to include arm span, girths, and limb lengths and bone breadths to describe whole body physique. Most commonly, skinfolds are reported as a sum of seven (or eight) sites rather than as a percentage body fat, as this avoids the use of prediction equations specific to different population groups and with the built-in assumption that the densities of the fat and FFM are the same between individuals. Since no equations to estimate percent body fat from skinfolds have been developed in a Paralympic athlete population, it remains appropriate to report a sum of skinfolds (plus or minus the technician's technical error of measurement, or TEM) and change over time. Further, since no normative data are available in this population, results must be interpreted individually.

Modifications in methodology may be required according to the nature of the impairment. Examples include:

a. Using the left-hand side of the body instead of the standard right-hand side for athletes with right-side hemiplegic CP or with right-sided amputees/limb deformities. The technician should decide whether this is done only for the affected limb (the remainder of the body resuming to the right-hand side) or for all measures, and should be clearly noted on the athlete's records.

b. Using only four skinfold sites (biceps, triceps, subscapular, and abdominal) for athletes with SCI. Remaining seated alters the position of supraspinale landmark, and it is likely that leg musculature is also substantially atrophied.

c. Stature may be more appropriately measured as a seated height, rather than as a standing or prone stature. However, this has not been shown to provide an accurate estimate of stretch stature, so should be used as a stand-alone measure.

d. Where muscle atrophy is present, it can be difficult to differentiate the body fat component of skinfold thickness, and other injuries (such as burns or the location of a stoma) can influence skinfold thickness. The technician may need to alter the location of the skinfold site (ensuring documentation of this is made for future reference), or leave a site out altogether.

Bioelectrical impedance analysis

Bioelectrical impedance analysis (BIA) uses the conductivity of an electrical current passed through the body to measure body composition, based on the assumption that fat and bone tissue are devoid of water and electrolytes and will therefore not carry current as opposed to lean tissue. Measurements are normalized for stature, and it is important to control testing conditions such as hydration status. The subject assumes a supine position for measurement with electrodes placed on various sites around the body. Consequently, stand-on scales that measure bioelectrical impedance are not as valid as they do not assess the whole body (rather, leg to leg). One important assumption of BIA is that tissue-specific resistivity is constant for all body segments, yet it is known that the composition of the fat-free body changes following SCI, potentially making BIA less valid in this athlete population.

Due to the lack of a reference population data and other limitations stated, the suitability of BIA to measure body composition in Paralympic athletes must be carefully considered, and if used must be undertaken by skilled technicians—using highly standardized conditions—who only report individual changes over time, rather than reporting against any normative data.

Physique traits in Paralympic athletes

The ISAK (International Society for the Advancement of Kinanthropometry) standard has been used to describe body composition and physique traits of various elite able-bodied athlete populations. As yet, very little has been published on the body composition and physique traits of Paralympic athletes, most likely due to the varied nature of this population and the small number of athletes related to classification. While some Paralympic athletes would not be expected to differ from able-bodied athletes (e.g., visually impaired and intellectual disabilities), the majority would be expected to have some unique physique traits. Consequently, there are no normative data available for Paralympic athletes. Recording time since onset of injury, the specific nature of impairment (e.g., level of spinal cord lesion, complete or incomplete lesion, amputation vs. congenital malformation) and considering the classification of the athlete is important when undertaking body composition assessments in Paralympic athletes so that, over time, the potential to pool data for analysis is possible.

Most reports of body composition in Paralympic athletes are from wheelchair-bound athletes. Early reports present skinfold measures (using techniques different from ISAK standards) and generally summarize that converting skinfolds to percent body fat, and using hydrodensitometry to estimate percent body fat, are inappropriate in this athlete population. Higher BMD, lean mass, and lower percent body fat (via DXA) have been reported in the upper body of female wheelchair users compared to nonexercising, age-matched controls, with the opposite occurring in the lower body. No comparison was made against exercising able-bodied athletes. In contrast, the sum of four skinfolds (using ISAK methodology), seated height, weight and arm span, has been reported in male wheelchair basketball players, subdivided into eight different sport classes in wheelchair basketball. If more researchers and practitioners can publish results using standard ISAK methodology, reporting a sum of skinfolds or individual skinfold measures along with disability classification, then collection of normative data will become more viable especially considering the greater practicality in the field of skinfold measures compared to DXA.

Body composition and performance in Paralympic athletes

As with the description of physique traits, very little has been published on body composition and performance in Paralympic athletes. Body density (hydrodensitometry), but not body mass, has been correlated to 10-km race time and a higher efficiency (speed at maximal oxygen consumption) in male paraplegic wheelchair racers. A case study of a Paralympic wheelchair tennis player reported a reduction in the sum of four skinfolds and body mass along with physiological adaptations (improved pushing economy) over an 18-month training period, although performance per se was not assessed.

Medication use in Paralympic athletes and its impact on athletic performance

Specific medical considerations to Paralympic athletes have been discussed in Chapter 4. Team physicians should indeed emphasize injury prevention techniques, including the importance of good muscle strength and coordination to provide better control over the body, on the application of appropriate training skills, and the use of good quality protective equipment. Of particular interest is the pharmacological management of Paralympic athletes. Paralympic athletes often have to be treated with medications due to their impairment or intensive sports participation, or due to secondary health problems affiliated with the impairment. This may vary from exercise-induced

bronchospasm over hypo- or hypertension, urinary tract infections, and muscle spasticity to diabetes mellitus and seizure disorders. Unfortunately, pharmacological literature does not offer much relevant information concerning the effects of medication on exercise performance in Paralympic athletes. Data on medication use by Paralympic athletes are not systematically available.

Based on a review of experiences and supported by the little scientific evidence available, most problems encountered by Paralympic athletes are essentially the same as in able-bodied athletes. Furthermore, the injury rate has generally been found to be within the same range. For example, the wide variety of movement disorders, including neurological deficit and disorders of muscle tone, may have a deleterious effect on an individual's ability to perform activities of daily living and participate in recreational activities and/or competitive sports. Medical treatment constitutes, besides non-pharmacological alternatives (e.g., physiotherapy, acupuncture, electrical stimulations, spinal cord stimulation, and desensitization), an appropriate "medical best practice."

Although limited to a (random) selection of Paralympic Games participants, a study on reported medication use in athletes who were selected for doping control gives some insight on medication use of Paralympic athletes. In the Athens 2004 Paralympic Games, two-thirds of the athletes subjected to doping control (436 of 680 athletes, which represents approximately 11% of the total number of Games participants) declared the use of medications or food supplements during the final 3 days before testing (Tsitsimpikou et al., 2009). Paralympic athletes' medication and supplement use pattern was similar to that of their Olympic counterparts, though dosages in general were smaller (with the exception of the reported use of creatine). Medication classes represented treatment plans for the major (expected) pathological conditions found in Paralympic athletes, with equal spread over treatment of disorders from the central nervous system, cardiovascular system, and urinary tract. Nonsteroidal anti-inflammatory medication (NSAIM) and analgesics were mostly found in in-competition testing samples, indicating that these preparations were not mainly for the use of chronic inflammatory or pathological conditions. NSAIM use was mainly reported in wheelchair athletes who place heavy workload on their upper limbs. The infrequent use of medication to treat urinary tract disorders was felt indicative for Paralympic athletes being able to manage neurogenic bladder very well.

Pharmacological classes

In the following section of this chapter, the most prevalent pharmacological classes are addressed in more detail by means of a typical single substance as an example of the corresponding substance group. Commonly, this allows for the characterization of a substance group. The reader is advised that within certain substance groups, effects can differ substantially from substance to substance, and from athlete to athlete. The listing specifies substances and methods, which will lead to an adverse analytical finding, once detected in an athlete and thus constitute a possible anti-doping rule violation.

Diclofenac (Voltaren®)

Diclofenac belongs to the group of NSAIM and is indicated for inflammatory and degenerative forms of rheumatism, painful inflammations, and swelling, as well as for acute pain in gout, dysmenorrhea, or migraine attacks. NSAIMs are often used by athletes to suppress pain of the musculoskeletal system in order to be able to compete. The ingestion of NSAIMs can lead to gastrointestinal bleeding or to somewhat severe allergic reactions of the skin. For long-term use, the control of kidney and hepatic function is recommended. NSAIMs are not listed as prohibited substance and a therapeutic use exemption (TUE) is not required when prescribed.

Tramadol (Tramal®)

Tramadol is a so-called opioid analgesic, which acts via the central nervous system. It is used in case of persistent strong pain, if NSAIMs (see above) show no satisfactory analgesic effects. Tramadol has an additional antitussive effect. Tramadol should not be used in the state of shock or reduced consciousness of unknown genesis. The adverse effects of tramadol on the cardiovascular system are minor, but vertigo, nausea, and vomiting as well as fatigue can appear. Tramadol is occasionally prescribed as an alternative for morphine because it is not prohibited and does not require a TUE.

Pregabaline (Lyrica®)

Pregabaline is an analogon of gamma-amino butyric acid (GABA) and reduces the release of different neurotransmitters. The neuronal excitation of the central nervous system is reduced. Pregabaline is prescribed for the treatment of neuropathic pain (e.g., in SCI) or as an adjuvant therapy in epilepsy and anxiety disorders. It is generally accepted that coping with activities of daily life is facilitated due to the analgesic working substance. Otherwise, physical activities might be strongly limited due to adverse effects such as weakness, sleepiness, and obnubilation. In few cases, disturbance of coordination and concentration has also been reported. Pregabaline is not prohibited and can be prescribed without TUE.

Tizanidine (Sirdalud®)

Tizanidine is a central acting myotonolytic and antispastic substance. Tizanidine is effective in acute and painful muscle spasms as well as in chronic spasticity of spinal or cerebral genesis. Adverse effects are dose-dependent, and may include sleepiness, fatigue, xerostomia, hypotension, and nausea, which are mostly of transient nature. After abrupt withdrawal of tizanidine, medication rebound effects were reported. It is recognized that while this medication can substantially enhance an individual's ability to function on a daily basis with everyday activities, it may simultaneously affect an individual's ability to excel in athletic performance. Due to the decreased muscle tone, resistance against passive movements (antagonist) is reduced, which in turn facilitates voluntary muscle contraction force. However, tizanidine is subject to large interindividual variability. Not listed as a prohibited substance, it is recommended that tizanidine can be prescribed by neurological specialists only and that periodic review of the individual's status is considered to ensure a correct treatment in appropriate doses. Therefore, it is imperative that the athlete and his specialist caretaker proceed with the spirit of sport in mind (see "Doping" section).

Baclofen (Lioresal®)

Baclofen is an antispastic medication acting on the spinal level, and reduces the reflex transmission in the spinal cord due to the stimulation of GABA-receptors. Neurological disorders in conjunction with spasticity are positively influenced by reducing muscle contractions, painful spasms, and clonii. Some athletes with SCI use baclofen intrathecally (medication pump), though should be aware that an inadequate dosage may undo the positive effects on motor function. Increased performance is documented in both human and animal studies. However, consideration should be given to what the impact is on a (reduced) quality of daily life in the absence of treatment. Baclofen should be used carefully in subjects with reduced liver or kidney function and amentia. Under the treatment with baclofen, sleepiness, obnubilation, vertigo, and impaired vision may occur. These effects are intensified if alcohol is consumed under baclofen treatment.

Triamcinolon (Kenacort®)

Triamcinolon is a substance of the group of glucocorticosteroids. Glucocorticosteroids act by inducing synthesis of specific proteins in the cell, which are responsible for multiple biological processes. With high doses, it is possible to achieve therapeutic effects such as inflammatory inhibition and immunosuppression. Indications of glucocorticosteroids treatments include rheumatic, allergic, pulmonary, and hematological disorders as well as neoplasms. It is known that in some sports, glucocorticosteroids are used for performance enhancement. However, most of the scientific studies failed to show an ergogenic effect. Notwithstanding, depending on the route of administration, glucocorticosteroids are prohibited substances and require a TUE or Declaration of Use (see "Doping" section). Additionally, due to potential adverse

effects in prolonged use (adrenalotropic insufficiency, loss of adrenal gland, Cushing Syndrome, osteoporosis, diabetes mellitus) and the contraindication to existing viral infections (e.g., herpes), the use of glucocorticosteroids requires a strictly controlled supervision by a physician as well as an accurate instruction to the athlete (to which the athlete is expected to adhere).

Methylphenidate (Ritalin®)

Methylphenidate is a stimulant, which acts at the central nervous level and shows distinctive effects on mental and motor function. The substance is used for the treatment of hyperkinetic abnormal behavior in children and adolescents and in case of narcolepsy, and often is prescribed to individuals with intellectual impairment. There exists no consensus among experts if the treatment with methylphenidate has to be stopped during physical activity as positive and negative influences on exercise performance have been reported. However, due to methylphenidate belonging to the category of stimulants, usage is prohibited during competition. A TUE is necessary. Furthermore, methylphenidate should not be used in case of hypertension or cardiovascular diseases, and chronic abuse of the substance may lead to psychical dependence with abnormal behavior.

Salbutamol (Ventolin®)

Salbutamol selectively stimulates the beta-receptors of the bronchial musculature (beta-2 agonist). This leads to a fast and intense bronchospasmolysis. The substance is applied for the treatment and prevention of asthma bronchiale and chronic bronchitis, and typically prescribed for exercise-induced asthma. Tremor, fast pulse, and palpitation often occur as adverse effects. In most of the cases, they disappear after long-term application or reduction of the salbutamol dose. The effect of salbutamol on exercise performance in non-asthmatic athletes is discussed controversially. Whereas some studies showed an increase in aerobic and anaerobic exercise capacity, others did not find any effect on exercise performance. Under the 2010 WADC Prohibited List, the presence of salbutamol in urine in excess of 1000 ng/ml is presumed not to be an intended therapeutic use of the substance and will be considered as an adverse analytical finding unless the athlete proves, through a controlled pharmacokinetic study, that the abnormal result was the consequence of the use of a therapeutic dose of inhaled salbutamol.

Metoprolol (Beloc ZOK®)

Metoprolol is a cardioselective blocker of beta-receptors. The substance is applied in case of hypertension, angina pectoris, chronic heart insufficiency, and arrhythmia. Bradycardia, orthostatic problems, cold hands and feet are commonly reported adverse effects. Further, dyspnea during exercise and nausea can occur. Because archery and shooting performances are significantly increased due to a reduction in tremor after metoprolol ingestion, beta-blockers are prohibited in these sports and thus would require a TUE, also for Paralympic athletes. However, it is very unlikely that on international levels such an approval will be given as the advantage for the athlete under beta-blocker prescription is too obvious. In endurance sports, ingestion of metoprolol reduces exercise performance as maximal heart rate, stroke volume, and maximal oxygen uptake are reduced due to the blockade of beta-receptors. This is why beta-blockers are not prohibited in biathlon, although shooting makes a substantial component of the sport.

Enalaprile (Reniten®)

Enalaprile is a long-acting inhibitor of angiotensin-converting enzyme (ACE). The substance modulates the renin–angiotensin–aldosterone system, which plays a key role in the regulation of blood pressure. Enalaprile provokes a reduction in the workload of the heart (preload and afterload) and as a consequence leads to an increased pumping capacity of the heart. Enalaprile is used for the treatment of hypertension and heart insufficiency. In contrast to beta-blockers, the application of enalaprile has no effect on aerobic exercise performance or metabolism during aerobic exercise in hypertensive subjects (and consequently its use is not prohibited). Therefore, ACE inhibitors are recommended as medication of

the first choice in hypertensive endurance athletes. Prescription of the substance is contraindicated in persons with idiopathic angioedema or if angio-neurotic edema occurred during a former treatment with ACE inhibitors.

Sildenafil (Viagra®)

Sildenafil is a selective inhibitor of phosphodiesterase type 5 and induces a pulmonary vasodilation. Experimentally, healthy athletes showed an increased exercise performance of more than 10% at high altitude (4000 m) as well as better oxygen saturation and cardiovascular function. For this reason, World Anti-Doping Agency (WADA) currently considers sildenafil on its Monitoring Program.

The adverse effects reported are mostly headache, flush, dyspepsia, impaired vision, nasal congestion, and vertigo. The hypotensive effect of nitrates is potentiated by sildenafil ingestion. Thus, the concomitant ingestion of sildenafil in subjects treated with coronary vasodilators containing nitrates is an absolute contraindication. Sildenafil also acts peripherally on penis erection. However, a sexual stimulus is necessary for the development of the desired positive pharmacological effect of sildenafil. This, in combination with WADA's interest to consider sildenafil for further investigation, has prompted experts on Paralympic athletes within the anti-doping community to take an increasing interest in this class of medications, even though research has not shown that they improve athletic performance at sea level or moderate altitudes. Many athletes with SCI use these medications to treat erectile dysfunction of neurologic origin. Therefore, it is important to understand what effects, if any, this class of medications has on athletic performance in athletes with SCI. It is plausible that sildenafil could have a deleterious effect on exercise performance by causing peripheral vasodilation. Because a large number of athletes with SCI use sildenafil for the treatment of erectile dysfunction of neurologic origin, this warrants investigation of the effect of this medication on athletic performance at low and moderate altitudes, where sports competition generally takes place. Such study is initiated by the International Paralympic Committee (IPC) under the WADA 2009 Scientific Program.

Botulinum toxin (Botox®)

Botulinum toxin A blocks the peripheral release of acetylcholine at the presynaptic site by disruption of synaptosomal-associated protein of 25 kDA (SNAP-25). The medical indications of botulinum toxin are infantile CP, focal spasticity (after cerebrovascular insult or after SCI), and cervical dystonia. Further, the substance is used for the treatment of disturbances in micturition after SCI. Commonly adverse effects appear within the first days after injections and disappear gradually, and include local muscle weakness, general fatigue, sleepiness, nausea, and influenza-like symptoms. Consequently, a treatment with botulinum toxin seems not to impact athletic performance (and thus is not prohibited), but it may be considered not to be prescribed shortly before important competitions.

Ciprofloxacine (Ciproxin®)

Ciprofloxacine is a representative of the group of antibiotics (subgroup: chinolones). Ciprofloxacine shows bactericidal effects over a wide spectrum of gram-negative and gram-positive bacteria. The substance is used namely in case of infections of the respiratory system, the kidney, and the urinary tract. Antibiotics are not prohibited substances and can be prescribed without a TUE. However, it is crucial that sick athletes suffering from such infection reduce physical activity and completely avoid intense exercise.

Atorvastatin (Sortis®)

Atorvastatin is a substance belonging to the group of statins. They reduce plasma cholesterol and lipoprotein levels by inhibition of HMG-CoA-reductase and hepatic cholesterol synthesis. Thus, a significant reduction of low-density lipoprotein cholesterol in patients with familial homozygotic hypercholesterolemia can be found. Moreover, statins are used to prevent coronary heart disease. Due to muscular side effects, a treatment with statins is poorly tolerated by elite athletes. Additional adverse effects that may occur include insomnia, headache, vertigo, pruritus, myalgia, and arthralgia. Hepatic diseases and myopathy are contraindications for a medical therapy with atorvastatin. There is no need for a TUE for the prescription of statins as they are not on the list of prohibited substances.

Loperamide (Imodium®)

Loperamide is a synthetic opioid, which is used for the symptomatic treatment of severe diarrhea of different genesis. The substance binds to the opiate receptor located in the intestinal wall and shows a fast and long-lasting therapeutic effect, without an influence on the central nervous system in the recommended application dose. The medication is popular for athletes who travel all over the world and have difficulty adapting to local food. Loperamide is not listed as a prohibited substance and can be prescribed without a TUE. Loperamide should not be used as primary therapy for the treatment of acute infectious or ulcerative colitis.

At present, a TUE is not necessary for many of the substances listed earlier. However, as with any medical treatment, it is recommended that individuals who may benefit from these medications be treated by a specialist with extensive knowledge of the individual's condition. Periodic review of the individual's status is necessary to ensure that the correct treatments are being administered in the correct doses. It is recognized that while some of the medications listed can substantially enhance an individual's ability to function on a daily basis with everyday activities, they may simultaneously affect an individual's ability to participate in sports. There is no clear or objective distinction between obtaining an improvement in activities of daily living versus obtaining enhanced sports performance. Therefore, it is imperative that the individual and their health-care provider proceed with the spirit of sport in mind.

Doping

The personal and financial rewards of modern-day sport to create an unhealthy desire to win at all costs also exists in the Paralympic Movement.

To gain a competitive advantage, some athletes therefore find their way to so-called ergogenic aids, which enhance sporting performance beyond that attainable through genetic ability and sustained effective training. Ergogenic aids including pharmacological (e.g., performance-enhancing drugs) and physiological (e.g., blood doping) supplies is commonly referred to as "doping." A discussion on pharmacology and medication use in Paralympic athletes, therefore, cannot go without consideration of prohibited substances and prohibited methods.

World Anti-Doping Code (WADC)

To ensure a level playing field, doping is controlled by sports governing bodies, including the IPC and its member Paralympic Sport Federations, who have agreed to abide by the rules established by the WADA and its WADC. WADA was created in 1999 because the International Federations (IFs) and the International Olympic Committee (IOC) realized that the war against substance abuse could not be won by sport alone. The IOC invited the governing bodies to join the fight and both parties, the Sports Federations and the governing bodies, set up an independent authority, named WADA. After a wide consultation round with all stakeholders involved, WADA approved the WADC in 2003 "to protect the athletes' fundamental right to participate in a doping-free sport and thus promote health, fairness, and equality for athletes worldwide, and to ensure harmonized, coordinated, and effective anti-doping programs at the international and national level with regard to detection, deterrence, and prevention of doping." The fundamental rationale of the WADC is that anti-doping programs seek to preserve what is intrinsically valuable about sport. This intrinsic value is often referred to as "spirit of sport." The spirit of sport is characterized by ethics, fair play and honesty, health, excellence in performance, and respect for the rules of the sport.

Doping therefore is fundamentally contrary to the spirit of sport. Within these premises, not only enhancing substances (and methods) should be considered as "doping," but also substances (and methods) that affect the health of an athlete or are against the spirit of the game. Indeed, WADA is very clear in its mission that the fight against doping equals the rights to protect:

• Clean athletes: protect their right to doping-free sport.
• Healthy and safe competition: protect athletes from being compelled to use unhealthy or dangerous methods in an attempt to be competitive.
• Spirit of sport: protect the spirit of sport and ensure that sport remains a worthy human activity.
• Society: protect youth and future athletes by providing them with doping-free role models.

As a stakeholder of WADA, IPC in its role as governing body of the Paralympic Movement has developed, accepted, and implemented the IPC Anti-Doping Code as the anti-doping rules for the Paralympic Movement. This implies that the IPC membership adheres to this code, and that this code applies to all IPC-sanctioned events and competitions (all competitions that fall under IPC jurisdiction, including Paralympic (Winter) Games, specified Regional Games and Competitions, and all sanctioned competitions in IPC sports). The actual version of the IPC Anti-Doping Code can be retrieved from the IPC Handbook (www.paralympic.org—IPC—IPC Handbook).

Anti-doping rule violations

The WADC defines three criteria under which a substance or method can be considered for inclusion on the Prohibited List: enhances performance, poses a threat to the athlete's health, and violates the spirit of sport.

The WADC lists a series of circumstances and conducts that constitute an anti-doping rule violation (WADC article 2). These are related to classes of pharmacological substances (articles 2.1 and 2.2; presence or use of a substance) or mechanisms of action (articles 2.3–2.8, e.g., refusal to deliver a sample, tampering, trafficking, failure to submit whereabouts information). The anti-doping rule violations due to mechanisms of action fall outside the scope of this chapter.

It is very difficult to determine the exact side effects that a substance or a method or combination thereof may have on an otherwise healthy athlete who is doping. This is partly because:
• the relevant studies cannot be conducted on individuals without a therapeutic reason to do so;

- the substances or methods used by doping athletes are usually developed for patients with well-defined disease conditions and are not intended for use by healthy people;
- volunteers in a therapeutic study are unlikely to be subjected to the same conditions of administration and dosage of a substance and/or method as those of an athlete who is doping;
- athletes who use prohibited substances often take them in significantly larger doses, and more frequently, than these substances would be prescribed for therapeutic purposes, and often use them in combination with other substances;
- substances that are sold to athletes as performance enhancers are often manufactured illegally and may therefore contain impurities or additives, which can cause serious health problems or may even be fatal.

Because the many combinations and/or doses of performance-enhancing substances used by athletes who "dope" have never undergone official trials, for an athlete to acquiesce to doping is to accept being a "guinea pig" (i.e., an experimental model) and to risk adverse effects of unknown nature and unknown gravity. Substances and methods indeed initially are meant for therapeutic use (to treat sick people or sick animals) and do not have the same effects on healthy athletes as they do on sick patients. Furthermore, adverse effects can be hard to determine in athletes because athletes who dope do not usually talk about it. Moreover, using combinations of several drugs means not simply adding but compounding the risks (e.g., the nontherapeutic use of any type of hormone risks creating an imbalance that affects several functions, and not only the function that is usually directly concerned by the given hormone). Additional health risks are present when the use of substances or methods involves injections. Nonsterile injection techniques, including sharing possibly contaminated needles, can increase the risk of transmission of infectious diseases such as hepatitis and HIV/AIDS. Finally, the use of any substance may also lead to addiction, whether psychological or physiological.

Once a laboratory has reported a positive test result to the relevant anti-doping agency, a result management process is initiated. This result management process makes up the major part of any anti-doping code and ensures that standardized and harmonized processes are followed throughout the sports community. The following main steps can be differentiated in the result management process:

- conducting an initial review to determine whether an applicable TUE has been granted or will be granted as provided in the International Standard for Therapeutic Use Exemptions, or whether there is any apparent departure from the International Standard for Testing or International Standard for Laboratories that caused the adverse analytical finding;
- disqualification of the athlete from the event in which the doping control leading to the positive test result occurred and eventual provisional suspension of the athlete;
- organization of the B-sample analysis and hearing, if not waived by the athlete;
- sanctioning of the athlete which may include imposing a period of ineligibility and eventual financial sanction;
- foresee appeal procedures.

It is only from the moment that the athlete accepted the anti-doping rule violation or, in view of the anti-doping agency, is not able to provide satisfactory explanation to the facts that constitute the investigation, that a positive laboratory result is considered an anti-doping rule violation. Until that time, the findings are reported as "adverse analytical finding" or "atypical finding," and the athlete is subject to a "possible" anti-doping rule violation.

Strict liability principle

Under the strict liability principle that is key to all anti-doping rules and regulations and that is adopted by the WADC signatories (all sporting bodies that accepted the WADC), only the athlete is responsible for whatever substance found in the body, independent of an intentional or unintentional intake. Therefore, besides properly educating himself/herself, it is of utmost importance that the athlete has full confidence in the team physician who must have a keen knowledge on the status of pharmacological substances and techniques. Within this relationship, the physician will play multiple roles to the athlete, including educator, healer, detective, and counselor.

Prohibited substances

There is a single list of prohibited substances and methods, which is published by the WADA. This list (WADC Prohibited List) applies to ALL sports in the Olympic and Paralympic Movement (and beyond) and is revised every year. As mentioned earlier, WADA considers three criteria under which a substance or method can be considered for inclusion on the Prohibited List: enhances performance, poses a threat to the athlete's health, and violates the spirit of sport. The inclusion of substances on the Prohibited List is the result of a wide consultative process and review of all available scientific literature. WADA actively supports the process of development of new analytical tools and strategies by spending 25% of its annual budget in scientific research. The annual list becomes effective from January 1 and is published 3 months before it comes into effect. The current version is always posted on WADA's website at www.wada-ama.org.

The prohibited substances (and methods) are classified in pharmacological groups. Further subdivision is made for substances and methods that are prohibited only in particular sports, and to distinguish substances that are prohibited out-of-competition from those prohibited in-competition. An overview of the prohibited substances and methods under the WADC 2010 Prohibited List is provided in Table 10.3 (for detailed and updated information, refer to www.wada-ama.org).

Prohibited substances should not be prescribed by physicians unless the athlete would experience a significant impairment to health if the prohibited substance or prohibited method were to be withheld in the course of treating an acute or chronic medical condition; unless the therapeutic use of the prohibited substance or prohibited method would produce no additional enhancement of performance other

Table 10.3 Prohibited substances under the WADC 2010 Prohibited List (retrieved from www.wada-ama.org).

Substances prohibited at all times

S1. Anabolic agents	– Anabolic androgenic steroids (AAS), both exogenous and endogenous – Other anabolic agents, including but not limited to clenbuterol, selective androgen receptor modulators (SARMs), tibolone, zeranol, zilpaterol	– Evidence may be obtained from metabolic profiles and/or isotope ratio measurements to differentiate between exogenous (ordinarily not produced by the body naturally) and endogenous (capable of being produced by the body naturally) agents. – It is important to note that some dermatological creams used for gynecological and urological reasons may include anabolic agents in their formula. – Some birth control pills may contain norentindrone, which may result in a positive test for 19-norandrosterone.
S2. Peptide hormones, growth factors and related substances	– Erythropoiesis-stimulating agents (EPO, CERA, hematide, etc.) – Chorionic gonadotrophin (CG) – Insuline – Corticotrophins – Growth hormones – Platelet-derived preparations (e.g., blood spinning) administered by intramuscular route	Insulin is permitted only to treat insulin-dependent diabetes and requires a therapeutic use exemption by the concerned anti-doping authority.
S3. Beta-2 agonists		All beta-2 agonists are prohibited except salbutamol (max. 1600 mg over 24 h) and salmeterol by inhalation, which required a Declaration of Use in accordance with the WADC International Standard for therapeutic use exemptions. The presence of salbutamol in urine in excess of 1000 ng/ml is presumed not to be intended therapeutic use of the substance and will be considered as an adverse analytical finding unless the athlete proves through a controlled pharmacokinetic study that the abnormal result was the consequence of the use of a therapeutic dose of inhaled salbutamol.

(continued)

Table 10.3 (*Continued*)

S4. Hormone antagonists and modulators	– Aromatase inhibitors – Selective estrogen receptor modulators (SERMs) – Other anti-estrogenic substances – Agents modifying myostatin functions	
S5. Diuretics and other masking agents		A TUE for diuretics and masking agents is not valid if an athlete's urine contains such substance(s) in association with threshold or subthreshold levels of an exogenous prohibited substance.
M1. Enhancement of oxygen transfer	– Blood doping, including the use of autologous, homologous, or heterologous blood or red blood cell products of any origin – Artificially enhancing the uptake, transport, or delivery of oxygen	In the case of blood transfusion for medical treatment (e.g., hemorrhage or acute anemia), a TUE is required.
M2. Chemical and physical manipulation	– Tampering or attempting to tamper in order to alter the integrity and validity of samples collected during doping controls is prohibited – Intravenous infusions are prohibited except for those legitimately received in the course of hospital admissions of clinical investigations	The use, or intention to use, substances or methods (e.g., catheterization—see "IPC Position Statement on Catheters" section) that affect the integrity and validity of urine samples is forbidden.
M3. Gene doping	– Transfer of cells or genetic elements (e.g., DNA, RNA) – Use of pharmacological or biological agents that alter gene expression	

Substances and methods prohibited in-competition

S6. Stimulants		All stimulants are prohibited, except imidazole derivatives for topical use and those stimulants included in the monitoring program*.
S7. Narcotics		
S8. Cannabinoids		
S9. Glucocorticosteroids	All glucocorticosteroids are prohibited when administered by oral, intravenous, intramuscular, or rectal routes	A Declaration of Use must be completed by the athlete for glucocorticosteroids administered by intra-articular, periarticular, peritendinous, epidural, intradermal, and inhalation routes. Topical preparations for auricular, buccal, dermatological, gingival, nasal, ophthalmic, and perianal disorders are not prohibited.

Substances prohibited in particular sports
(NOTE: only Paralympic sports listed)

P1. Alcohol	Prohibited in archery (FITA)	Detection will be conducted by analysis of breath and/or blood. The doping violation threshold (hematological values) is 0.10 g/l.
P2. Beta-blockers	Prohibited in archery (FITA), curling (WCF), shooting (IPC)	In these Paralympic sports, the use of beta-blockers is prohibited both in-competition and out-of-competition.

*Monitoring program.

than that which might be anticipated by a return to a state of normal health following the treatment of a legitimate medical condition; or unless there is no reasonable therapeutic alternative to the use of the otherwise prohibited substance or prohibited method. At all times, (team) physicians should stress the medical risks associated with their use. Athletes have the right to know all the risks related to (wrong) choices, and addressing these topics with them is an important responsibility of the athlete support personnel, in particular the (team) physician.

International Standards

To ensure that due processes and procedures are followed, the WADC is complemented with "International Standards" for different technical and operational areas for testing, TUE management, laboratory analysis, and protection of privacy and personal information. All these International Standards are mandatory complementary parts to the WADC and adhered to by all WADA stakeholders. Without entering into too much detail, it implies that selection of athletes and sample-taking procedures are done following standardized procedures. The same applies for TUE management and the analysis of samples at a WADA-accredited laboratory. Additionally, appropriate, sufficient, and effective privacy protections to personal information stored by anti-doping authorities are also scoped.

Athletes may be selected for doping control at any given moment in time, both in-competition and out-of-competition, and without any advance notice. An accredited doping control officer (DCO) (or blood collecting officer) must be able to identify himself/herself as well as show a letter of authorization of the respective anti-doping agency (International Federation, National Federation, National Anti-Doping Agency, or WADA are entitled to direct doping controls on athletes who fall under the respective jurisdiction).

As soon as the athlete is notified of selection for doping control, he/she will have to proceed with the sample collection immediately, either in a (temporary) doping control station or in his accommodation/residential facility. An athlete is entitled to a representative assisting him/her throughout the administrative processes, and should receive a copy of all paperwork (notification, doping control form, event reporting sheets) at the end of the procedure.

The DCO and his agency are responsible for following the samples to a WADA-accredited laboratory and to submit the paperwork to the anti-doping agency that directed the testing. In accordance with the WADC, only WADA-accredited laboratories are entitled to analyze samples for anti-doping agencies. The laboratory is obliged to report test results to the agency that directed the testing with a copy to WADA. In the case of a positive laboratory result, the laboratory shall also send a copy of the report to the concerned International Sports Federation.

Incidence of positive cases in the Paralympic Movement

An overview of the incidence of positive cases in past Paralympic Summer and Winter Games and detailed statistics by sport and substance are presented in Figure 10.5.

The data apply only to anti-doping rule violations that fall under the jurisdiction of the IPC. This implies all Paralympic and Regional Para-Games, some major multisports events that are recognized by IPC, and for anti-doping rule violations that occurred through in- and out-of-competition testing by the IPC and WADA (on behalf of IPC) on athletes in IPC Sports. To have a full picture of incidence of anti-doping rule violations in the Paralympic Movement, the data presented in Figure 10.5 need to be complemented with the statistics from the different International Sports Federations (IFs and International Organizations of Sport for the Disabled) that have para-sport athletes under their jurisdiction, and with statistics from national testing programs. In the absence of a centralized management of anti-doping rule violations, it is however impossible to report correct data to reflect the real incidence of anti-doping rule violations in Paralympic athletes.

Besides an increase in overall testing, it is worth mentioning that increased importance ought to be given to out-of-competition testing. Some experts believe that in-competition testing is illogical since the athlete can anticipate testing. Out-of-competition

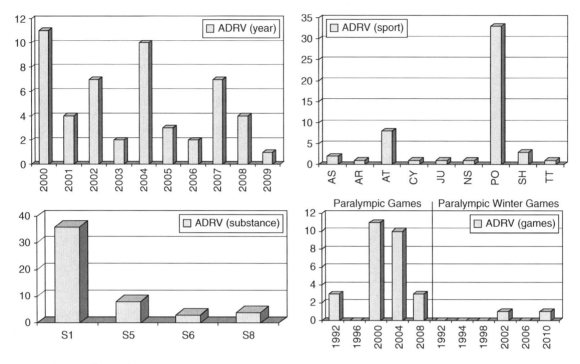

Figure 10.5 Incidence of anti-doping rule violations (ADRV) under IPC jurisdiction (number by year, sport, substance, and Paralympic Summer and Winter Games). AS, Alpine ski; AR, archery; AT, athletics; CY, cycling; JU, judo; NS, Nordic ski; PO, powerlifting; SH, shooting; TT, table tennis; S1, anabolic agents; S5, diuretics and masking agents; S6, stimulants; S8, cannabinoids.

testing therefore seems to be a smarter approach to catch potential cheaters, but has significant challenges related to locating athletes, availability of resources, and logistics of testing. In recent years, increased attention has been paid to so-called intelligence testing in which the primary focus lies in investigating the proof of "use" of a prohibited substance or method (e.g., blood profiles, biological passport) over the "classical" approach of investigations that follow from the proof of "presence" of a prohibited substance or method in an athlete's bodily specimen.

Anti-doping and TUE management in the Paralympic Movement

Anti-doping agencies, including the IPC and its membership, have a responsibility to ensure that athletes and their support staff are provided with updated and accurate information on at least the following issues:
- substances and methods on the prohibited list,
- health consequences of doping,
- doping control procedures,
- athletes' rights and responsibilities.

The programs should promote the spirit of sport in order to establish an anti-doping environment that influences behavior among all involved. Anti-doping education is a primary responsibility of the National Federations and National anti-doping agencies, as they are the closest to the athletes. However, there is no doubt that all parties will benefit from coordinated efforts at supranational level and in close cooperation with concerned International Federations.

Additionally, athlete outreach booths in which athletes can familiarize themselves with anti-doping matters are set up at major competitions and events (Figure 10.6). Outreach booths are exhibition stands in a high-visibility area that receives a great deal of athlete traffic throughout the sporting

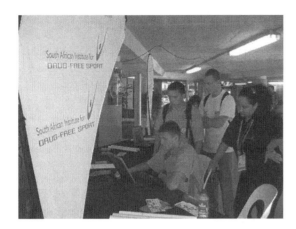

Figure 10.6 Athlete outreach booths at major competitions and events are popular for athletes to familiarize themselves with anti-doping matters (Photo: IPC).

event. Anti-doping outreach booths are staffed by anti-doping experts and aim to create an environment in which athletes feel comfortable asking questions about anti-doping issues. A very popular facet of the outreach booth is the WADA doping quiz, which also can be assessed online through www.wada-ama.org.

Therapeutic use exemptions

Besides being informed on the prohibited substances and methods on the WADC Prohibited List, athletes need to familiarize themselves with the TUE process. Athletes must obtain a TUE in accordance with the rules of the National or International Federation. Athletes are not allowed to apply to more than one anti-doping organization for a TUE. Athletes should also be aware that they remain vulnerable to a positive laboratory result and possible anti-doping rule violation until the TUE has been granted. Medical treatment therefore should not be started before the start date of the TUE certificate.

Therapeutic use exemption applications will not be considered for retroactive approval except in cases where the conditions set forth in the WADC International Standard for Therapeutic Use Exemptions apply (e.g., emergency medical treatment or treatment of an acute medical condition, or in the exceptional circumstance of insufficient time or opportunity for an athlete to submit, or a TUE Committee to consider, an application prior to doping control).

Modifications for testing Paralympic athletes

The WADC International Standard for Testing provides the opportunity to modify standard doping control procedures (WADC IS Testing, Appendix B). A DCO has the authority to make modifications to the standard procedures for collecting samples from athletes with a disability as long as such modifications will not compromise the integrity, security, or identity of the sample and are authorized by the athlete and/or his/her representative. This may be the case when athletes:

• have restricted mobility or coordination that prevents application of the standard sample collection procedure (e.g., if the athlete is unable to handle the collection vessel, carry the sample, split the sample into the A and B bottles, or seal the A and B bottles, either the athlete representative (preferably) or the DCO may perform these tasks if requested by the athlete);

• have visual impairment (e.g., the athlete representative may sign the Doping Control Form or Supplementary Report Form on behalf of the athlete; the athlete is provided the opportunity to inspect sample collection equipment by touch; the athlete representative should be afforded the opportunity to inspect the sample collection kit);

• have neurological or developmental disabilities (e.g., an athlete with a neurological or developmental disability should be accompanied at all times during the sample collection session by an athlete representative, preferably of the athlete's choice);

• have a catheter or condom device to allow for urine production.

In the latter condition, athletes who are using urine collection or drainage systems should, when practical, choose one of the following means for provision of their samples:

If indwelling catheter or condom drainage is used, the athlete should ideally discard the collection bag in use and attach a new, unused bag to the catheter. The urine collected in this new bag will be drained into the collection vessel as the sample to be processed.

• If replacing/disconnecting the bag already in use is difficult due to the type of catheter used, the existing bag must be fully emptied, and a fresh sample collected in the bag. The fresh urine collected in the bag is drained into the collection vessel as the sample to be processed.

• The sample may also be taken directly through the catheter into the collection vessel. The athlete or attendant, under the athlete's instruction, may temporarily clamp off the catheter to the leg bag.

• As is the case with all sample collection procedures, the catheterization process is witnessed. The collection bag should be drained and replaced (if possible) as soon as practical following notification. Using the contents of the sample collection bag prior to notification is not an acceptable sample.

In the case of an inability to collect a blood sample by puncture in the arm veins, the blood collecting officer will try to retrieve a blood sample from a vein in the foot or groin. Any special accommodations made for an athlete with a disability should be noted on a Supplementary Report Form.

IPC position statement on the use of catheters

Following a decision taken with regard to an anti-doping rule violation in Canada (2008, Canadian Sports Disputes Panel of Athletics Canada vs. Adams), the IPC has considered its position on the use of catheters by Paralympic athletes subject to doping controls. This resulted in a position statement that applies for all situations in which the anti-doping program falls under the jurisdiction of the IPC. The IPC position statement stipulates that the catheter used by an athlete with need for self-catheterization is to be considered as "personal equipment." Athletes might react adversely to different brands and models, potentially leading to infections and/or allergic reactions. Therefore, athletes mainly use one particular type of catheter. Furthermore, due to the variety of brands, models, and sizes, it cannot be expected that Organizing Committees or DCOs will supply catheters that meet the individual requirements of each athlete. Within this perspective, and giving absolute priority to the athlete's health, the catheter used is the responsibility of the athlete. Although not mandatory, it is recommended that athletes use sterile catheters for hygienic reasons.

In particular cases (e.g., Paralympic Games), the doping control stations may be equipped with a number of sealed, sterile catheters; however, this would never include all brands, sizes, and/or materials available worldwide. This must be regarded as a complimentary service offered to the athletes in such a particular competition. Even in those cases, experience has shown that it is very rare for an athlete to choose a catheter supplied by the DCO over the use of his/her own catheter.

The IPC is not directly responsible for the training of DCOs. However, in preparation of IPC-sanctioned events, workshops for Organizing Committee members are often held in which IPC stresses the importance for DCOs to comply with the WADA International Standard for Testing Annex B "Modifications for Athletes with a Disability," and the IPC Position Statement on the Use of Catheters.

Conclusion

Despite the lack of published literature on nutrition and body composition for Paralympic athletes, sports scientists rely heavily on the array of evidence available for able-bodied athletes. There is good reason to believe that this remains valid for the Paralympic population, since skeletal muscle does not differ between exercising humans. The successful application of this information to individual Paralympic athletes requires a thorough understanding of physiological processes and the impact of any impairment on this, as well as an understanding of the practical challenges that the athlete may face. Paralympic athletes often have to be treated with medications due to their impairment or intensive sports participation, or due to secondary health problems affiliated with the impairment. Unfortunately, pharmacological literature does not offer relevant information concerning effects of medication on exercise performance in Paralympic athletes. It is recognized that while some of the medications listed can substantially enhance an individual's ability to function on a daily basis with everyday activities, they may simultaneously affect an individual's ability to participate in sports. There is no clear or objective distinction between obtaining an improvement in activities of daily living versus obtaining enhanced sports performance. Therefore, it is imperative that athletes and their support staff familiarize themselves with the prohibited substances and TUEs, as well as all other doping control procedures and that all proceed with the spirit of sport in mind. To conclude, it is important to understand that nutrition and pharmacology in Paralympic athletes are highly dynamic subjects, and it is the responsibility of the athlete to be very well informed and up to date. This calls for a major effort to surround the athlete with a multidisciplinary and professional team of athlete support staff, and increased efforts to focus on Paralympic specific research in these areas.

Acknowledgments: Elizabeth Broad would like to thank Greg Shaw for his assistance in preparing the nutrition section of this chapter.

References

Abel, T., Platen, P., Rojas Vega, S., Schneider, S. & Struder, H.K. (2008). Energy expenditure in ball games for wheelchair users. *Spinal Cord*, **46**, 785–790.

Burke, L. & Deakin, V. (2010). *Clinical Sports Nutrition*, 4th edition. McGraw-Hill. Sydney, Australia.

Tsitsimpikou, C., Jamurtas, A.Z., Fitch, K., Papalexis, P. & Tsarouhas, K. (2009). Medication use by athletes during the Athens 2004 Paralympic Games. *British Journal of Sports Medicine*, **43(13)**, 1062–1066.

Recommended readings

ACSM/ADA/DC Joint Position Statement (2009). Nutrition and athletic performance. *Medicine and Science in Sports and Exercise*, **41**, 709–731.

American College of Sports Medicine (2007). Position stand: exercise and fluid replacement. *Medicine and Science in Sports and Exercise*, **39**, 377–390.

Chan, K.M., et al. (eds.) *FIMS Team Physician Manual*, 2nd edition, pp. 184–203. International Federation of Sports Medicine. Hong Kong 2006.

Dec, K.L., Sparrow, K.J. & McKeag, D.B. (2000). The physically-challenged athlete. Medical issues and assessment. *Sports Medicine*, **29**, 245–258.

De Rose, E.H., da Nobrega, A.C.L. & de Castro, R.R.T. (2006). Drug testing and doping. In International Paralympic Committee (2009). IPC Anti-Doping Code. International Paralympic Committee (retrieved from www.paralympic.org).

Maughan, R.J., Burke, L.M. & Coyle, E.F. (2004). Sports nutrition. *Journal of Sports Nutrition*, **22**, 1–145.

McArdle, W.D., Katch, F.I. & Katch, V.L. (2009). *Exercise Physiology: Energy, Nutrition and Human Performance*, 7th edition. Lippincott, Williams & Wilkins. Philadelphia, PA, USA.

World Anti-Doping Agency (2008). World anti-doping code. World Anti-Doping Agency. Available at: www.wada-ama.org.

World Anti-Doping Agency Toolkits. Available at: www.wada-ama.org.

www.isakonline.com.

www.ausport.gov.au/ais/nutrition/supplements.

Chapter 11
Mental preparation

Dietmar Martin Samulski[1], Franco Noce and Varley[2] Teoldo da Costa[2]

[1]Department of Physical Education, Federal University of Minas Gerais, Belo Horizonte, Minas Gerais, Brazil
[2]Department of Physical Education, University of Belo Horizonte, Belo Horizonte, Minas Gerais, Brazil

Introduction

According to the Instituto Brasileiro de Geografia (IBGE), in the Brazilian census for 2000, about 24,600,256 people in the country had some form of disability. This figure may have changed recently due to the number of people who have been affected by some cause of disability.

Studies conducted in the field of sports show that sports participation can play an important role in the recovery of people affected by disability and in their reintegration into society. It is an effective instrument in the process of rehabilitation, socialization, and improvement of quality of life, leisure, and pushing the limits of physical performance. Its importance has been stressed since the 1940s. According to the neurosurgeon Gutmann, "sports can help disabled people to restore the connection with the surrounding world" (Samulski, 2003). Gutmann believed in the value of sports for disabled people, both as a means of overcoming depression and of gaining a new purpose in life, because, for him, the practice of sports is essential for socialization. The practice of sports can achieve far more than social integration, as it restores self-esteem and develops the awareness of one's true capacity. Many institutions that have investigated physical activity and high-performance sports have focused on the process of rehabilitation in acknowledgment of their importance, since physical activity is a beneficial and efficient method for reintegration, socialization, quality of life improvement, and leisure for the disabled people in society.

Paralympic sports have grown worldwide and increasingly more people in a range of scientific fields are paying attention to this area. According to the International Paralympic Committee (IPC), the number of athletes participating in the 2004 Athens Paralympic Games increased significantly when compared to the first event in Rome (1960), when only 400 athletes from 23 countries participated. In Athens, this number rose to about 4000 participants from 143 countries (20 more than in Sydney in 2000), competing in 19 sports, which shows how Paralympic sports have progressed over the recent years.

In Brazil, Paralympic sports are one of the most successful proposals directed at this population, with the goal of using participation in a range of adapted sports to help disabled people develop in different aspects of their lives. The action of the disabled people associations, along with those of the Comitê Paraolímpico Brasileiro (CPB, Brazilian Paralympic Committee), is fundamental for making this fact a reality today. In this context, many aspects of sports psychology are now being directed to disabled people. Sports psychology is becoming relevant for sports professionals in specific ways.

In the last few years, sport psychology has contributed effectively to a better understanding of how psychological factors influence athletic performance, especially elite performance as demonstrated

The Paralympic Athlete, 1st edition. Edited by Yves C. Vanlandewijck and Walter R. Thompson. Published 2011 by Blackwell Publishing Ltd.

in the Olympic Games and Paralympic Games. Gould et al. (1998) once said, "Successful Olympic Performance is a complex, multifaceted, fragile and long-term process that requires extensive planning and implementation. Attention to detail counts, but must also be accompanied by flexibility to deal with numerous unexpected events."

Sport psychology research has consistently shown that for optimal performance to occur, elite athletes must achieve an ideal performance state (IPS) or an emotional zone of optimal functioning. This optimal performance state is a complex, multivariate combination and interaction of cognitions, emotional states, and physiological conditions. The most common elements include optimal arousal level, anxiety and stress control, self-confidence, goal setting, attention control, and perceptions of self-control.

According to Hackfort and Munzert (2005), physical preconditions, physiological states, and motor skills are not the exclusive fundamentals required for peak performance in sports. Hackfort (2006) also considers that mental abilities, as well as various psychological factors, are necessary for attaining excellence. Gould et al. (2002) investigated Olympic champions' psychological characteristics and their development. Olympic champions exhibited the following characteristics: coping with and control anxiety, confidence, sport intelligence, the ability to focus and block out distractions, competitiveness, hard work, ethics, ability to set and achieve goals, "coachability," high levels of dispositional hope, optimism, adaptive perfectionism, and mental toughness. Jones et al. (2002) defined mental toughness as an important characteristic of an expert athlete as, "Having the natural or developed psychological edge that enables you to, generally, cope better than your opponents with many demands (competition, training, life style) that sport provoke. Specially, be more consistent and better than your opponents in remaining determined, focused, confident and in control under pressure" (p. 209).

Athletes can acquire and train psychological skills by systematic and long-term psychological training oriented and supervised by an expert in sport psychology. Thus, it is important to know how to coach and counsel athletes at the same time. Psychology is a fundamental element of an athlete's good performance.

Basic concepts

Concept of counseling

The objective of counseling is to help coaches and athletes understand and solve their psychological and social problems. The function of counseling is to provide emotional support to athletes in critical situations. Sport psychologists, as counselors, through interaction with the athlete, provide the environment that allows self-actualization to emerge from within the person. According to Henschen (2005), the characteristics of excellent counselor/athlete relationships are genuineness, empathy, confidence, respect, positive attitude, positive emotional support, social perception, and effective listening and communication.

Concept of psychological training

The purpose of mental training (MT) is to develop and improve psychological skills and competencies (cognitive, motivational, emotional, and social) of athletes, coaches, and teams by applying psychological techniques and MT programs. The main goals of psychological training are to develop and improve cognitive, emotional, motivational, and social skills of athletes and coaches; stabilize emotional behavior during competition (emotional self-control); accelerate and optimize the process of rehabilitation and recovery; improve communication processes (leadership and communication); and develop cohesion and team building.

Psychological techniques

Mental training can be applied through different forms of psychological techniques, such as imagery, attention control, stress control, and self-motivation. Imagery is the systematic and repetitive visualization of motor skills, techniques, strategies, or complex situations. The purpose of attention control training is to develop and apply different styles of attention control depending on the situation. Concentration is the ability to focus the attention on relevant stimuli and to maintain high concentration levels during a certain period of time. The aim of stress control training is to develop and maintain an optimal activation level before and during competition. The purpose of self-motivation training is to learn and apply motivational techniques in order to regulate one's own level of motivation, to overcome obstacles, and to persist in critical situations.

Model of peak performance

The pyramid model of peak performance consists of five sets of factors, all of which reciprocally interact to influence athlete's performance. Specifically, the top of the pyramid represents a task-specific IPS that leads to peak performance and results from three sets of internal factors:

a. fundamental personality, motivational and philosophical characteristics, and dispositions;

b. psychological skills/strategies for facilitating peak performance;

c. coping with adversity strategies.

The area surrounding the pyramid is the physical, social, psychological, and organizational environment in which the athletes perform and train (Figure 11.1).

The personality and motivational characteristics of the athletes included their level of trait confidence, goal orientation, trait anxiety, attention style, perfectionism, hope, and optimism. The philosophical orientation already emphasized the importance of the athletes' understanding of their own reasons for athletic involvement.

Included in the psychological skills/strategies for facilitating peak performance are factors such as focusing on process or performance goals at the moment of competition, using imagery, applying

relaxation techniques, and developing specific mental preparation routines. The application of these strategies increases the probability of success by helping to create an IPS.

Elite athletes can learn to cope with stress resulting from their own and others' performance expectations, the media, injury, time demands, and general life concerns. Thus, they must also have the psychological skills (e.g., imagery, goal setting process, relaxation) to cope with those adversities that could interfere with achieving their IPS.

Elite athletes compete and train in a physical, social, psychological, and organizational environment that can both facilitate and disrupt their psychological state. Situations such as national sport organization policy, team selection controversies, bad officiating, lack of finances, and family/friends concerns disrupt their psychological state. Therefore, coaches, trainers, athletes, clinicians, and sport scientists must recognize and consider these factors when planning interventions or designing investigations. Gould (2001) suggested that the pyramid model for peak performance could be used by athletes and coaches to guide professional practice in an effort to request their opinions on what areas they need to develop.

Model of the interdisciplinary cooperation

The contribution of sport science to modern sport is unquestionable. The involvement of specialized professionals, such as physiologists, nutritionists, physiotherapists, biomechanists, and physicians, is of great importance because of the increasing competitiveness within Paralympic sports. The sport psychologist used to be attached, but not integrated, in this context. In the model of interdisciplinary cooperation, the sport psychologist has to provide various types of support to the team (Figure 11.2). The sport psychologist can create interventions (athlete, coach, and team oriented) in various aspects of training in order to enhance and maintain performance. In order to accelerate the rehabilitation process of injured athletes, sports psychologists cooperate with physiotherapists, applying mental techniques for rehabilitation. It is recommended that sport psychologists develop a good working relationship

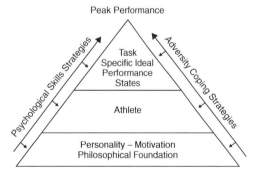

Figure 11.1 Model of peak performance.

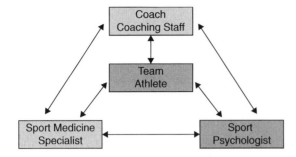

Figure 11.2 Model of interdisciplinary cooperation.

and communication with the head coach and other members of the coaching staff.

Diagnosing psychological abilities for action takes into consideration the cognitive, behavioral, and social aspects. A method for applying these aspects in practice is presented in the following section as an example. Practical diagnosis and intervention measures are also considered.

Diagnosis: the first step

Diagnosis is a determining factor for the success of the work in sports psychology as a whole. Its function is to indicate to the coaching team the areas requiring MT. The characteristics of each modality of sports are taken into consideration in deciding which tests should be applied. At the outset, the use of interviews and basic psychometric tools is recommended to establish a profile for each athlete, as well as to obtain initial information about the individual and collective requirements of the group.

The diagnosis may also be organized into cognitive, behavioral, and social areas. The real need for and appropriateness of the information generated should be evaluated with the aim of improving the intervention process in the future. From the cognitive point of view, decision-making, attentional and perception processes, and tactical thinking and behavior can be evaluated. There is ample opportunity for the evaluation of the behavioral aspect, including stress, motivation, overtraining, mood, discipline, among others. The social aspect is evaluated by the components of communication, leadership, and sociometric factors.

Intervention: developing abilities and minimizing problems

As explained earlier, intervention is tailored to the requirements identified in the diagnosis for each modality or athlete. Accordingly, examples of applications to some Paralympic modalities, as well as supporting theories that help to elaborate new intervention methods, will be presented.

Psychological routines for competition

According to Samulski (2009), "a psychological routine represents a combination of different physiological and psychological techniques with the aim of stabilising the emotional behavior of athletes and helping them to direct their attention to the stimuli relevant to the task to be carried out." Studies show that athletes who apply mental preparation routines before or during competition perform better than athletes who do not. The elements of a psychological routine may be:

- goal setting,
- regulation of stress and activation levels,
- imagery and visualization techniques,
- mental attention and concentration techniques,
- positive self-motivational statements in decisive situations.

The psychological routines can be developed and applied in individual and group sports, such as psychological routines for swimming (Table 11.1) and table tennis (Table 11.2), as presented here.

As can be seen from these tables, the function of the psychological routine in swimming is to help the athletes to maintain focus on the goal. Athletes report that it is very common to be preoccupied with the adversary's performance or to feel insecure because an adversary with a better time is in the same competition. Above all, psychological routine (see Table 11.1) helps the athletes to avoid negative thoughts (Table 11.3).

The routine for table tennis (see Table 11.2) has a specific aim, which is to help athletes make decisions and define the best strategy to be employed in the match. A basic aspect in this modality is the attitude to adopt before the beginning of each athletic contest.

Table 11.1 Psychological routine for swimming.

Swimming competition routine

Before (1 day)

Care with quality of sleep, light food at night, warm bath to relax, and calm music (at low volume) to induce relaxation

Before (on the day)

Wake on time (mentalize success)
Breakfast without excess
At the venue: warm-up routine (free swimming and positive self-talk)
Check in: 15 min before start
In the preparation room: psychoregulation routine, visualization of the competition, motivation through self-talk, and positive thinking

During

On the chair: psychoregulation routine followed by visualizing the competition.
On the starting block: psychoregulation routine, mentalization of the goal, state of alertness (maximum concentration for the starting shot)

After

Rest
Physical and mental relaxation
Postcompetition analysis: positive (reinforce) and negative (what to improve) aspects
Precompetition analysis: determination and analysis for the next competition

Table 11.2 Psychological routine for table tennis.

Table tennis competition routine

Before

20 min before start
Check and analyze adversary (mentalization of style, strengths, and weaknesses)
Planning of tactical behavior (A, offensive; B, defensive)
2 min—physical and mental warm-up—motivation routine

During

Between sets (2 min)
Between points (A, serving; B, receiving)
1 time per set (1 min)

After

Physical and mental relaxation
Postmatch analysis positive (reinforce) and negative (what to improve) aspects
Prematch analysis determination and analysis of next adversary

The athletes' awareness of factors such as their level of alertness, emotional and cognitive aspects (particularly their ability to concentrate), as well as of their technical capacity, helps to decide the tactics to be employed (Figure 11.3). Hence, the athletes evaluate their condition in the moment and choose their tactic for either offense or defense. In sports such as table tennis, an error can be decisive for the match outcome. Figure 11.4 shows important considerations about the relationship between the technical demand level and concentration level. An error is a relationship between the task demand level and an incompatible concentration level. The athletes must be capable of perceiving the concentration level oscillations and adjusting to the demands of the task to be performed to minimize the possibility of error.

Table 11.3 presents a set of important complementary techniques for athletes in a range of situations. MT is a very useful technique that enables athletes to plan and rehearse the procedures to be performed in competition. Negative thoughts are, normally, a problem in various competitive situations, and keeping the athletes focused on productive factors or on problem solving is a challenge. Finally, developing and improving the state of alertness is a necessary ability in many modalities of sports.

Finally, psychoregulation is a type of routine that aims to maintain the athletes at optimum

Table 11.3 Complementary techniques for competition.

Complementary techniques

Visualization of the competition (mental training)

The athlete must, in first place, induce a state of relaxation. For this, the athlete may use one of the described psychoregulation techniques (Figure 11.5). An optimal low activation level is ideal for cognitive tasks.

After achieving the state of relaxation, the athlete must, with closed eyes, imagine the participation in the competition in real time. Normally, the imagery time is very close to the athlete's time in the competition.

The visualization of the trial has several functions, depending on the sports modality. In sports such as artistic gymnastics, for example, visualization may boost the confidence and concentration capacity before the competition.

Block out negative thinking

Athletes commonly have negative thoughts, particularly after poor performance or when they find themselves under some type of pressure. The best way to block out negative thoughts is to make the athletes occupy the mind with productive things, such as tactical planning, elaboration of a plan for solving problems, among others.

When affected by negative thoughts, the athletes must first think of something else to block them out (e.g., imagine a road sign =STOP=). Next, the athletes must mentalize positive images, followed by productive thoughts (as described earlier).

State of alertness

The maximum point of concentration that enables the athletes to respond optimally to the stimuli that arise in the environment. Depending on the situation, the athletes must know how to manipulate their state of alertness, because if the stimulus delays too much, or appears too quickly, the athletes will lose out in responding.

To achieve the state of alertness, a specific amount of time is necessary. A gradual increase in the concentration level takes place, and this may be sustained for a specific time. After this time, the concentration level gradually falls.

The time that each athlete succeeds in maintaining the state of alertness varies. In practice, it is possible to increase the time that the state of alertness is maintained.

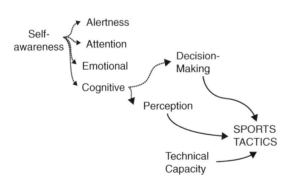

Figure 11.3 Factors that interfere in defining sports tactics.

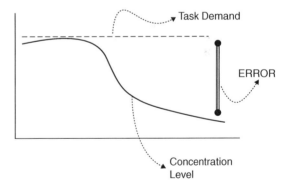

Figure 11.4 Influence of psychological factors on the occurrence of an error.

performance level. Figure 11.5 shows that for the best performance, there is an optimum concentration of activation energy. Athletes' performance level decreases either above or below this optimum level of performance. The gray area represents the region of optimum activation. The optimum activation zone is circled on the diagram. When the energy level fluctuates, whether to a higher or lower level, athletes must apply psychoregulation techniques.

Work is done with four basic indicators to achieve psychoregulation: respiration, language, thinking,

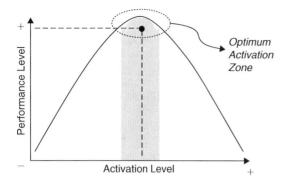

Figure 11.5 The importance of psychoregulation.

and movement, which are manipulated as required (activation or relaxation):

a. activation

Respiration: increasing breathing frequency

Language: verbalization of reinforcement words or phrases ("Power!," "Go for it!," etc.)

Thinking: visualization of images of speed, power, and encouragement

Movement: moving more quickly

b. relaxation

Respiration: reductions of breathing frequency (breathe in deeply and expire slowly)

Language: verbalizations of calming words or phrases ("calm down!," "relax!," etc.)

Thinking: visualization of calming images (a lake, the sea, mountains, etc.)

Movement: moving more slowly

Technical–tactical behavior in team sports

Technical–tactical behavior is a determining factor of team success. Its results are important in helping the coaching team make decisions to increase team effectiveness in different areas. The aim is also to motivate the athletes, serving as an objective element of evaluation of their performance. Decision-making, the foundation of technical–tactical behavior, is a complex process that involves many variables. In competitive sports, failure in making decisions can lead to errors and loss of performance.

The athletes' decision-making procedure begins, in truth, very early (Figure 11.6). There is a period of response readiness that starts with the perception of a stimulus for readiness, which activates the decision-making system. The next step is the selection of the relevant stimulus that guides decision-making and triggers the response (motor action). Feedback is an inherent mechanism in the decision-making process, informing the individual of the quality and effectiveness of the action.

The quality of the perception is fundamental to the process. Further details of the decision-making process are given in Figure 11.7. One of the biggest differences between novices and experienced athletes usually begins in their overview of the situation. The correct selection of stimuli enables faster decision-making as a whole and allows the athletes to anticipate actions more effectively. Athletes make decisions about their action based on sensory information and then perform it. Another important aspect is to have alternative actions on standby for any potential action. The process ends with the evaluation of the action, and the next process begins immediately with the search for new sensory information.

Naturally, decision-making may suffer various interferences that lead to error. The most common interferences are fatigue, distraction, and an incompatibility between concentration and the demands of the task. According to Noce and Samulski (2001), it is very difficult for athletes to maintain a high level of concentration during an entire match or competition (depending, of course, on factors such as the duration of the task). The level of concentration must be sufficient to maintain the quality of technical performance required by each action. An error occurs when athletes fail to perceive that the concentration level has declined and do not attain the level required by the task (see Figure 11.4).

It is important that athletes understand and recognize the importance of the perception of their own attentional capacity. The more refined and precise a movement is, the greater the need for conscious control and, normally, the greater the amount of energy required by the task. To minimize the frequency of errors, athletes have to only adjust

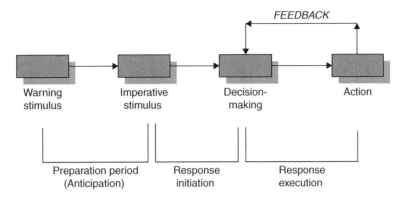

Figure 11.6 Response cognitive procedures (adapted from Tenenbaum, 2001).

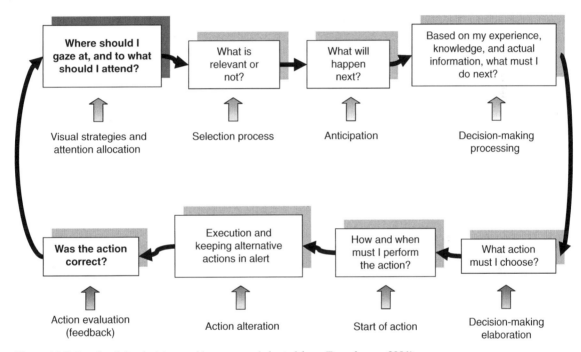

Figure 11.7 Details of the decision-making process (adapted from Tenenbaum, 2001).

the action demands to the level of concentration available at the time.

Mental training

Mental training is a very useful tool for improving the performance of athletes, whether in learning new techniques and tactics or in stabilizing and optimizing performance for competition through the application of specific strategies.

Samulski (2009) identified MT as "imagining motor skills, sports techniques, and tactical strategies in a planned, repeated, and conscious way." For Eberspächer (1995), MT is "the planned repetition of the conscious imagining of an action in a practical way."

There are different concepts and visions of MT; some see MT as a complex of different mental skills, such as goal setting, increasing self-confidence, development of concentration, visualization and imagination, activation and anxiety control, and mental routines for competition. It should be clear that the latter concept of MT as a complex of different mental skills is being used in this chapter.

According to Eberspächer (1995), MT can be implemented in three ways:

1. Training by self-talk: Mentally repeating the practice of the movement in a conscious way using self-talk.

2. Training by self-observation: Individuals must use "mental eyes" to observe a detailed film of them practicing the movement, or trying to imagine themselves appearing in a film about practicing movements. Here, individuals assume the role of spectators of themselves, i.e., they observe themselves from an *external perspective.*

3. Ideomotor training: Individuals must update, constantly and in detail, their internal perspective of the physical movement; they must seek to transfer themselves into the movement so that they can feel and live the sensation of the internal processes that occur when carrying out the movement. It is advisable to use self-verbalization training to gradually improve the athletes' ability to imagine the movement, particularly for athletes who, at the beginning of ideomotor training, have difficulty in identifying with the internal perspective of the movement, or for those who do not have experience of MT. The second methodological step is then self-observation. The goal of ideomotor training consists of entering into a mental state that enables the real development of performance potential. According to Weinberg and Gould (1999), "athletes can reconstruct, by the imagination, positive past experiences or visualise future events with the objective of mentally preparing themselves for the performance."

Mental training is directed at two objectives in sports: movements and situations. Movements are specific motor skills developed in sports (techniques) and situations, and the tactical and strategic sports actions within a specific context (Figure 11.8).

The imagery in these objectives can be achieved in three temporal strategies: anticipatory, integrative, and retroactive.

In *anticipatory imagery*, the aim is to imagine an action to be conducted so as to analyze it, seeking to control the internal and external factors, and

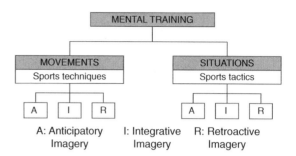

Figure 11.8 Mental training strategies.

optimize the technical, tactical, and psychological conditions for performing the action.

In *integrative imagery*, the aim is to imagine the action during the competition as a way to integrate the cognitive, motor, and psychological stimuli, seeking to achieve improved performance.

In *retroactive imagery* (*mental replay*), i.e., the visualization of any action already conducted, the basic function is to analyze and evaluate past actions, so as to enable positive *feedback* for the regulation of the motor, technical, and psychological aspects of future actions.

Requirements for implementing a program

According to Eberspächer (1995), the requirements for MT are:

- state of relaxation,
- one's own experience,
- one's own perspective,
- profound experiences.

At the start of any MT session, the athletes must first enter a state of relaxation, because it is only in this state, with the mind free of thoughts that disturb or distract their concentration, that it is possible to work at 100%. The concentration capacity must be maintained.

Motor skills and sports techniques must have been tried in advance, because something that has never been tried cannot be mentally trained. The imagined movement to be used as the basis for the MT must be inserted in the movement that the individual is capable of executing. Of course, it is possible for anyone to adopt specific aspects or characteristics of the movement, from a model, transform them into one's level of possibilities and, later, direct one's imagination to the movement.

Mental training works when one can experience and naturally update the performance of the movement that is to be trained. To succeed in passing every detail of the movement from thoughts into the correct form, the colors must be "seen," the sounds "heard," the smells "smelt," "feeling" the movement in its entirety and in each of its components mentally (Figure 11.9). This type of "experiencing in the imagination" enables, as various scientific experiments and studies have proven, physiological reactions such as increased heart rate, perspiration, and muscle contraction.

In practice, it has been proven extremely effective to practice the movement first as a "self-talk," i.e., to mark by means of self-talk the path of the movement, as long as the self-talk does not "rewind" or jump from one part to another, and does not distract from other training contents. In this way, training can be more effectively controlled.

Four-step training model

Eberspächer (1995) developed a four-step MT program.

Step 1:
The practice of the movement to be trained must be stimulated in the brain through the different senses. The athletes are required to describe the experience acquired in the imagination, i.e., describe the progress of the movement in words, so that the coach

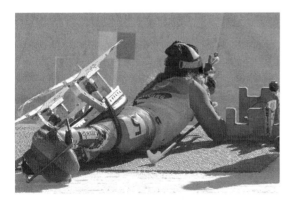

Figure 11.9 The biathlon takes great concentration that can be enhanced by mental training. Reproduced courtesy of Lieven Coudenys.

can judge whether the imagery of the movement in question is correct or not. In this way, possible failure or weaknesses in the process are eliminated immediately. The description of the movement may be either oral or written.

Step 2:
Athletes must learn the correct progression of the movement continuously recited by the coach. In this way, they are able to repeat the progress of the movement subvocally using "self-talk," updating it during the action. In other words, individuals explain the phases and principle characteristics of the moment to be trained to themselves and then repeat them internally. When these phrases can be imagined without difficulty, it is possible to proceed to step 3.

Step 3:
This consists of systematizing the individual elements of each phase of the movement and making them available in a structure. Here it is necessary to stress the so-called key points of the movement, i.e., the moments that are decisive for its performance. For example, key points of movement in tennis are:
1. throwing the ball into the air;
2. contraction arc;
3. pulling the racquet back;
4. fully extending the body;
5. hitting the ball with the racquet.

If the ball is not thrown in an optimal way above the head, it is not possible to carry out the serve correctly (Figure 11.10). If the first key point is not mastered, it is not possible to establish correct foundations for the movement to progress successfully. When the different key points of the movement are well defined, it is possible to continue to the next MT step.

Step 4:
The key points of the movement must be marked symbolically. These symbols encompass the different steps/key points of the action in a summary in such a way that the motor program for executing the movement can be recalled quickly and accurately.

A discus thrower symbolically marked the key points of the throw movement in the following way: rotate, take position for the throw, throw. By means of this symbolic marking of the key point

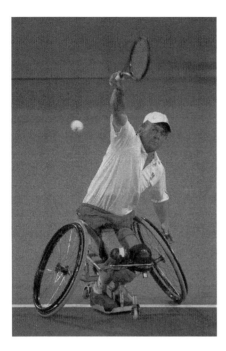

Figure 11.10 In wheelchair tennis, if the ball is not thrown in an optimal way above the head, it is not possible to carry out the serve correctly. If this first key point is not mastered, it is not possible to establish correct foundations for the movement to progress successfully. Reproduced courtesy of Lieven Coudenys.

of the movement, the athlete is able to emphasize the rhythm of the movement, and, hence, reinforce its execution in a simpler way. When athletes have reached step 4, they can already recall the movement in their imagination at any moment. Progressing correctly through the four steps allows the athlete to remember one or more steps without committing errors as needed, i.e., assimilating corrections from the coach.

Practical procedures

The acquisition of the technique of MT, according to Eberspächer (1995), happens in eight steps.

Step 1:
Choice of the sports technique that one wishes to mentally train.

Step 2:
Writing in a detailed and concrete way the development of the complete movement and what is necessary for the execution of the sports technique, including the inner sensations of the movement.

Step 3:
Reading and analyzing what has been written and described regarding the movement over the following 3 days, for half an hour each day; trying to memorize the progress of the movement very intensely; trying to imagine, while reading, that the movement is being executed. If this level of perfection is achieved, next is trying to obtain the first and detailed "analysis from the perspective of the internal camera lens"; observing this "internal perspective" over several days, for 15 min, very intensely.

Step 4:
When the "internal perspective" is reproduced without any problem, one can identify five or six core or "key" points of the movement considered, determining the correct execution of the movement. Trying to move, in one's thoughts, from one key point to another, in such a way that imagining the technique occupies a time period similar to that necessary in practice, exercising the "reduced internal perspective" until one feels confident to master it.

Step 5:
Describing and classifying the key points of the movement with short words; trying to adapt oneself to the rhythm of the movement using these words as supporting points. Exercising the use of this approach (for not more than 15 min at a time), until it has an internal duration similar to the effective motor performance of the technique.

Step 6:
Mentally exercising this level for another two or three sessions. If one has difficulty in imagining the movement, return to step 2 or 3, as required.

Step 7:
Combining (after agreement with one's coach) the MT with the performance (e.g., two mental repetitions, 10 motor performances), in accordance with the proposed technique or combined technique.

Step 8:
Subsequent MT of the pre- and postpreparation phases in short pauses or interruptions in a competition or match.

When using these techniques, athletes and coaches should take the following into consideration:

• Only movements in which one has prior experience should be trained, i.e., those performed at least once before.
• Principally at the beginning, exercise must be detailed and accurate. MT must be started only in a relaxed state.
• Deep concentration must be maintained during training.
• Always exercise from one's own perspective.
• MT must not be longer than performing the action itself.
• The situation must be updated to be as real as possible (using all of the senses).

The following should be avoided:

• Overdoing its application.
• Skipping phases of the movement in steps 2 and 3.
• Negative thoughts (e.g., thinking of poor actions).
• Blocking your thoughts.
• Measuring the total time of the duration of the technique (mental or actual) inaccurately.

The main objectives of MT are to develop mental performance abilities, to create an emotional state suitable for training and competitions, and, finally, to develop a good quality of life for the athletes, coaching staff, and other people involved in the sport. MT must be considered an element of the daily training of athletes and coaches (Figure 11.11). Before applying MT, a precise diagnosis of the initial mental conditions of the athletes is necessary. The MT must be carried out with permanent evaluation and monitoring to assess and control the processes and their effects. The MT must be applied by professionals who are well qualified in the different methods and programs. The MT should be applied to the athletes, coaches, directors, referees, athletes' parents, sports reporters, and other people connected to competitive sports, being important to apply MT before, during, and after the competition. MT should be applied at the start of sports practice so as to create a work culture in this area and to stimulate mental abilities in the young, and develop specific MT programs for each modality and situation. MT can be applied to accelerate the recovery from injuries, and improve the performance, health, and quality of life of athletes.

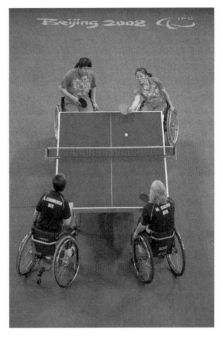

Figure 11.11 Mental training can become complicated in team sports. Reproduced courtesy of Lieven Coudenys.

The Brazilian model of counseling Olympic athletes

In 2004, a team of 10 sport psychologists were responsible for the psychological preparation of Brazilian Olympic athletes and teams (242 athletes and 7 teams). The actions of psychological evaluation and intervention were oriented and supervised by the consultant in sport psychology of the Brazilian Olympic Committee (COB), Dr. Dietmar Samulski. The psychological evaluation was an important part of the interdisciplinary evaluation of the Brazilian athletes. Before the application of intervention techniques, consent forms were obtained from all athletes and coaches.

Psychological strategies and intervention techniques applied in the preparation period

During the preparation period from January to August 2004, the following psychological strategies were applied:

• individual-oriented preparation of athletes (MT and emotional control);

• team-oriented preparation (group cohesion and group dynamics);
• psychological support of the coaches (leadership, motivation, and communication strategies);
• psychological support of the Brazilian Olympic delegation (concept of Brazilian Olympic family, psychological guidelines of behavior during Olympics, code of ethics: no doping and fair play).

The most frequently applied intervention techniques in this period were confidence building; self-motivation and goal setting; relaxation techniques; anxiety control and stress management; attention control; self-verbalization, imagery, and MT; coping strategies; and pain control. The consultant in sport psychology was integrated in the Brazilian delegation as a member of the medical staff. He was responsible for the psychological assistance and support of the athletes and the teams during the Olympic Games.

Psychological problems and intervention techniques applied during the Games

The psychological problems most frequently detected in athletes during the Games were adaptation problems, concentration problems, precompetitive anxiety, psychological pressure of the media, and emotional problems during competition, frustration after losing, and injuries (Table 11.4).

One of the main objectives of the psychological support was to develop and optimize psychological routines to be applied by the athletes before and during competition. Most of the athletes applied their own routines and rituals developed during their sports careers. Psychological routines are critical for maintaining mental concentration and emotional stability and control during competition,

Table 11.4 Selected examples of psychological problems and applied intervention techniques in Brazilian athletes during the Olympic Games in Athens 2004—Individual sports.

Athletes	Sports	Psychological problems	Intervention techniques
1	Judo	Lock of self-esteem Competitive anxiety	Relaxation and deep respiration Positive attitude and concentration
2	Tae-kwon-do	Pre-competitive anxiety Physical debility	Relaxation and recovery Competitive routines
3	Wrestling	Pre-competitive anxiety	Relaxation and deep respiration Concentration successful
4	Swimming (50 m)	Anxiety and humor changes Emotional instability	Deep respiration and visualization of the competition Activation, motivation, and verbalization
5	Diving	Recovery problems Anxiety and insecurity	Relaxation and deep respiration Competitive routines
6	Synchronized swimming	Pre-competitive anxiety Worry about refereeing	Relaxation and deep respiration Visualization of the routine
7	Sailing	Lack of self-confidence Signs of stress	Relaxation and deep respiration Positive verbalization
8	Triathlon	Adaptation problems Problems of recovery	Concentration before/between competitions Relaxation and recovery between competitions
9	Mountain bike	Competitive anxiety Insecurity about performance	Relaxation and positive attitude Mental rountines and concentration
10	Athletics(marathon)	Pre-competitive anxiety Stress and insomnia	Relaxation and deep respiration Strees control and competitive routines
11	Table tennis	Concentration problems Pre-competitive anxiety	Concentration and visualization techniques Mental routines
12	Shooting	Concentration	Deep respiration and concentration

especially in situations of decision-making and high psychological pressure. Thus, the intervention techniques applied during the competition were mainly competitive routines, besides others like confidence building, relaxation techniques, anxiety control, stress management, imagery and MT, coping strategies, and psychological pain control (see Table 11.4).

Conclusions

Most of the athletes and coaches gave positive feedback on the psychological support during the Games. There was an excellent cooperation and interaction between the sport psychologist and other members of the medical staff, especially with the physiotherapist regarding the rehabilitation and recovery of injured athletes. In the next Paralympic Games, it was recommended to integrate more sport psychologists into the delegation in order to more effectively support the athletes, coaches, and teams.

It was also observed during the Games that some of the national coaches demonstrated problems related to effective leadership, team building, motivation, and communication. For this reason, it was recommended that the Brazilian Paralympic Committee should offer coaches' education programs in the future in order to develop psychological and social skills. The coaches' education programs should consider topics such as philosophy of coaching, human values, motivation, leadership, and communication skills.

Psychological preparation has to be an integrated and long-term preparation process, oriented and supervised by an expert in coaching and counseling. Specially, young athletes need more intensive mental preparation and emotional support. There was also a recommendation to integrate the Olympic and Paralympic actions and the development of international cooperation with international governing bodies such as the International Olympic Committee (IOC) and the IPC. Sport psychology is not the only key to sport excellence, but it is one of the most important and crucial elements for success.

References

Eberspächer, H. (1995). *Mental Training: A Manual for Trainers and Athletes* (Spanish). INDE Publicaciones, Zaragoza.

Gould, D. (2001). The psychology of Olympic excellence and its development. In: A. Papaioannou, M. Goudas & Y. Theodorakis (eds.) *Proceedings of the 10th World Congress on Sport Psychology*, pp. 51–61. Christodoulidi Publications, Thessaloniki/Hellas.

Gould, D., Greenleaf, C., Guinan, D., et al. (1998). Factors influencing Atlanta Olympian performance. *Olympic Coach*, **8(4)**, 9–11.

Gould, D., Dieffenbach, K. & Moffet, A. (2002). Psychological characteristics and their development in Olympic champions. *Journal of Applied Sport Psychology*, **14(3)**, 172–204.

Hackfort, D. (2006). A conceptual framework and fundamental issues for investigating the development of peak performance in sports. In: D. Hackfort & G. Tenenbaum (eds.) *Essential Processes for Attaining Peak Performance*, pp. 10–25. Meyer & Meyer Sport, Oxford.

Hackfort, D. & Munzert, J. (2005). Mental simulation. In: D. Hackfort, J. Duda & R. Lidor (eds.) *Handbook of Research in Applied Sport and Exercise Psychology: International Perspectives*, pp. 3–18. Fitness Information Technology, Morgantown, WV.

Henschen, K. (2005). Mental practice—skill oriented. In: D. Hackfort, J. Duda & R. Lidor (eds.) *Handbook of Research in Applied Sport and Exercise Psychology: International Perspectives*, pp. 19–36. Fitness Information Technology, Morgantown, WV.

Jones, G., Hanton, S. & Connaughton, D. (2002). What is this thing called mental toughness? An investigation of elite sport performers. *Journal of Applied Sport Psychology*, **14**, 205–218.

Noce, F. & Samulski, D. (2001). Attention and athlete performance. In: K. Lemos & E. Silami-Garcia (eds.) *Temas Atuais em EF e esportes VI* (Portuguese), pp. 173–182. Belo Horizonte, Editora UFMG.

Samulski, D. (2003). Psychological support for paralympians. In: IOC Medical Commission (ed.) *Abstract of the VII IOC Olympic World Congress on Sport Sciences*. Athens, October 7–11, 2003. Behavioral Section, 3A.

Samulski, D. (2009). *Sports Psychology: Concepts and New Perspectives* (Portuguese). Manole, São Paulo.

Tenenbaum, G. (2001). Cognition and expertise in sport. *9th Brazilian Conference of Sports Psychology* (Portuguese). School of Physical Education, Belo Horizonte.

Weinberg, R. & Gould, D. (1999). *Psychological Foundations of Sport Psychology*. Human Kinetics, Champaign, IL.

Recommended readings

Anjos, D.R. (2005). *Elaboration and Validation of an Instrument of Subjective Perception of Stressing Factors in Physically Disabled Athletes* (Master's Dissertation in Portuguese). School of Physical Education of UFMG, Belo Horizonte.

Anshel, M. (2005). Strategies for preventing and managing stress and anxiety in sport. In: D. Hackfort, J. Duda & R. Lidor (eds.) *Handbook of Research in Applied Sport and Exercise Psychology: International Perspectives*, pp. 199–216. Fitness Information Technology, Morgantown, WV.

Brazilian Paralympic Committee (Comitê Paraolímpico Brasileiro, CPB) (2004). Paralympics: Evolution 2004 (Portuguese). Available at: www.brasilparaolimpico.org.br (accessed on November 10, 2005).

Crews, D. (1993). Self regulation strategies in sport and exercise. In: R. Singer (ed.) *Handbook of Research on Sport Psychology*, pp. 557–568. Macmillan, New York.

Gordon, S. (2005). Identification and development of mental toughness. In: *Proceedings of the 11th World Congress of Sport Psychology*. CD-ROM, Sydney, Australia.

Gould, D. & Damarjian, N. (2000). Mental training in sports. In: B. Elliott & J. Mester (eds.) *Sports Training*, pp. 99–152. Phorte Editora, São Paulo.

Greco, P. & Benda, R. (2001). *Universal Sports Initiation*, Vol. 1 (Portuguese). Health, Belo Horizonte.

Grosser, M. & Neumaier, A. (1982). *Techniktraining*. BLV Sportwissen, München.

Hanin, Y. (1999). Individual zones of optimal functioning (IZOF) model: emotion–performance relationships in sport. In: Y. Hanin (ed.) *Emotions in Sport*. Human Kinetics, Champaign, IL.

Jackson, S. & Csikszentmihalyi, M. (1999). *Flow in Sports: The Keys to Optimal Experiences and Performances*. Human Kinetics, Champaign, IL.

Kröger, C. & Roth, K. (2002). *Ball School: Essential Education for Beginners in Sports Games* (Portuguese). Phorte, São Paulo.

Loehr, J. (1982). *Athletic Excellence: Mental Toughness Training for Sports*. Forum, New York.

Loehr, J. (1986). *Mental Toughness Training for Sports: Achieving Athletic Excellence*. Stephen Greene Press, Lexington, MA.

Loehr, J. (1990). *The Mental Game*. Penguin Books, London.

Mello, M.T. (2002). *Paralympics of Sidney 2000: Evaluation and Prescription of Training of Brazilian Athletes*. Atheneu, São Paulo.

Mello, M.T. (2004). *Clinical Evaluation and Aptitude of Brazilian Paralympic Athletes: Concepts, Methods, and Results*. Atheneu, São Paulo.

Moran, A. (2005). Training attention and concentration skills in athletes. In: D. Hackfort, J. Duda & R. Lidor (eds.) *Handbook of Research in Applied Sport and Exercise Psychology: International Perspectives*, pp. 61–74. Fitness Information Technology, Morgantown, WV.

Nideffer, R. (1985). *Athlete's Guide to Mental Training*. Human Kinetics, Champaign, IL.

Nideffer, R. (1992). *Psyched to Win*. Leisure Press, Champaign, IL.

Nideffer, R. (1993). Attention control training. In: R. Singer, M. Murphey & L. Tennant (eds.) *Handbook of Research on Sport Psychology*, 542–553. Macmillan Publishing Company, New York.

Noce, F. (1999). *Analysis of Psychological Stress in Elite Volleyball Athletes: A Comparative Study of Sex* (Master's Dissertation in Physical Education/Sports Training—Portuguese). Physical Education School of UFMG, Belo Horizonte.

Noce, F. & Samulski, D. (1996). Psychological balance can define the winning team. *Revista Vôlei Técnico*, Rio de Janeiro, **7**, 19–27 (Portuguese).

Noce, F. & Samulski, D. (2002). Analysis of psychological stress in elite volleyball setters. *Revista Paulista de Educação Física*, **16**(2), 113–129 (Portuguese).

Orlick, T. (1986). *Coaches Training Manual to Psyching for Sport*. Human Kinetics, Champaign, IL.

Orlick, T. (2000). *In Pursuit of Excellence*. Human Kinetics, Champaign, IL.

Paivo, A. (1985). Cognitive and motivational functions of imagery in human performance. *Canadian Journal of Applied Sport Sciences*, **10**, 22–28.

Samulski, D. & Anjos, D. (2005). Contributions of sports psychology to the development of Paralympic sports. In: *Proceedings of the 2nd International Symposium of Sports Psychology and 3rd III Parana Symposium of Sports Psychology*. Curitiba, 95–97.

Samulski, D. & Noce, F. (2002a). Psychological evaluation of sports. In: M.T. Mello (ed.) *Paralympics of Sidney 2000: Evaluation and Prescription of Training of Brazilian Athletes*, pp. 99–133. Atheneu, São Paulo.

Samulski, D. & Noce, F. (2002b). Psychological profile of Brazilian paralympic athletes. *Revista Brasileira de Medicina do Esporte*, **8**(4), 157–166 (Portuguese).

Samulski, D., Noce, F., Anjos, D. & Lopes, M. (2004). Psychological evaluation. In: M.T. Mello (ed.) *Clinical Evaluation and Physical Aptitude of Brazilian Paralympic Athletes: Concepts, Methods, and Results*, pp. 135–158. Atheneu, São Paulo.

Samulski, D., Noce, F. & Raboni, M. (2005). Psychological support of Brazilian athletes during the Athens 2004 Paralympics: a practical experience report.

In: E. Silami-Garcia & K. Lemos (eds.) *Temas Atuais X em Educação Física e Esportes* (Portuguese). Saúde, Belo Horizonte.

Schmidt, R. & Wrisberg, C. (2001). *Learning and Performance: A Problem-Based Approach of Learning* (Portuguese). ArtMed, Porto Alegre.

Starkes, L. & Ericsson, A. (2003). *Expert Performance in Sports*. Human Kinetics, Champaign, IL.

Suinn, R. (1993). Imagery. In: R. Singer (ed.) *Handbook of Research on Sport Psychology*. Macmillan, New York.

Ugrinowitsch, H. (2003). *Effect of the Level of Stabilization on the Performance and Type of Disturbance of the Adaptative Process in Motor Learning* (Doctorate Thesis—Portuguese). School of Physical Education and Sports of Universidade de São Paulo, São Paulo.

Unestahl, L. (1989). Mental skills for sports and life. In: *Proceedings of the 7th World Congress in Sport Psychology*. Singapore, 109–113.

PART 4
BEST PRACTICES

Chapter 12
Preparation for the Paralympic Summer Games: heat, humidity, pollution

Marco Túlio de Mello[1], Sílvio de Araújo Fernandes Jr[1], Andressa da Silva[1], Luiz Oswaldo Carneiro Rodrigues[2], Emilson Colantonio[3], Marcos Gonçalves de Santana[4] and Sergio Tufik[1]

[1]Departamento de Psicobiologia, Universidade Federal de Sao Paulo, São Paulo, Brazil
[2]Departamento de Educação Física, Universidade Federal de Minas Gerais, Belo Horizonte, Brazil
[3]Departamento de Biociências, Universidade Federal de Sao Paulo, Santos, Brazil
[4]Campus Jataí, Universidade Federal de Goiás, Jataí, Brazil

Introduction

The personal and the sports success of people with disabilities (PWDs) require a combination of motivation, work, training, sacrifice, encouragement, and opportunities. Health-care professionals assist PWDs overcome their difficulties and promote their rehabilitation from congenital and acquired lesions, including medullar lesions, traumas, amputations, blindness, and hearing impairment, among many others.

In the postwar period (after 1945), systematic encouragement toward the practice of adapted sports became an essential part of the medical and social rehabilitation of these patients. The inclusion of sports activities into the daily life of PWDs provides them with the challenges of overcoming their limitations, engages their opponents, and achieves records at the highest levels, and thus increases their competitive intensity. A demand arose for the creation of specific training and competitions at increasingly higher levels.

As a result, Paralympic sports have gained importance every year, and researchers all over the world have been contributing to improve the safety and

The Paralympic Athlete, 1st edition. Edited by Yves C. Vanlandewijck and Walter R. Thompson. Published 2011 by Blackwell Publishing Ltd.

the performance of Paralympic athletes. Among the relevant issues, scientists studied the effects of environmental conditions on the health and performance of the athletes. This chapter will discuss the questions related to body temperature, heat and pollution, as well as the influence of these factors on the performance of athletes with medullar lesions and cerebral palsy who seem to have the greatest sensitivities.

Physical exercise for the general population

The regular practice of physical exercise results in benefits to health, since there is evidence that it reduces the rates of early mortality from certain diseases associated with sedentary living and poor nutritional habits. The beneficial changes can be observed in all individuals, including those with physical and mental disabilities, as long as the exercises are prescribed according to some well-established principles. In effect, all people regardless of ability or disability will benefit from regular exercise.

Physical activity generates heat that needs to be dissipated into the environment for body temperature to remain stable. In this regard, the large size of the human brain presents an additional thermoregulatory challenge, because adequate neurological functioning only takes place within a very narrow temperature range (±2°C). In fact, natural selection resulted in the unique human capacity to keep their body temperature stable during the performance of physical exercises in hot and dry environments.

Nevertheless, even with effective physiological regulation and adaptation, the performance of physical exercise generates a gradual increase in body temperature, which has critical limits for the adequate functioning of physiological systems and the resulting maintenance of good health. The speed at which body heat intensifies depends on the ability of the central nervous system to administer heat dissipation relative to the aerobic and cardiovascular capacities, the states of acclimatization and hydration, the time of day, the quality of sleep the previous night, the presence of pathologies and the use of certain medications. This set of factors is in turn influenced, to a lesser or an advanced degree, by the temperature, humidity, and ventilation within the environment.

Therefore, to optimize the health and sports performance of Paralympic athletes, it is important to understand how the physiological neural control of body temperature occurs during physical exercise under many different environmental conditions. Then, there can be a greater understanding of how this control may be affected by diseases or conditions that have chronic physical manifestations.

The levels of physical or mental impairment of each athlete must be compatible with a sport-related blindness, limb amputations, spinal cord injuries (SCIs), and cerebral palsy. The last two conditions might lead to some degree of uncontrolled thermoregulation (Figure 12.1).

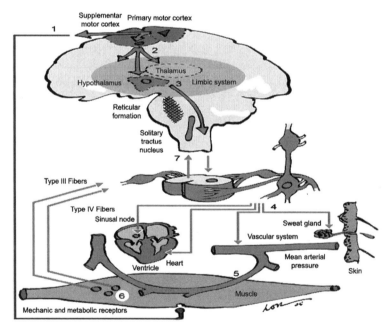

Figure 12.1 Neural mechanism of body temperature regulation during exercise—(1) motor commands sent to muscles are generated simultaneously with stimuli (2) targeted to other areas of the central nervous system that (3) integrate the information and activate (4) the autonomous nervous system to increase heart rate and blood pressure, regulate the vasomotor tonus and produce sweat, supplying (5) blood flow to the muscles. In case the perfusion is inadequate, (6) local temperature sensors and metabolism products inform the central nervous system, (7) which readjusts the autonomic stimulus continuously.

BOX 12.1 Heat Production and Dissipation

Conduction: exchange of heat by direct transfer of energy from one matter to another.

Convection: exchange of heat by replacement of a layer of fluid (air, water, etc.) that is already in thermal balance with a surface with another layer at a different temperature.

Radiation: exchange of heat between two bodies at different temperatures through electromagnetic waves.

Phase change: exchange of heat by change of phase, for instance, from liquid to gas (evaporation) or from gas to liquid (condensation).

Evaporation of sweat: constitutes the main mechanism of heat exchange in humans during exercise. Cooling of the skin takes place and sweat reaches its surface and evaporates, transferring heat to the vapor that dissipates into the environment.

Body temperature

The human body is continuously producing heat and exchanging it with the environment through five mechanisms: conduction, convection, radiation, phase change, and evaporation of sweat (Box 12.1). The temporary result of these exchanges is that the body temperature is kept as consistent as possible so that physiological processes take place adequately. Temperature varies in each part of the body, and what is known as "body temperature" is the average temperature of all the different tissues, and it is usually expressed as an adjusted combination of the central temperature and the skin temperature.

The central temperature corresponds to the temperature of structures and organs located in deeper areas, mainly the brain, and in humans it should remain between 35.0°C and 39.0°C for those organs to function correctly. Physiological regulation works to keep the internal temperature stable within this range, even when the external

temperature varies within some limits, depending upon the duration of the exposure, the air speed, the power of the heat source and other thermodynamic factors, and the health condition of the individuals. Another factor of temperature tolerance is the acclimation level: for instance, the Khoisans live in the Kalahari Desert (southern Africa including much of Botswana and part of Namibia and South Africa) where the temperature can drop to 5°C at night and rise to 50°C during the day. However, they are fully adapted to the variations in that dry weather.

Body temperature, then, fluctuates in response to physical activities, emotions, and variations in room temperature. In addition, there is a circadian variation of about 1°C in the central (i.e., core) temperature of the human body. The lowest temperatures happen during sleep, and slightly higher temperatures occur during waking hours, more specifically at the end of the afternoon and the beginning of night (Figure 12.2).

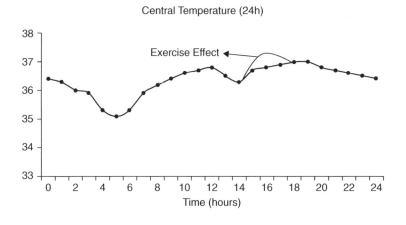

Figure 12.2 Oscillation of body temperature over the day and an inductor effect of heating up as a response to exercise (adapted from Marques, N., Menna-Barreto, L. Available at: http://www. crono.icb. usp.br).

The body temperature stabilization mechanisms are autonomic and behavioral nervous that work through systems of forward and feedback signals. They are linked to complex connections of several areas of the central nervous system, mainly the hypothalamic thermoregulation centers.

Temperature sensors are found over the human body to continuously inform the central nervous system about the thermal condition of the skin and other tissues. The peripheral information is integrated with central indicators of the rate of heat accumulation in the body, and then certain responses are triggered to keep the body temperature stable, such as behavioral changes (staying away from the sun, looking for shade, use of clothes, etc.).

When behavioral regulations are impossible or insufficient, there is skin vasodilation associated with sweating to dissipate heat, or vasoconstriction to preserve heat. When vasoconstriction is insufficient, shivering might occur, which is an involuntary way to produce heat. If these mechanisms are effective, the temperature remains stable; otherwise, there is an increase (hyperthermia) or a decrease (hypothermia) of the central temperature. Both of these challenge the functioning of physiological systems and might lead to health impairment or even death could result after prolonged exposure.

Physical exercise and the heat and the humidity

An increase in room temperature or in the metabolic production of heat (exercise) or both results in an increase in the body temperature, which in turn triggers heat dissipation mechanisms (including behavioral mechanisms, vasodilation, and sweating). If these mechanisms are insufficient or impaired, heat accumulates within the body, leading to hyperthermia. Hyperthermia decreases performance (by precipitating fatigue and reducing strength, concentration, and motor coordination) and might endanger the athlete's health.

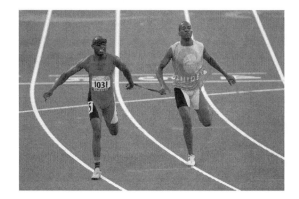

Figure 12.3 Blind athletes competing in the Summer Paralympic Games. Reproduced courtesy of Lieven Coudenys.

Considering that sweat evaporation is the main cooling mechanism of the human body, the relative humidity of air exerts a strong impact on the efficacy of heat loss by evaporation, since cooling only happens if the sweat evaporates. If humidity is high, the pressure of the vapor in the room air is close to that of the wet skin, reducing evaporation and therefore the loss of heat (Figure 12.3). As a consequence of the higher humidity, the athlete experiences a lower efficacy of heat loss to the environment. In that scenario, much sweat is produced without effective heat dissipation, causing a useless loss of water that might result in dehydration and overheating.

Even though most Paralympic athletes do not reach the same increase in body metabolism as do other athletes (e.g., up to 20 times the basal metabolism), any factors that interfere in the body cooling of people with medullar lesions or cerebral palsy can potentially cause hyperthermia. The most important factors are:

1. Neurological disturbances that reduce the ability of the individual to perceive increases in body temperature and to adopt adequate behavior (including sensory or motor disorders that result in locomotive incapacity and inability to stay away from the heat source).

2. Dissociation between the perception of thirst (which automatically reflects the state of hydration) and the ingestion of water, including the use of medication that interferes in thirst

or in the instinctive behavior of protection against heat.

3. Neurological damages that prevent sympathetic autonomic cardiovascular regulation, which is responsible for the cardiac output and distribution of blood to cool the skin.

4. Autonomic neurological disorders that alter the sympathetic sweating response.

5. Reduced aerobic capacity as a result of lower regular physical activity.

6. Low acclimatization to heat as a result of physical activity performed only in sheltered environments.

7. Disorders in body mass (in relation to its surface) that make the individual more vulnerable to the gain or loss of heat from the environment.

8. Dysfunction in the response to skin vasodilation that reduces the direction of heat into the surface.

Considering the specific conditions mentioned above, athletes can use a number of strategies to prevent or reduce the associated risk with exercise at high temperatures, including preexercise cooling, acclimatization, and the correct ingestion of liquids for volume replacement.

Moistening and heating the air that is inspired causes heat loss in the airways, contributing to a reduction of body heat in hot environments. However, the same mechanism can lead to hypothermia during physical activities that increase ventilation in very cold environments.

Recommendations

The following are some practical recommendations to trainers and athletes targeting the minimization of impairment caused by high ambient temperatures during competitions, mainly related to preventive measures before competitions and emergencies while and after competitions.

Before competitions

– Respect a minimal period for acclimatization of athletes. Some authors recommend exposing athletes to environments of competitions from 2 to 6 days before competitions.

– Promote a perfect state of body hydration. High temperatures and calorie loss due to exercises promote a dangerous state of dehydration. If these conditions are related to high air humidity, the loss of body fluids is even higher.

– Appropriate electrolyte replacement. The reduction of sodium intake can result in diminution of muscular strength and premature fatigue. Therefore, on prolonged activities (2 h or more), under hot climates and high humidity, it would be recommended the athlete ingest drinks containing electrolytes 2 h before physical activity.

– Body cooling. Methods of precooling before competitions have been used mainly for endurance tests. The likely benefits refer to the increase of capacity to store heat, in which would permit the athlete to complete the physical task before body temperature gets to a critical condition, therefore slowing fatigue.

During competitions

– Use adequate clothing. Wearing adequate clothing guarantees sweat evaporation as the right measure to promote thermoregulation during exercise (Figure 12.4). This is possible only if the sportswear is adequate to this purpose. Light clothing and clothes with special fabrics that guarantee heat exchange with the environment make a difference in the final results.

– Sustain hydration. For long duration competitions, it is necessary to ingest drinks both for body cooling and to guarantee hydration.

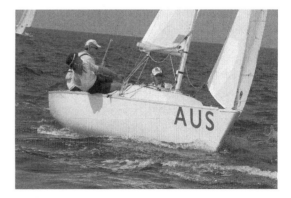

Figure 12.4 Sailing athletes must be especially concerned with adequate clothing and sunscreen protection. Reproduced courtesy of Lieven Coudenys.

After competitions

– Promote rehydration. After the competition has ended, hydration must be reestablished.
– Promote body cooling. The main methods used in recent studies both before and after exercises are body exposure to cold air and cold water immersion. The necessary time to obtain a physiological cooling seems to be 130 min to reduce tremors and sudden changes in the metabolism. The discomfort that such techniques cause can be a deterring factor for applying those techniques on elite athletes. Some researchers suggest that, for elite athletes, the immersion in water with gradual reduction of temperature is the most adequate method.

Physical exercise and air pollution

The pollutants that appear to cause the greatest concern to both amateur and professional athletes are nitrogen dioxide (NO_2) and ozone (O_3). Even at high concentrations, NO_2 does not seem to significantly affect individuals performing submaximal exercise, even though it might cause significant effects during high-intensity exercises (James et al., 2004). The deleterious effects of exposure to O_3 seem to be similar in different populations, such as children, young adults, women and older adults, as long as the dose of exposure is proportional to the body size.

Photochemical pollution or "atmospheric pollution" is the product of the action of sun rays on chemical elements resulting mostly from fuel combustion. "Photochemical oxidants" are the mixture of secondary pollutants formed by reactions between nitrogen oxides and volatile organic compounds released during incomplete fuel combustion and the evaporation of fuels and solvents in the presence of solar light.

One can imagine the losses caused to both the performance and the health of any athlete who needs to compete in an environment with high levels of pollutants. During athletic effort, the need to elevate the cellular absorption of oxygen causes the entire respiratory system and ventilator mechanics to work to increase the exposure of lung tissue to the environment and inhaled air. Therefore, the greater the respiratory capacity of an athlete has, the greater is the absorption per minute of particles in the atmosphere.

The lungs have various defense mechanisms against pollutants, including the action of antioxidants through the mucociliary movement (mucociliary escalator) and phagocytosis by cells of the immunological system such as macrophages. The oxidative stress arises in the lungs after they are exposed to pollution and it is a signal for the beginning of an inflammatory process. According to studies that relate exercise to the inflammatory response in polluted environments, the harm done to the health and performance of athletes is related to the type of pollutant and time of exposure to it.

NO_2 is a product of industrial activities and fuel combustion and can also be released by power plants and motor vehicles. This type of pollution affects mostly the population of industrialized countries but it is also found in any country with a large number of vehicles. According to the Environmental Protection Agency (EPA), diesel engines produce 25% of all nitrogen oxides, which are the main component for the formation of acid rain and a principal source of urban atmospheric pollution. Carbon monoxide (CO) is a colorless and odorless gas that results from incomplete fuel combustion, released by both cars and factories. High CO concentrations are found in areas of intense vehicle traffic. PM_{10} pollutants can be defined in a simple way as those with aerodynamic diameter lesser than 10 μm. Inhalable particles are classified as fine, $PM_{2.5}$ (<2.5 μm), and coarse (2.5–10 μm). Due to their small size, the fine particles may reach the alveoli of the lungs, but the coarse ones are retained in the upper tract of the respiratory system, causing oxidative stress in a way similar to O_3. Sulfur dioxide (SO_2) is the main sulfur-containing by-product from the combustion of fuels, such as diesel, industrial fuel oil, and gasoline. It is one of the main elements in acid rain formation. SO_2 can react with other substances present in the air and form sulfate particles that are responsible for reducing the atmospheric visibility. The damages caused to human health by this pollutant are associated to its solubility on the walls of the respiratory tract. It dissolves in the wet secretions and reaches the lower respiratory tract, causing bronchiole spasms, even in small concentrations. In larger quantities, it irritates the entire respiratory system and damages lung tissues. For small-to-moderate volumes and nasal respiration, penetration into the lungs is minimal, but for large volumes and oral inhalation, the segmental bronchi are affected and the respiratory tracts are burned, resulting in tissue inflammation, hemorrhaging, and necrosis. In the presence of SO_2, preexisting respiratory diseases worsen and new ones may also appear. When the mucociliary system is harmed, SO_2 causes chronic tracheobronchitis and greater susceptible to respiratory infections. Asthmatic or allergic athletes may be 10 times more reactive than healthy individuals.

The main product of the reaction of photochemical oxidants, however, is O_3, which is used as an indicator of the presence of such oxidants in the atmosphere. Of all the major pollutants, the impact of O_3 on health and physical exercise has received the most attention in literature. The O_3 that is found in the atmosphere layer is closest to the ground, where people breathe. It is toxic and therefore is called "bad ozone." In the stratosphere, however, at around 25 km elevation, it has the important function of protecting the planet of the ultraviolet rays emitted by the sun.

The ozone may cause irritation in the airways and impair pulmonary function. The harmful effect of ozone is related to the effective dose to which the individual is exposed. The "effective dose" is a combination of the ozone concentration, the duration of exposure to it, and the volume of ventilated air (James et al., 2004). The exposure to O_3 causes symptoms such as persistent and nonproductive cough, chest pain, headaches, and irritation in the eyes, and it also leads to higher perceived effort during submaximal exercise, reinforcing the idea that it might significantly hinder athletic performance. Furthermore, the reduction in pulmonary function and the resulting impairment of performance are related to the subjective respiratory discomfort, and this might reduce tolerance to exercise. Obviously, elite athletes are more predisposed to receiving a high dose of O_3 since their pulmonary volumes inhaled every minute (i.e., their minute ventilations) are higher when compared to nonexercising subjects.

Maximal physical performance depends directly on the effective transport of oxygen through the pulmonary system to the skeletal muscles. Therefore, high performance is related to optimum functioning of the respiratory muscles, the airways, and the pulmonary parenchyma. However, exposure to harmful particles in polluted environments leads to a restriction in the flow of air in the airways and a resulting reduction in oxygen saturation. This hypoxemia has a negative effect on the maximum aerobic capacity of a high-performance athlete. On average, a reduction of approximately 1% of the arterial oxygen saturation might reduce the maximal aerobic capacity by 1%. Evidence available in the literature suggests that continuous exposure to ozone might promote physiological adaptation, so that performance would be partially recovered during reexposure, thus reducing the deleterious effects on health. However, this adaptation was not observed in all the studies on this topic, and seems to be dependent on various factors, including the initial sensitivity of the individual to O_3 (James et al., 2004). However, exercise in environments with high concentrations of pollutants is not recommended for any individuals, athletes or not, since it might negatively affect performance and health, and may also be related to increased cardiovascular, morbidity and mortality (Sharman et al., 2004).

Doctors and health professionals are unanimous when it comes to indicate the practice of exercises outdoors. Elite athletes benefit from this practice, but general recommendations to amateur and professional athletes who do their training sessions in the open air are to avoid areas of big urban concentration or next to highways (Figure 12.5). Athletes who need to do their training in polluted cities must concentrate their outdoor training sessions in the early hours of the day, which is the period of the day when the concentration of pollutants is low.

It is important to mention that the athletes who participated in the last Olympic Games in the cities of Sydney in 2000, Athens in 2004, and Beijing in 2008 were exposed to environments with different levels of pollution. The Australian government made combating pollution a priority beginning in November 2007 and in 2008, it signed the ratified Kyoto Protocol. In 2009, Australia released 553 million metric

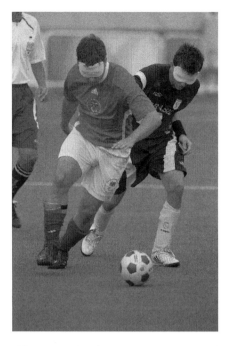

Figure 12.5 Recent Paralympic Games organizers had to be concerned about pollution for all outdoor events including five-a-side football. Reproduced courtesy of Lieven Coudenys.

tons of greenhouse gases, which represents 1.5% of the global emissions. However, its 28.6 metric tons per inhabitant is five times greater than China's and ranks Australia first in the world as the per capita polluter. One of the reasons is Australia's dependence on coal. Australia is not only the number one world exporter of coal, but also uses this fossil energy to produce 84% of its electricity. To solve the problem, the government is striving for a reduction in the CO_2 emissions between 5% and 25% in relation to 2000 data by 2020.

In a review, James et al. (2004) studied the association between the polluted atmosphere and the performance of athletes in the Athens Olympic Games in order to assess whether there would be a loss in their final results. Various authors have reported on the difficulty of making this relationship, considering that the studies used models based on pulmonary ventilation rates much lower than those of athletes who participated in the Athens Olympic Games in 2004. Furthermore, it is known that the response to O_3 may vary between individuals.

Those authors reported that many research groups tested countless models to evaluate the quality of air in Athens during the Games. The city of Athens lies in a drainage basin with approximately 450 km^2 of surface surrounded by mountains and open sea. This topography, along with the local weather conditions, results typically in high levels of air pollution in Athens. In the last few years, great historical monuments have suffered the effects of acid rain. One very well-known example is that of the Acropolis; the effects of acid rain in the last 40 years are equivalent to those of the previous 2,000 years.

These characteristics might entail a negative impact on performance. However, according to some observers, the information available, and models to predict the effects of O_3 and other pollutants on elite athletes are not reliable since it is a known fact that the response to ozone might vary among individuals.

In the Olympic and Paralympic Games recently held in Beijing, around 10,000 athletes competed in one of the most polluted capitals in the world. According to data from the Chinese Environment Ministry, in June 2007, the average concentration of polluting substances per square meter in the largest Chinese cities, including Beijing, resulting from the automobile traffic and industrial activity was 0.053 mg of SO_2, 0.035 mg of NO_2, and 0.1 mg of suspended particles. This led the International Olympic Committee (IOC) to admit the existence of "some risks" for the athletes participating in open air competitions, especially those requiring high levels of continuous effort, such as triathlon, race walking, cycling, and especially the marathon. The heat and humidity posed a clear threat to the optimal performance of competitors in different modalities, so much so that some delegations took their athletes to acclimatize in countries with similar weather, such as Singapore, Japan, or Australia. Nevertheless, the greatest concern of the IOC was the health of the athletes, rather than their performance. The fast urbanization of China since 1980 resulted in a lower quality of air in that country, which is corroborated by the fact that 16 out of the 20 most polluted cities in the world are in China.

The next Olympic Games, in 2012, will be held in London, the British capital, and the concerns with the air quality of this city are already evident. Although less polluted than Beijing, London is among the most polluted capitals in the world. A British television station measured the air particle concentrations in Beijing in 2008 and found that close to the Olympic Stadium, the level was always greater than 100 $\mu g/m^3$. A peak of 532 $\mu g/m^3$ was recorded for a few days. In order to perceive the magnitude of this level of pollution, the amounts in London recorded during the same time were between 30 and 40 $\mu g/m^3$.

Today, British authorities are studying ways to control the emission of pollutants in order to ameliorate the situation before the Games begin. The King's College Environmental Research Group announced that some of the measures that London should adopt if the city wants to ensure better conditions for the athletes are to prohibit car traffic and reschedule events during the competitions in 2012. The capital of the United Kingdom is in a "new age" of atmospheric pollution. With 7.5 million inhabitants, it ranks the worst among the European capitals for nitrogen dioxide and one of the worst for dangerous suspended particles.

The fight against environmental pollution should be one of the greatest concerns of all for governments and sports authorities for the next Olympic and Paralympic Games of this century in order to ensure better health to all professionals, spectators, and the population in general who along with the athletes really do desire to breathe truly "pure air" in consonance with the spirit of the Games.

Athletes with medullary lesions

Medullar lesion is a traumatic event that brings about great unpredictability, since irreversible changes block the individual's capacity to carry out their most basic tasks. SCI is a trauma that might result in the loss of voluntary movements and/or sensitivity of the upper and/or lower limbs in many respects, including tactility, sensitivity to pain, and deep sensitivity. It can also lead to alterations in the functioning of the urinary, intestinal, respiratory, circulatory, sexual and reproductive systems.

In addition to the physical and sensory dysfunctions, there are many sequels of medullar lesion, including atrophy of the muscle–skeletal system,

spasticity, autonomic dysfunction, hormonal and neuromuscular changes, and reductions in respiratory capacity, blood circulation and the physical dimensions of the cardiac structure. These factors taken together may lead to cardiovascular and respiratory diseases. These alterations curb the physiological responses to motor activity leading to a faster onset of fatigue. The reduction in respiratory capacity might be related to a weakness or a certain degree of paralysis of the respiratory muscles. It could also be due to a low extensibility of the lungs and the thoracic cage, since the motor root takes place between C3 and C5 for the diaphragm, between T7 and T12 for the abdominal muscles, and between T8 and T12 for the thoracic and intercostal muscles.

There is an increase in the heart rate and systolic blood pressure among individuals with medullar lesion even though they may present a vasoconstriction response below the level of the lesion (lower limbs and abdominal area). This may result in blood concentration (i.e., pooling) in the lower limbs and hypotension during exercise in the upper limbs or orthostatism (being seated or having a passive upright position). Furthermore, individuals with medullar lesion, especially those with lesions above T6, might present a loss of sympathetic control of the heart, a loss of adrenal medullar and vasomotor response, in addition to a loss of the thermoregulatory response.

Active individuals or athletes with medullar lesion participate mainly in wheelchair sports, where the biomechanics and the motor act of the sport are concentrated in the upper limbs. During intense exercise, energy metabolism in the upper limbs increases substantially. Similarly, the brain triggers mechanisms for the loss of accumulated heat, such as blood redistribution to the skin, sweating, and an increase in the blood flow to the active muscles.

However, temperature regulation is impaired in these individuals. Their thermoregulatory capacity is lower due to reduced control by the autonomic and somatic nervous systems near and below the level of the lesion. This directly affects the distribution of blood to the skin and reduces sweating. A consequence of this limited peripheral vascular control is an increase in body temperature, both during activity and at rest (which negatively affects the performance of the wheelchair athlete), and will present early fatigue, among other characteristics.

These athletes demonstrate an inability to maintain cardiac output for prolonged periods of time. This characteristic hinders the cardiac control of the redistribution of blood both to the skin and to the deeper organs. An associated factor is the afferent feedback reduction that would stimulate sweating, causing an increase in body temperature. It is clearly established that the reduction in the thermoregulatory control of individuals with medullar lesion is inversely proportional to the level of the lesion (i.e., there is less control with higher lesions).

Some of the physiological impairments athletes with medullar lesion might exhibit include the denervation of sympathetic, spinal and ganglionar sensitivity as well as of that in the areas of the peripheral receptors; the loss of supraspinal inhibitory control; and the formation of abnormal sympathetic connections. These alterations are present in individuals with autonomic dysreflexia. One of the worst consequences of dysreflexia is the inability to control blood pressure. During prolonged physical exercise under unfavorable weather conditions, the increased metabolism and the excessive increase of body temperature are paralleled by an increase in blood pressure. In an attempt to control this increase, the carotid and aortic baroreceptors are stimulated, which in turn activates the parasympathetic nervous system. However, descendent impulses that go from the vasodilation center to the spinal cord are unable to continue their route beyond the level of the lesion, and therefore they do not adequately regulate peripheral vasoconstriction and the systemic hypertension that results from exercise.

Regarding hypothermia, individuals with medullar lesion above T1 are unable to respond to a reduction of internal temperature with vasoconstriction since in these cases there is a disconnection between the peripheral sympathetic system (starting from T1) and the more central parts of the central nervous system. In lesions below T1, a certain degree of vasoconstriction will be preserved, inversely proportional to the level of the lesion. However, when the internal temperature rises, vasodilation should occur from the suspension of the sympathetic tonus (present or absent in individuals with medullar lesion, again depending on the level of the lesion). The "active" vasodilation that should also happen (in addition to the suspension of the sympathetic tonus) in turn depends on sympathetic stimulation of the exocrine sweat glands. Again, the sympathetic system is responsible for vasodilation, but indirectly: acetylcholine is released to the sympathetic terminations of the sweat gland, along with vasoactive peptides that promote vasodilation near the gland to increase the flow of warm blood (and hence, the skin temperature) and transfer this heat to the environment through the evaporation of sweat. In this sense, the same medullar lesion that prevents vasoconstriction in hypothermia will prevent sweating and vasodilation in hyperthermia. Therefore, depending on the level of the lesion, the individual with medullar lesion can be a victim of both hot and cold environments.

Arm movements are especially important for athletes with SCI. However, paraplegic or tetraplegic athletes might have their heat dissipation concentrated mainly in their upper limbs and head. Some evidence suggests that the loss of heat through the head of these athletes represents a significant part of their thermoregulatory mechanism. Consequently, some procedures are necessary to allow the adequate thermoregulatory control, since excessive increases of temperature might have consequences that impair performance of the athlete and affect their health.

Athletes with cerebral palsy

Cerebral palsy is a nonprogressive disease that compromises movement and posture. It presents multiple etiologies that result in damage to the central nervous system, most of the times characterized by hypoxia of the neurological tissue in the perinatal period. Cerebral palsy is nonprogressive from the perspective of its etiopathogeny.

The incidence of cerebral palsy is around 2 in 1,000 babies born alive in developed countries, a frequency that has been changing in recent years. Evidence points to an increase in premature babies who are underweight at birth. The clinical condition varies greatly, ranging from a mild monoplegia with normal intellectual capacity to severe spasticity of the whole body associated with mental retardation. In general, individuals with cerebral palsy have at least one additional deficiency (secondary to the main condition) resulting from damage to the central nervous system, such as cognitive impairment, sensory loss (sight and/or hearing), convulsions, behavioral alterations, thermoregulatory alterations, and/or systemic chronic diseases (orthopedic, gastrointestinal, and respiratory).

Cerebral palsy is classified as spastic, ataxic, dyskinetic, hypotonic, or mixed, according to the kind of neuromuscular impairment. Based on its topographic distribution, spastic cerebral palsy can be classified into quadriplegia (affecting all four limbs, but more the upper ones), diplegia (affecting the lower limbs, with minimal impairment of the upper ones), and hemiplegia (spasticity reaches the lower and upper limb on one side, usually the most impaired). Temperature control in these individuals might be impaired if there is hypothalamic dysfunction with resulting hypothermia, which is commonly observed in individuals with cerebral palsy.

Therefore, Paralympic athletes with cerebral palsy might present intolerance to extreme temperatures, mainly cold, depending on the degree of impairment. However, in specific modalities where the exchange of heat with the environment is fundamental for performance, individuals with less hypothalamic impairment will present less reduction in their final results.

Effects of hydration level and the combined effects of heat stress and dehydration on physical performance

Appropriate hydration levels are necessary for the full attainment of aerobic capacity and of muscular potency. Separately, dehydration is interpreted by the central nervous system as a threat to the physiological stability of the organism and results in reduction of effort intensity or precocious interruption of exercise—in other words, in the anticipation of fatigue. If dehydration is added to hyperthermia or increased thermal stress, the effects are potentially more dangerous putting the individuals' health at risk because the dissipation of body heat in humans requires the production of perspiration, which depends on reserves of existent liquids. The eventual

reduction of body mass in Paralympic athletes, due to neurological lesions, results in smaller levels of total body water and greater vulnerability to dehydration.

Effects of energy stores depletion on thermoregulation and physical performance

The central nervous system is capable of continually evaluating available energy pools, especially the level of carbohydrates indispensable for appropriate brain functioning. Therefore, prolonged fasting, inadequate feeding, or excessive energy expense in physical activities can result in reduction of hepatic levels of glycogen, which would constitute an indicator for the nervous system that exercise should be reduced or interrupted. If to this indicator are added, for example, physiological signs of corporal temperature, increase of the resulting perception of threatening conditions to the individuals' health engages fatigue earlier as a protection mechanism. Paralympic athletes can exhibit reduction of muscular mass and consequently possess lower muscular glycogen reserves, which in turn makes them more dependent on hepatic glycogen, while reducing their functional capacity in situations of prolonged fasting or deficient caloric replacement. Some practical recommendations for athletes are to watch one's nutrition to prevent muscle mass loss and be sure to eat carbohydrates before sports activities.

Effects of electrolyte imbalance on physical performance

The main electrolytic imbalance related to physical activities is the reduction of serum sodium levels due to its loss through perspiration that creates an output higher than its intake from food ingestion. A drop in body sodium levels of moderate amounts results in the decrease of muscular strength, premature fatigues, and eventually cramps. At more serious levels, it can cause cerebral edema that potentially results in coma and occasionally in death. The habit of trying to restore in a forceful and complete way the losses from sweating through the ingestion of pure water has resulted in cases of drops of sodium levels in the plasma (hyponatremia). Electrolytic beverages are only necessary in very prolonged activities (greater than 2 h), in hot environments and with high level of perspiration production. Practical recommendations include drinking 500 ml of pure water 2 h before the activity and replace liquids adequately when thirsty.

Differences between heat exhaustion, heat cramps and heat stroke and what are the treatments for these conditions

The international literature presents these concepts in an imprecise way. It is known that there is a progression in the severity of signs and symptoms of hyperthermia from the physiological thermoregulatory signs in response to a situation of corporal temperature increase to a state of shock, to coma, and finally death. Table 12.1 can be useful in the separation of different phases between protective fatigue and the irreversible failure of organs.

The treatments corresponding to each one of the severity levels are:

Fatigue: interrupt the exercise, remove the individual from the hot place or away from the source of heat, and promote hydration and rest. As a prevention measure, monitor the environment and adopt measures of acclimatization and physical conditioning.

Exhaustion: needs medical observation for several hours because it can develop in an unexpected way toward the following phase—shock. Exercise should be immediately interrupted, and the individual removed away from any hot environmental source and the body should be cooled with fans, ice packs, or air-conditioning. Furthermore, oral or intravenous hydration should be provided if necessary. Supplying supplemental oxygen and monitoring renal function is also suggested. As a prevention measure, monitor the environment and evaluate predisposing factors for hyperthermia while also promoting information for heat acclimatization and increasing physical conditioning before subsequent exposure to exercise under hot conditions.

Shock: shock constitutes a medical emergency, because it presents high mortality and complications in survivors. It should be treated in specialized centers with intensive care units. For reasons still unknown, survivors constitute preferential victims for new cases of hyperthermia. As a prevention measure, monitor the environment and the level of acclimatization and increase individuals' conditioning so that increased exposure to exercise in the heat can be experienced by the athlete.

Table 12.1 Levels of hyperthermia severity during physical exercise under hot conditions.

Level of severity	Signs and symptoms
Fatigue	Desire to interrupt the activity
	Inattention
	Loss of efficiency
	Increase in mistakes
Exhaustion	Syncope (transitory hypotension)
	Tachycardia
	Cephalea
	Nausea
	Loss of muscular endurance
	Ataxia or difficulty in movement coordination
	Muscular cramps
	Hyperventilation
	Sweating dysfunction
Shock	Prolonged hypotension up to acute circulation insufficiency
	Neurologic dysfunction up to coma
	Oliguria (reduction in the urinary volume) up to renal insufficiency
	Hepatic insufficiency
	Septicemia
	Death

Monitoring the environment

The most commonly internationally used indicator is the temperature WBGT (wet bulb globe temperature), which gathers the measures of three temperatures of the environment (dry, humid, and global, this last related to the intensity of solar radiation). WBGT represents the potential impact of thermal stress on the organism and its use is only complete when involving the expense of energy (therefore the production of corporal heat) occurring from physical training in a certain environment. The WBGT index was developed by the US Marine Corps at Parris Island in 1956 to reduce heat stress injuries in recruits and has since been revised several times.

The WBGT is a composite temperature used to estimate the effect of temperature, humidity, wind speed, and solar radiation on humans. It is used by industrial hygienists, athletes, and the military to determine appropriate exposure levels to high temperatures. It is derived from the following formula:

$$WBGT = 0.7T_w + 0.2T_g + 0.1T_d$$

where T_w = temperature measured with a humidity indicator; T_g = temperature measured with a black globe thermometer, to measure solar radiation; T_d = normal air temperature in degree Celsius).

The American Conference of Governmental Industrial Hygienists publishes threshold limit values (TLVs) that have been adopted by many governments for use in the workplace. The process for determining the WBGT is also described in ISO 7243, Hot Environments—Estimation of the Heat Stress on Working Man, Based on the WBGT Index (http://www.iso.org/iso).

In hot areas, some US military installations and sports organizations display a flag to indicate the heat category based on the WBGT.

Category	WBGT (°C)	Flag color
1	≤26.6	No flag
2	26.7–29.3	Green
3	29.4–31.0	Yellow
4	31.1–32.1	Red
5	≥32.2	Black

Modifications in hot, humid, or polluted environments

Heat and humidity can be monitored by the WBGT index and the levels of different polluting agents

can be determined. Furthermore, as a general recommendation in addition to care taken with environment temperature, be it cold or hot, no sport should be practiced in polluted environments, since physical activity increases the inhalation of air and all its elements. Table 12.2 lists personal factors such as medications, supplements, sleep, and recent illness that affect the risk of thermoregulatory disturbances during physical activity.

Table 12.2 Factors that affect the risk of thermoregulation disturbances during physical activity.

Factor	Mechanisms
Genetic	Polymorphisms selected during human migrations generate genes that confer a greater resistance to heat in some individuals
Acclimatization	Promotes neurohumoral adjustments Increases cardiovascular capacity Can increase the synthesis of thermal stress proteins
Age (children and elderly)	The relationship mass/volume varies according to age, as does thermoregulatory capacity as a function of alterations in aerobic capacity
Aerobic capacity	Cardiovascular availability for thermoregulation
State of hydration	Plasmatic volume Interference in sweating capacity
Sex	Factors related to aerobics capacity and corporal/volume mass relation
Social–economic level	The costs of technological resources for home protection increase the risk in poorer individuals
Educational level	Related to the social economical level influences job status
Diseases	Most cardiovascular and psychiatric conditions as well as diabetes for its own physiopathology and for the eventual use of medications that affect the perspiration or hydration levels
Widowhood	Age effect, loneliness, and income level
Sleep	Restriction of sleep produces reduction in night cerebral cooling and work in shifts affects thermoregulatory capacity
Urbanization	Big cities produce "islands of heat"; radiation is higher in the top of high buildings

Athlete education

Every trainer and coach should possess the necessary basic knowledge to inform athletes about the major risk factors to their health, and especially to teach them to distinguish the signs of fatigue and to respect them, and to recognize that thirst is an efficient instrument of natural maintenance of the normal state of hydration.

Hyperthermia induces a reduction of peripheral muscle activation due to decreased central activation (brain fatigue)

One of the possible mechanisms related to the reduction of muscular endurance in the heat would be the possible decrease of muscular activation by central nervous system neurons. Although this has been partially observed in laboratory animals, its application to human fatigue is still subject to debate.

Summary

Under unfavorable environmental conditions, a lower efficacy of thermoregulation might pose an extra risk to the health of Paralympic athletes that might lead to dehydration, hyperthermia, or an increase in blood pressure. These conditions have potentially serious negative consequences far beyond the loss of medals and records, including aphasia, brain hemorrhage, blindness, cardiac arrhythmia, and even death. In general, the influence of environmental factors such as heat, humidity, and pollution on sports performance has always been a challenging question. This challenge is even greater with Paralympic athletes because of their specific thermoregulatory mechanisms and their different responses to stressing factors. Within this context, elucidation of the physiological mechanisms that control body temperature under thermal stress and environmental conditions helps the understanding of how such alterations might influence performance, and could represent the difference between winning and losing.

References

James, G.F., Donaldson, K. & Stone, V. (2004). Athens 2004: the pollution climate and athletic performance. *Journal of Sports Science*, **22**, 967–980.

Sharman, J.E., Cockcroft, J.R. & Coombes, J.S. (2004). Cardiovascular implications of exposure to traffic air pollution during exercise. *Quarterly Journal of Medicine*, **97**, 637–643.

Recommended readings

American College of Sports Medicine and American Heart Association: Recommendations for cardiovascular screening, staffing, and emergency policies at health/fitness facilities (1998). *Medicine Science Sports Exercise*, **30**, 1009–1018.

American College of Sports Medicine (2007). Exertional heat illness during training and competition. *Medicine and Science in Sports & Exercise*. Available at www.acsm-msse.org

American College of Sports Medicine (2010). *Guidelines for Exercise Testing and Prescription*, 8th edition. Lippincott Williams & Wilkins, Philadelphia, PA.

Bar-Or, O. (1980). Climate and the exercising child—a review. *International Journal of Sports Medicine*, **1**, 53–65.

Febbraio, M.A. (2000). Does muscle function and metabolism affect exercise performance in the heat? *Exercise & Sport Science Review*, **28**, 171–176.

Maughan, R.J. & Shirreffs, S. (2004). Exercise in the heat: challenges and opportunities. *Journal of Sports Science*, **22**, 917–927.

Chapter 13

Preparation for the Paralympic Winter Games: cold, altitude

Marco Bernardi[1] and Federico Schena[2]

[1]School of Specialization in Sports Medicine, Department of Physiology and Pharmacology "V. Erspamer", "Sapienza", Università di Roma, Rome, Italy and Italian Paralympic Committee

[2]Department of Neuroscience & Faculty of Exercise and Sport Science, University of Verona, and Center of Bioengineering and Sport Science, Verona, Italy

Introduction

Winter Paralympic sports include Ice Sledge Hockey, Wheelchair Curling, Alpine skiing and Nordic skiing, where skiers compete both in cross-country skiing events and Biathlon. In both Alpine and Nordic skiing, athletes are divided into three main groups: standing, sitting, and visually impaired skiers, each one competing for the same medal event. Because the impairments within each group can vary widely and because the characteristics of each impairment, and therefore the severity, vary from a physiological, biomechanical, and medical point of view, an integrative approach, which gathers athletes together on the basis of their degree of residual functionality (functional classification), has been developed. Classes, indicated with the acronym LW and a number, range from LW1 to LW9 for standing skiers, from LW10 (the most impaired) to LW12 (the least impaired) for sitting skiers and from B1 (blind) to B3 (least impaired) for visually impaired skiers. A performance-based statistical approach, which takes into account previous season results, has been developed to group skiers, correcting the time spent to complete the race depending on the class (the less impaired class will have either the smallest or no reduction

of the actual time, while the most impaired class will have the smallest multiplying correction factor determining the highest time reduction).

Alpine skiing physiology

Alpine skiing includes four main specialties: slalom (in which male racers, for example, negotiate from 55 to 75 gates with best times after two runs determining ranking), giant slalom (two runs, longer than slalom but with fewer gates and allowing for smoother and wider turns), super giant slalom (a speed event with a minimum of 30 direction changes and gates at least 25 m apart), downhill (one run down a long steep course with turns and jumps), plus "combined," which includes two of the aforementioned specialties. Alpine elite skiing requires all components of physical fitness (PF): muscular strength, anaerobic power and capacity, aerobic power, flexibility, reactivity, balance and coordination. In the Alpine Paralympic world, skiers usually compete in all four specialties. The kind of specialty and the duration of a race, ranging from 1 to 3 min, determine the relative contribution of the three metabolic energy pathways, and the relative importance of the main physiological PF components. Table 13.1 shows the corrected time results of the four specialties of the Turin 2006 Paralympic Games for men and women divided by classes.

When the impairment only partially prejudices the biomechanics of the skiing performance (e.g., standing athletes with below elbow amputation

The Paralympic Athlete, 1st edition. Edited by Yves C. Vanlandewijck and Walter R. Thompson. Published 2011 by Blackwell Publishing Ltd.

Table 13.1 Time results (mean and standard deviation SD values, and ranges) of the four specialties of Turin 2006 Paralympic Games for men and women divided by groups (standing, sitting, and visually impaired skiers). Within each group the classes (LW and following number) of the athletes who scored the best and the worst results (lowest and highest real time) are also indicated.

		Time (s) Standing Skiers		Time (s) Sitting Skiers		Time (s) Visually Impaired Skiers	
Men							
Downhill	Mean ± SD	88.89 ± 5.681		101.85 ± 4.143		93.86 ± 5.049	
	Range	79.861	107.051	96.001	114.081	86.891	101.061
	Class	LW5/7-2	LW1	LW12-1	LW10-1	B2	B2
Super-G	Mean ± SD	79.74 ± 5.230		96.42 ± 4.370		92.04 ± 7.703	
	Range	73.230	100.131	89.381	104.441	87.031	102.741
	Class	LW6/8-2	LW1	LW10-2	LW10-1	B3	B2
Giant slalom	Mean ± SD	129.01 ± 15.982		158.81 ± 42.591		148.79 ± 34.264	
	Range	76.100	163.861	132.721	405.383	123.811	231.091
	Class	LW5/7-2	LW1	LW10-2	LW11	B2	B1
Slalom	Mean ± SD	95.77 ± 12.997		131.26 ± 20.054		115.49 ± 10.546	
	Range	83.201	151.841	70.950	168.591	123.811	231.091
	Class	LW4	LW2	LW10-2	LW11	B2	B2
Women							
Downhill	Mean ± SD	99.30 ± 6.576		110.15 ± 4.683		123.51 ± 26.763	
	Range	90.231	103.361	106.701	116.711	103.171	168.421
	Class	LW4	LW2	LW12-1	LW11	B3	B1
Super-G	Mean ± SD	86.73 ± 5.184		101.33 ± 5.283		116.29 ± 21.437	
	Range	79.491	96.131	97.801	107.351	94.641	153.461
	Class	LW9-2	LW2	LW12-1	LW10-2	B3	B1
Giant slalom	Mean ± SD	137.54 ± 12.656		173.39 ± 33.509		197.31 ± 62.888	
	Range	119.421	170.061	144.181	257.472	157.511	322.842
	Class	LW3-1	LW2	LW12-2	LW11	B1	B1
Slalom	Mean ± SD	102.98 ± 8.468		153.18 ± 12.671		156.47 ± 40.916	
	Range	95.761	123.231	136.691	180.881	133.161	233.971
	Class	LW2	LW3-2	LW12-2	LW11	B3	B1

or visually impaired skiers), the physiology of the able-bodied Alpine skiers (Andersen & Montgomery, 1988) is applicable to Paralympic athletes. LW2 skiers (above knee amputated standing athletes who ski on one leg and stabilize their body center of mass holding outriggers) and LW10–12 skiers (sitting athletes whose movement is due to the upper part of the body) show unique characteristics which affect not only physiology and biomechanics but also the physical adaptations to the sport.

This paragraph will deal preferentially with the physiology of LW2 skiers and some technical information will be provided on sitting skiers, whose PF will be described in a separate paragraph. Data presented have been collected on four LW2 skiers (mean age 29 ± 4.8 years) and are compared, as appropriate, with five sitting skiers (32 ± 3.0 years) and three visually impaired skiers (30 ± 8.7 years). From an anthropometric point of view, as in able-bodied Alpine skiers, successful LW2 athletes are today taller and heavier than in the past and are characterized by having higher lean mass. Indeed, measuring fat mass in Italian Alpine skiers, we found the lowest values (14.5 ± 0.66%) in our best LW2 skiers (mean height 183 ± 4.2 cm, body mass 69.5 ± 0.71 kg).

In able-bodied Alpine skiers, leg strength correlates significantly with performance. Indeed both in able-bodied and in disabled skiers, the sport is characterized by high levels of eccentric forces, applied when changing direction, and high isometric forces, due to the long-lasting crouched position and to combat gravitational and centrifugal forces. Therefore, increased isometric leg strength is one distinguishing adaptation of elite Alpine skiers when compared to nonelite skiers. Indeed, measuring quadriceps muscles isometric force, we found in LW2 athletes very high values during leg extension (891 ± 107.1 N). Top level visually impaired skiers reached, at the same test and with their best lower limb, values corresponding to $75 \pm 11.4\%$ of the LW2 skiers.

When comparing international level able-bodied Alpine skiers, fastest athletes are characterized by the best performances in single vertical jump tests. Indeed, maximal explosive power is a significant predictor of Alpine skiing performance. We measured peak power during simulation of squatting and countermovement jumps in standing and visually impaired Alpine skiers. LW2 skiers jumping with one leg showed the best results. Peak power was equal to 805 ± 29.7 and 948 ± 46.6 W in squatting and countermovement tests, respectively. These figures corresponded to 67.3 ± 0.34 and $68.5 \pm 1.24\%$ of the values found in our best B3 Alpine skiers jumping with two legs. Anaerobic capacity (maximal mechanical work carried out in a high-intensity exercise) was studied with the same instrument, asking the athletes to execute 10 consecutive jumps at maximal power. We found in LW2 skiers a mean power decrease of 14% (the final values were $86.4 \pm 6.38\%$ of the first jump). Visually impaired skiers decreased their power of about 17% (the final values were $83.1 \pm 7.57\%$ of the first jump). Considering that the test is carried out with one leg, LW2 skiers show excellent results. These results on disabled skiers support the findings that able-bodied Alpine skiers have the highest activity of lactate dehydrogenase (related to anaerobic lactic metabolism) and creatine phosphokinase (related to anaerobic alactic metabolism) in their thigh muscles compared to athletes from other sports.

To obtain specific insights about energy expenditure of Alpine skiing, we measured through a wearable metabolimeter (K4, Cosmed, Italy) pulmonary ventilation (VE), oxygen consumption (VO_2), carbon dioxide production (VCO_2), and heart rate (HR) during simulated giant slalom races. Blood lactate (BL) was measured before and after the race. To validate the results, HR and BL were measured in the same skiers during the Italian Championships. Giant slalom race simulation lasted 75 ± 0.9 s. VE reached 89 ± 9.7 l/min, VO_2 increased up to top values of 2.26 ± 0.389 l/min and HR peaked at 183 ± 7.1 beats/min. All parameters did reach the highest values at the end of the race as it occurs usually in all disciplines. BL peak values during recovery were equal to 7.8 ± 0.96 mmol/l. Peak values measured in the same athletes in incremental up to exhaustion exercise tests, carried out on a rowing ergometer, were equal to 3.07 ± 0.390 l/min, 47 ± 8.5 ml/kg/min, 187 ± 11.9 beats/min and 8.6 ± 1.13 mmol, respectively, for VO_{2peak} in absolute and relative values, HR_{max} and BL_{peak}. The VO_2 kinetics during and after the simulated race (fast and slow excess postexercise oxygen consumption—EPOC) and BL highest value was analyzed to assess the total energy expenditure of the race. In detail, the increase of VO_2 over the basal value during the race was used to assess the energy deriving from the aerobic metabolism. The fast EPOC subtracted from the slow EPOC was used to assess the energy deriving from the alactic anaerobic metabolism. Each mmol of BL increment over the basal value was multiplied by 3 ml of oxygen and by the body mass (kg) to estimate the oxygen equivalent of the energy derived from glycolisis (anaerobic metabolism). We measured a total energy expenditure of 100.2 ± 9.94 kJ (4.77 ± 0.473 l of O_2) corresponding to VO_2 values of 53.4 ± 1.41 ml/kg/min. The aerobic, alactic anaerobic, and lactic anaerobic metabolisms contributed for $41 \pm 2.1\%$, $27 \pm 3.3\%$, and $31.7 \pm 2.75\%$, respectively. These metabolic patterns, just with lower energy volumes, do not differ significantly from those we measured in sitting skiers during the same race simulation.

Studies carried out on able-bodied top level skiers (Veicsteinas et al., 1984) do not substantially differ from our results, showing that anaerobic lactic metabolism during the race contributes up to 40% of the total energy expenditure, but VO_2 may increase to 75–100% of maximal aerobic power (giant slalom probably relies the most upon aerobic energy metabolism). The contribution of both aerobic and anaerobic metabolisms to the performance and therefore the recruitment of both slow and fast twitch muscle fibers are probably the reasons why the muscles of Alpine skiers do not possess a distinct fiber-type composition. According to the glycogen depletion pattern found in the slow twitch fibers of skilled able-bodied athletes when compared to unskilled athletes, it can be assumed that aerobic metabolism is crucial in elite athletes, which present in muscle biopsie a greater glycogen depletion. Based on these results, not only strength and anaerobic power and capacity but also aerobic power plays a very important role in the Alpine skier's performance. Indeed, in both sitting and standing skiers followed during three consecutive Paralympic Winter Games, we found that success in the Games was related to VO_{2peak}. High VO_{2peak} values, as in able-bodied skiers, may reflect the kind of training programs of the athletes and not the actual demand of the sport. Furthermore high-altitude training performed during summer and fall months, with the intermittent exposure to hypoxia, affects positively this parameter. Aerobic fitness (high VO_{2peak} and anaerobic threshold) would have at least a twofold advantage in elite Alpine skiers. First, aerobic energy contribution during the race would be higher, because of the more rapid increase in VO_2, (faster O_2 onset kinetics) than in skiers with low aerobic fitness levels, allowing a lower reliance on lactic anaerobic metabolism which is especially useful for the two-run races. Second, the increase of the recovery capacity (reduced time after each exercise bout), due to high aerobic fitness, is very useful during each training session allowing higher training volumes. This in turn determines greater physiological adaptations than in skiers with low aerobic fitness.

In conclusion, Alpine skier must be specifically trained for strength, maximal explosive power, anaerobic power and capacity, and aerobic power to be successful. Preseason training should be focused on improving energy systems (aerobic power and anaerobic capacity), by high amounts of endurance training. Approaching the season period, training should privilege strength, maximal explosive power, and anaerobic power with increased muscle coordination exercises during concentric and eccentric muscle activities. Intense eccentric exercise training on specific devices seems to be promising to improve performance.

From a technical point of view, LW2 athletes as well as all other Alpine skiers get maximum advantage from using carving skis. These skis are characterized by the side cut, reduced length, and presence of binding plates (risers) with the final effect of reducing the turning radius, increasing speed, and the probability of driving along the ski-edge. LW2 athletes use a pair of stabilizers (outriggers) to help them in changing direction and for propulsion at the start of the race. Due to their impairment, LW2 skiers behave differently when making turns on the side of the amputation (internal turn) compared to the other side ("blind" turn). In the internal turn the body weight is completely loaded on the uphill edge of the ski, which allows the skier to reduce turning radius and skidding, increasing the load on the ski with the final result of increasing the speed. While performing the blind turn, an excessive load on the external edge would result in the contact loss of the edge with the slope. To counteract this possibility and to maximize speed, the skier has to compensate with pelvis, trunk, and the arm of the side of the amputation.

Alpine sitting skiers use a sit-ski and hold an outrigger in each hand (Figure 13.1). The sitting device consists of a special seat whose height can be regulated depending on the level of impairment and type of control on the ski. The seat is attached to the ski through a suspension mechanism which includes a shock absorber with a light and strong frame. Athletes use a carving ski, taking the same advantages of carving in standing athletes. The upper part of the body has a key role in passing from one edge to the other and therefore to change direction. To enable skiers with high level of lesion (LW10

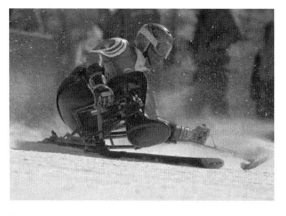

Figure 13.1 Alpine sit-skier holding outriggers.
Reproduced courtesy of the Italian Paralympic Committee.

classes) to maneuver the ski and change direction, the body center of gravity shift is increased by the arm movement, which is amplified by the outriggers. When approaching a turn, the skier moves his uphill arm bringing his body's center of gravity on the uphill edge of the ski. The crouched position kept by standing athletes is simulated in sit-skiing by the shock absorber, allowing sitting skiers to increase their speed and load on the ski with minimum skidding.

Nordic skiing physiology

Cross-country skiing is a high-energy expenditure aerobic exercise which combines the actions of arms and legs. It consists of a classical technique, in which propulsion is guaranteed by arm and leg movement alternated in a rhythmic fashion, and a freestyle technique, that incorporates a lateral pushing action with one ski while the opposite ski maintains a forward glide. Standing and visually impaired cross-country skiers compete in races of each technique. Nordic skiing also includes biathlon (cross-country races interspersed by shooting with a target of 30 mm for visually impaired skiers

and 20 mm for motor impaired skiers). Specific equipments are, for locomotor impaired skiers, the "sit-skis" (slightly shorter than standard skis with a chair attached to a cross-country binding), and for visually impaired skiers, a five-shot clip, conventional, air or carbon dioxide rifle, with a laser optronic system that allows aiming by auditory signal. Up to the Turin 2006 Paralympic Winter Games, cross-country skiers competed in the following events: short, middle, and long distance races. In male events short distance races were 5 km long, middle distance 10 km, long distance 15 km for sitting while 20 km for visually impaired and standing skiers. In female events short distance races were 2.5 km long for sitting and 5 km long for visually impaired and standing, middle distance 5 km for sitting and 10 km for standing and visually impaired, long distance 10 km for sitting and 15 km for standing and visually impaired skiers. Currently the short distance race has been substituted by the "sprint" race. The latter consists of a very short distance race (range between 0.8 and 1.2 km) in a "technically easy" course to warrant very high speeds. Table 13.2 shows the results of the Pragelato cross-country races held during the Turin Games.

Table 13.2 Results (mean and standard deviation, SD, values, and ranges) of the Turin 2006 Winter Paralympic cross-country ski races held in Pragelato are shown for the three groups of athletes, for men and women and for the three distances.

		Standing skiers Time (min)		Sitting skiers Time (min)		Visually impaired skiers Time (min)	
Men							
Short distance	Mean ± SD	15.72 ± 3.99		18.36 ± 1.77		14.66 ± 2.18	
	Range	13.08	33.41	15.97	22.57	11.59	18.91
Middle distance	Mean ± SD	33.05 ± 2.42		30.58 ± 2.60		31.86 ± 3.89	
	Range	28.52	38.01	27.19	37.61	26.16	40.73
Long distance	Mean ± SD	72.78 ± 10.52		48.41 ± 3.93		72.48 ± 14.71	
	Range	61.19	116.81	43.50	59.39	59.33	117.13
Women							
Short distance	Mean ± SD	17.91 ± 1.50		10.02 ± 1.16		17.87 ± 3.26	
	Range	15.56	21.80	8.27	12.29	14.55	26.54
Middle distance	Mean ± SD	40.72 ± 3.00		19.04 ± 1.57		37.20 ± 3.44	
	Range	37.10	45.13	16.39	21.35	33.20	44.31
Long distance	Mean ± SD	65.44 ± 4.11		35.14 ± 2.57		59.19 ± 5.48	
	Range	59.13	72.50	31.50	39.51	53.57.6	1.10.19

Biathlon consists of either a 7.5 km (short distance) or 12.5 km (long distance) loop/route divided into three or five 2.5 km stages, respectively. Between each stage athletes stop for two or four shooting sessions along the course and are allowed to hit a target located at a distance of 10 m with five shots. The penalty for a missed shot can be a time penalty added to the total time, or a penalty loop (150 m) to ski once per missed shot. Recently the short distance is sometimes substituted by the "pursuit," which consists of two sprint races within about 2 h. The first race, in which actual time is corrected by the class and the shooting penalties, serves as ranking for the second race in which penalty loops are applied for missed shots. The most important success factor during competition depends on the capability of alternating endurance performance, which depends on maximal aerobic power and anaerobic lactic capacity, and the shooting accuracy, which is affected by this specific skill but which is also related to the maximal aerobic power (the faster the HR declines the better the shooting accuracy). The total biathlon performance is therefore the result of skiing performance, which depends on both technical and athletic capabilities, and shooting performance, which consists of duration of shooting (shooting time) and shooting results (penalty time).

It has been shown in able-bodied Nordic skiers that about 85–90% of the energy for the shorter races is being provided aerobically and for the longer races, the aerobic energy contribution exceeds 98% (Eisenman et al., 1989). These figures certainly apply to disabled skiers but we can expect in standing Paralympic skiers a slightly higher taxing of the lactic anaerobic metabolism because of their greater strength effort. Aerobic fitness (VO_{2max} in ml/kg/min), together with technical skill (economy of motion) and the ability to work at a high percentage of VO_{2max} (and therefore the steady-state maximal lactate) are the predictors of success in able-bodied Nordic skiing. During able-bodied racing conditions, indeed, oxygen uptake rarely operates below 85% VO_{2max} and it is often higher than 90% VO_{2max} in spite of relatively high BL levels because of the high numbers of mixed oxidative muscle fibers. A large oxidative power is essential to maintain high speeds throughout the race and to allow a powerful

anaerobic sprint at the end of the race. BL increases quickly in the first minutes of the races, thereafter reach a balance between production and clearance and increases during short uphill sections of the course. As elite able-bodied cross-country ski racers, disabled Nordic skiers have some of the highest aerobic power values reported for endurance athletes as a result of a combination of both genetics and rigorous multiyear, year-round, training programs.

Because of their unique responses to exercise and adaptations to training, this part of the chapter will deal with Nordic sitting skiers (NSS), who compete, using only the upper part of the body, sitting on a sledge mounted on two skis. In these skiers propulsion is obtained by pushing through two poles. NSS are divided into five classes (LW10, LW10.5, LW11, LW11.5, and LW12), depending on the level of functionality regardless the kind of motor impairment and compete together for the same medals. The biomechanics of the movement slightly differs among classes, because LW10 NSS do not have trunk stability (control of abdominal muscles), while LW11 NSS have no control over hip flexion nor lower limbs control. In spite of the individual functional characteristics and the consequent different best performances, NSS compete usually in all three distance races. As it can be calculated from Table 13.2, mean speeds are very similar in these three races because the course is slightly "easier" when it becomes longer. However, when exactly the same course is utilized, the initial speed of the longer races (e.g., the speed of the first lap of a 3 lap 10 km race) is similar to the initial speed of a short race (e.g., the speed of the first lap of a 2 lap 5 km race) and then speed decreases throughout the race. This strategy pattern was verified in a study, approved by the International Paralympic Committee (IPC) and Turin Organizing Committee (TOROC), aiming at describing the gross kinematics of NSS (speed, cycle length and duration, duty cycle) during actual races. To accomplish this purpose, all NSS competing in the Turin Winter Paralympic Games 2006 were video-recorded during short, middle, and long distance races on two sections of the track with different slopes (a flat and an uphill section). With the aim of studying fatigue in NSS, we also tested the hypothesis that this sort of "all-out" performance model was typical for all NSS and therefore that the athlete was able to maintain the same absolute intensity (i.e., to counteract fatigue as better as possible) would be the winner of the race. Figure 13.2 shows the course of the 15 km (4 laps). The long distance race,

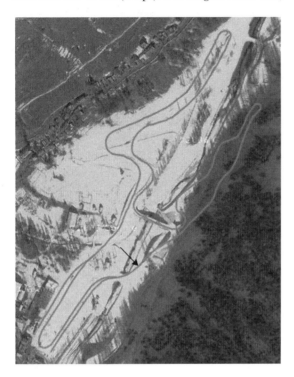

Figure 13.2 In the course of the 15 km (4 laps) in Pragelato during the Torino 2006 Winter Paralympic Games is indicated. The section of the course where the video-images were recorded is shown with an arrow.

indeed, was selected as the most appropriate race to study the physiological characteristics of NSS.

Besides the movement patterns, video-recording data were processed to measure the following parameters: cycle duration, cycle length, and duty cycle (percentage ratio between pushing and total cycle duration). From these parameters, sledge speeds during push and recovery phases of the cycle were calculated. In accordance with the final rank of the 15 km race, data collected were processed in 10 NSS, selected among the best and the worst classified, to obtain two groups in which one skier of each class was included. The group of the best NSS has been called G1 and that of the worst classified was called G2. In both groups, cycle speed showed a decreasing trend from the first to the last lap of the race during both flat and uphill sections. In the flat section of the course it decreased from 6.4 ± 0.15 to 5.5 ± 0.15 m/s in G1 and from 5.81 ± 0.48 to 4.57 ± 0.19 m/s in G2. G1 speed was significantly higher than G2 speed in the second, third, and last laps. The second-order polynomial curves of the graph of Figure 13.3 show this decreasing speed. These data are confirmed by the same kinematics analysis carried out to assess actual sledge speeds during the push and recovery phases of the cycle in both flat tracts and uphill tracts.

The average speed of the first lap, equal to 5.7 ± 0.27 m/s in G1 and 5.1 ± 0.35 m/s in G2,

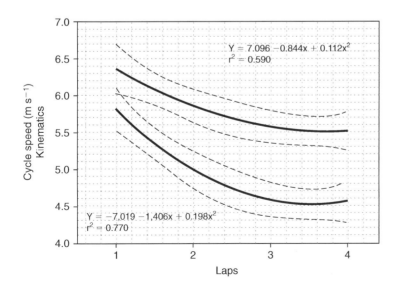

$$Y = 7.096 - 0.844x + 0.112x^2$$
$$r^2 = 0.590$$

$$Y = -7.019 - 1.406x + 0.198x^2$$
$$r^2 = 0.770$$

Figure 13.3 Speeds in the 4 laps of the 15 km race calculated from the cycle kinematics analysis obtained through video-recordings in a flat part of the course. Second-order polynomial curves, equations, and confidence intervals are shown for first (top lines) and last arrived Nordic sitting skiers (bottom lines).

decreased up to 5.4 ± 0.29 and 4.6 ± 0.42 m/s in G1 and G2, respectively, thus confirming the actual speeds obtained through the video-recording analyses of the flat and uphill sections. Considering that between the groups there were no significant differences in speed (flat, uphill, average) in the first lap but significant differences occurred at the last lap for all three speeds, a more pronounced fatigue effect was evident in G2. In conclusion, the strategy pattern is simply the attempt to keep speed as high as possible throughout the whole race, from the start to the end. Consequently, speed decreases from the first to the last lap of the race. This energy management strategy is used by all athletes. Both G1 and G2 NSS try to utilize all available energy sources from beginning to end. High levels of PF and therefore the ability to supply high amounts of energy throughout the race, at near equal intensity, seem to be the key to winning.

Energy expenditure and HR measurements during the three distances races confirm the performance pattern of the kinematics study. Data presented in this part of the chapter are related to athletes who competed in at least one of the following three Paralympic Winter Games: Nagano '98, Salt Lake City 2002, and Turin 2006. In this 10-year period, the authors followed, for at least 5 consecutive years, six top-level NSS, four male and two female athletes, with classes ranging between LW10 and LW12, who were studied both on field and in laboratory, to assess, respectively, their acute cardiorespiratory responses to different length races and their aerobic fitness. Field measurements were carried out in three experimental setups: during international level competitions (Paralympic Games or world championships), during Italian championships and in the Paralympic course of Pragelato few months before Turin 2006 Games. In the latter two occasions, we used a telemetric system (K4, Cosmed, Italy) to measure VE, VO_2, VCO_2 and HR. Figure 13.4 shows an NSS with a K4 apparatus during an Italian championship test.

BL peak was assessed at the end of the races (in Pragelato BL was collected also during a 10 km race, with few seconds of stops after each lap). HR and BL measurements were taken during world championships, while only HR measurements were taken during Paralympic Games. Laboratory sessions were

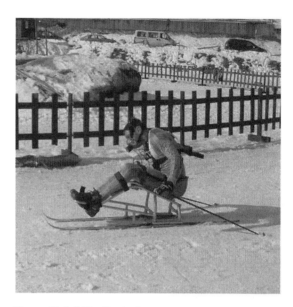

Figure 13.4 A Nordic sit-skier wearing a K4 apparatus during an Italian championship test.

carried out within a 2-week period with respect to the field measurements (for all measurements with the exclusion of the Paralympic Games that could also occur 1 month after the laboratory test). In the laboratory session, each athlete completed an incremental exercise test prolonged up to exhaustion to determine ventilatory threshold (VT) and VO_{2peak} under standardized laboratory conditions (see the methodology details in the section on the "general PF assessment"). Figure 13.5 shows typical metabolic and cardiac responses during the 5 km race of a very fit NSS.

As documented by Bernardi et al. (2010), mean VO_2 values during this race ranged in men, depending on the classes and the PF levels, between 32 and 50 ml/kg/min, corresponding in absolute values to 2.33 and 3.17 l/min. In three male NSS, the authors found VO_2 values for the 10 km race only slightly lower (39±5.9 ml/kg/min) and mean HR values slightly higher (175±9.3 beats/min). In both races, mean VO_2 corresponded to values higher than those found at the VT. The top values found in the most fatiguing phases of the race are about 95% of the maximal we observed during the laboratory exercise tests. Indeed, BL at the end of a 10 km race reaches mean values similar to the

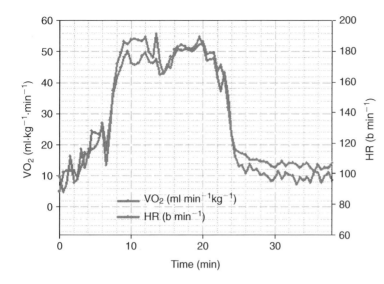

Figure 13.5 Oxygen uptake (VO_2) and heart rate (HR) responses during a 5-km-long Nordic sitting skiing race of an elite NSS. HR reaches peak values of 188 beats per minute, while VO_2 reaches 56 ml·kg^{-1}·min^{-1}.

maximal that can be found in these athletes in the laboratory maximal exercise tests (12–14 mmol). During the race the fittest NSS can show BL values around 5–7 mmol, confirming that the race intensity is just below the respiratory compensation levels. VO_2, HR, and BL do not differ significantly from data collected during the 15 km race. However, even when the PF of the NSS is very high, with the length of the race VO_2 decreases and HR increases.

A wide range of HR among Italian NSS was found in all distance races. This high standard deviation (about 11 beats/min) is explained by the difference in PF (only when the NSS are very fit they can maintain high HR values) and by the kind of impairment. NSS with spinal cord injury (SCI) tend to have about 10–15 beats/min higher values than NSS with poliomyelitis (PL) to counteract the lower venous return to the heart and the consequent lower stroke volume due to the Frank–Starling law.

Nordic sit-skiing locomotion energy costs (mean values) vary widely ranging from 2.7 to 4.5 j/kg/m depending on the mean speed during the race. This variability in energy cost is only partially due to the different technical skill of the NSS (economy of locomotion) but it is mainly due to the characteristics of the course (number and slope of downhill and uphill sections) and to the environmental conditions (which affects the gliding on the snow).

It is useful to know that, when the PF level is high, HR strictly mirrors the VO_2, being for the athlete an effective way to monitor the exercise intensity. At the end of the race if the intensity is kept high (little decrease of average speed), HR tend to increase slightly with respect to VO_2. As fatigue occurs in these athletes, HR tends to decrease. If HR is actually lower than the typical values for that athlete, this is an evidence of lower mechanical work due to poor effort or lower PF status. The graph of Figure 13.6 shows the HR during three distance races of the same NSS. The athlete won gold medals in both the 5 and 10 km races but was not as much successful in the long distance race. It is evident that mean HR (straight horizontal line) was significantly lower in the 15 km race.

Ice Sledge Hockey

Ice Sledge Hockey (ISH) is a high-intensity, intermittent game played on an ice surface by six athletes (three forwards, two defensemen, and one goalkeeper), strapped on a two-blade sledge. ISH players use sticks during competition that have a spike-end for propulsion and a blade-end for handling a puck of vulcanized rubber (weight up to 170 g). Because body contact is an integral part of the game, athletes wear protective gear including helmet with full cage, padding, and gloves. The sledge allows

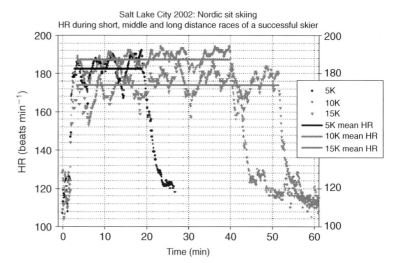

Figure 13.6 Heart rate (HR) of an NSS during three distance races of the Paralympic Winter Games of Salt lake City 2002. Actual values and mean values (horizontal lines) are in black, for the 5 km race, and in gray for both 10 km (top line) and 15 km (bottom line).

the puck to pass underneath. Athletes must have an impairment of permanent nature in the lower part of the body of such degree that it is obvious and easily recognizable, and consequently makes ordinary able-bodied standing ice hockey playing impossible. At the Paralympic level, each game consists of three 15-min periods of actual play and two rest intervals of 15 min. In case of parity in the finals for medals, there is a 10-min "overtime" period. If no goal is scored in this period, the winner will be decided through penalty scores. To play at an elite level, ISH requires a wide range of motor skills such as speed, coordination, balance, and agility to allow coordinated, creative, and reactive responses, as well as a high level of all the components of PF. Indeed, ISH is characterized by brief sprints of maximal acceleration, lower-intensity skating, checking and fighting for position, shooting and passing.

Total actual playing time per game ranges approximately from 11 to 19 min for forwards and 15 to 25 min for defensemen. The "shift" between player lines spent on the ice, which includes about two parts of uninterrupted play (approximately 30–50 s) followed by official play stoppage (approximately 20–35 s), lasts between 50 and 90 s. Depending on the number of player lines in the team (usually two for defensemen and three for forwards), the time between shifts ranges from 2 to 3 min. The best and most physically fit players are obliged to spend more time on the ice if few good substitutes are available. This causes an obvious performance detriment for the team.

A German time motion analysis study shows that during a line shift researchers can distinguish between phases of different intensities. Approximately 30–35% of the time the players skate slowly (speed lower than 2 m/s) and glide (especially when making turns). These low-intensity phases account for the majority of the distance covered during the match; however, a large variability among players exists. The distance covered as result of the line shift during the low-intensity phases averages about 6–700 m. Approximately 25% and 10% of the playing time is spent in body contact and puck handling, respectively. Phases of high intensity can be divided into sprints that are either longer or shorter than 10 m. Considering that the average period of hard skating during a shift is less than 5 s and that players have to change direction to avoid other players or make a move on the ice, there is usually not enough time to reach full speed. For this reason and for the obvious inertia of the system composed by sledge plus player, in short sprints speed ranges between 2 and 4 m/s and in long sprints it ranges between 4 and 5 m/s. In a match we can observe about 20 short (distance covered ranges between 5 and 6 m) and 20 long (distance covered renges between 14 and 24 m) sprints. Each one accounts for about 17% of the match time. Canadian time motion analyses partially confirm these data. According to them, in a single shift maximum effort sprints, which last about 3 s and are repeated four to six times, account for only 10% of total match time. Almost 40% of the match is spent doing light (mild intensity) skating or fast gliding, 25% for resting and slow gliding and 25% for moderate skating. These differences can be explained by game strategies and technical schemes as well as by the actual number of player lines used during the match.

These biomechanical evaluations are confirmed by physiological measurements (German and personal Italian data are averaged). Average HR during shifts (actual playing) is 147 ± 15 beats/min with lower values for defensemen and an increasing trend during the third period. HR shows an up and down trend, depending on the phases of the game, peaking at about 90% of the maximal HR values and rarely going below 120 beats/min. Based on a comparison from HR measurements on the ice with VO_2 measurements collected during arm cranking ergometry (ACE) incremental maximal exercise tests, we estimate an average intensity level of about 71 ± 5% of the maximal aerobic power. BL measurements confirm these figures ranging from 4 to 6 mmol.

From biomechanical and physiological measurements, the German study concludes that aerobic and anaerobic metabolisms account for 65% and 35%, respectively, of the energy provision. We can assume therefore that the relatively low lactate levels are due to frequent play stoppages and shift changes which, as with able-bodied hockey players, help to conserve glycogen allowing higher-energy production from aerobic metabolism. This suggests that an all-out intense shift with little stoppage would mean that anaerobic lactic metabolism would provide the majority of the energy, whereas in a shift composed of starts and stops, energy supply would be dependent mostly from the anaerobic alactic metabolism and the high-energy phosphagens would be replenished by aerobic processes. In the latter case, or when the recovery time during shifts is longer, the levels of BL would result lower.

Training should be focused on developing high levels of aerobic stamina, explosive power, anaerobic capacity, strength, and flexibility. Aerobic metabolism will allow the players to counteract fatigue as much as possible, especially important when players cannot be easily substituted. High-intensity interval training on ice with hockey sledges and on treadmill with sledge-rolls (or with ACEs if a treadmill is not available) is highly recommended for this purpose. Explosive power will allow them to propel themselves as fast as possible (the ability to change direction and to accelerate the sledge as quickly as possible play a fundamental role in ISH). Short sprints of different length on ice both in a linear path and with specific changes of directions will be useful to increase explosive power. Anaerobic capacity must be developed to tax the lactic anaerobic metabolism as effectively as possible and to be able to bear high levels of BL. Repetitions of high-intensity exercises as those typical for interval training and repetitions of long sprints can be useful for this purpose. Strength will be fundamental during body contact, will help in preventing both contact and noncontact injuries, and is a determinant factor of high explosive power. The latter is important not only to accelerate and decelerate body weight but is also a requisite for shooting as powerful as possible. High-resistance weight training of both trunk and upper limb muscles is recommended for this purpose. Flexibility will allow them to perform the skills of the game (balance and agility) more effectively and resist injury during contact and collisions, and therefore should be part of each training session.

Finally it is important to stress that it is highly recommended for an effective training and a successful performance that fluid loss should be minimized through a careful practice of rehydration. Since ISH is played in a seemingly cool environment, there may be a misconception that players do not encounter thermoregulatory problems. The combination of heavy padding, neutral thermal environment, and high metabolic activity contributes to a significant heat load. Since the primary mechanism of heat dissipation is through sweating, appropriate volumes of water should be drunk.

Thermoregulation and responses to hypoxia in athletes with SCI

Several winter sports disciplines are performed normally in special environmental conditions characterized by low temperature and reduced oxygen content in the air. These extreme conditions will challenge the winter Paralympic athletes.

Body cooling results when metabolic heat production is not sufficient to offset the body heat loss to the environment. The response to cold stress involves primarily the increase in tissue insulation by peripheral vasoconstriction and then the increase in metabolic rate by nonshivering and shivering thermogenesis. The body can be divided into two macroregions with different temperatures: the core and peripheral tissues outside the core. There is a temperature profile from the distal to proximal and from surface to deep regions of the body. When the body is exposed to a temperature gradient, there is a flux of heat. The body mass acts as a buffer, affecting the rate of body cooling during initial period of heat flux. Muscles (40% of the body mass) and subcutaneous fat (15% of the body mass) have the major influence on body heat loss. Many studies have shown that individuals with a bigger layer of subcutaneous fat cool more slowly than those with less fat. Comparing individuals with similar subcutaneous fat but with different muscle mass, it has been found that smaller people cool faster than larger ones. Normal healthy individuals are able to maintain a stable body temperature under normal ambient conditions, while individuals with SCI may have abnormal regulation of body temperature or may be less able to respond to changes in environment. People with SCI may have higher core temperatures in heat and lower core temperatures in the cold. They also present a very large portion of the skin that is insentient to changes in cold and heat, because the thermal-sensitive receptors in the skin require an intact spinal cord and its hypothalamic feedback. This condition leads to a loss in hypothalamic control, a poor vasomotor reaction, and an inability to sweat. For these reasons individuals with SCI have a substantial reduction of the heat production rate that may increase only 10–15% in response to a drop in ambient temperature, whereas in able-bodied a similar change of ambient temperature leads to an increase in heat production rate from 200% to 500%. The magnitude of impairment in thermoregulation is related to the level and completeness of the lesion.

The higher and more complete the SCI, the greater the thermoregulation impairment. Boot et al. (2006) showed that there are no differences in upper body skin temperature at rest between spinal cord injured and able-bodied controls. Instead they found a significantly cooler lower-body skin and core temperature in spinal cord injured compared to able-bodied controls. The possible explanations for these findings are muscle atrophy below the lesion and a shivering response that can take place only above the lesion level.

During ACE exercise in 10°C ambient conditions, individuals with SCI are not able to maintain their heat balance. The imbalance between heat production and heat storage may be related to the fact that the active muscle mass involved in ACE exercise is small because they are not able, due to their paralysis, to use their legs and trunk muscles for stabilization. In conclusion, despite the exercise, the heat balance in the cold is negative, which suggests a potential danger of hypothermia for athletes with SCI when exercising in the cold. Indeed, also at rest the lack of sympathetic vasoregulation below the level of the lesion may impede adequate vasoconstriction, in order to prevent heat loss in a cold environment. This mechanism could also impair the physiological responses to exercise in a hypoxic environment. For this reason it is very interesting to note that in chronic hypoxia conditions, some degree of sympathetic overreactivity that leads to vasoconstriction is necessary to maintain an adequate match between O_2 delivery and O_2 demand at the microvascular level in the exercising muscles. The sympathetic vasoconstrictor tone is greater in the less active muscles while it is attenuated in the more active muscles, providing an optimal balance of vasodilation and perfusion pressure for the muscles fibers with the greatest oxygen demand.

Regarding the physiological responses of spinal cord injured to exercise in hypoxic environments, there is a lack of studies in the scientific literature, but we can argue that the impaired mechanism due to the lesion could limitate the hypoxic response of the body. It has been demonstrated that the ventilatory response to hypoxia in individuals with SCI was not impaired by the interruption of the motor traffic running down to the spinal cord to respiratory muscle motoneurons. Despite no limitation of the ventilatory responses to hypoxia, the breathing pattern is different in spinal cord injured compared to able-bodied. Pokorski et al. (1995) have shown that the mean inspiratory flow (tidal volume divided by the time of inspiration) is the same, both in normoxia and hypoxia, in spinal cord injured compared to able-bodied controls; however, single components of mean inspiratory flow change with a smaller increase in tidal volume and a shorter time of inspiration. These results show that ventilation in spinal cord injured is more superficial and rapid.

The peripheral chemoreflex sensitivity to hypoxia is increased during exercise in able-bodied. This increase is determined by a neural drive from cortical irradiation during voluntary exercise, humoral factors carried in the bloodstream, and afferent neural information from exercising limbs. Pandit et al. (1994) demonstrated that electrically induced leg exercise (stimulation of the quadriceps muscles, in order to obtain the extension of the leg at the knee against gravity) in paraplegics during a brief period of hypoxia was able to cause an increase in hypoxic sensitivity during exercise. They concluded that afferent neural inputs from the limbs and volitional control are unnecessary for the increase in the acute ventilator response to hypoxia which occurs during steady exercise in paraplegics, and that the acute ventilator response to exercise in acute hypoxia is mediated only by humoral factors.

The interest in spinal cord injured athletes performing exercise in an altitude environment also leads to the question whether these individuals experience similar symptoms or have a similar occurrence of illness in altitude (acute mountain sickness—AMS) as able-bodied individuals. Dicianno et al. (2008) found that the occurrence and severity of AMS in individuals with neurological impairments (SCI, traumatic brain injury, and polytrauma) are at least as high and as severe as in those without disabilities and that the most common symptoms are fatigue and weakness.

In conclusion both in cold and hypoxic environments, individuals with SCI should take precautions to counteract possible adverse reactions especially during exercise. The advantage of the intermittent exposure to hypoxia at high altitude (increases submaximal aerobic efficiency) seen in able-bodied individuals could be aspired by individuals with SCI to improve VO_{2max}. To accomplish this purpose during high-altitude training, individuals with SCI should take extreme care in appropriate clothing and monitoring body temperature in the part of the body without sensory input.

General physical PF assessment

From the above described analyses of the physiological characteristics of each winter sport and of the consequences of SCI, it is evident that disabled athletes should have high levels of both technical abilities and PF to be successful in their performance. In Italy, to exclude possible risks due to high-level sport participation and to reduce injuries and diseases, besides the mandatory eligibility visit requested by the Italian Law, a health and fitness screening before the Paralympic Games is compulsory, in accordance with the rules of Italian Olympic and Paralympic Committees, for all athletes who may be involved in the following Games. For Paralympic athletes, the examinations of this preparticipation screening include a comprehensive health and fitness evaluation to assess their sport eligibility to compete at the Paralympic level. In this context, a norm of best practice is to globally evaluate, along with pulmonary, cardiovascular and metabolic health, all the physiological components of PF. To accomplish this PF assessment, all winter sports athletes (WSAs), regardless the practiced sport discipline, are functionally evaluated through the same nonspecific tests to compare possible differences among athletes of the same sport group. The PF assessment also compares sport groups to one another to assess specific adaptations induced by the sport discipline. This general PF evaluation should be carried out at least once a year, preferably at the beginning of the season, and should be used to assess the basal level of the athletes to improve the interpretation of the results of both sport performance and field evaluations (e.g., energy expenditure during sport simulation) and to give directions on the training prescriptions to coaches, athletic trainers, and obviously the athletes. Later in the season, the PF components of the specific sport should be assessed through a specific functional evaluation based on ergometers designed to simulate the typical gestures of the practiced sport.

The comprehensive general PF assessment carried out during this preparticipation screening includes the following physiological components: body composition, maximal aerobic power, strength and anaerobic power and capacity. For visually impaired skiers, PF can be carried out using routine tests used for able-bodied individuals. PF reference values are not available for sitting WSAs, including individuals with SCI, PL, lower limb amputation (LLA), and other neurological and orthopedic disorders. Obviously these PF reference values are necessary to substantiate basal assessments and document progression of training. To accomplish this purpose, in this section of the chapter we aggregated the PF evaluation results of the most successful Italian male WSA. PF tests were carried out before the last four Paralympic Winter Games, from Nagano 1998 to Vancouver 2010, using, for the athletes who competed in more than one Paralympic Winter Game, only the results of the period of their best performance.

WSA groups included 4 Curlers (3 individuals with SCI and 1 with lower limb dysmelia), 5 Alpine skiers (4 with SCI and 1 with spina bifida), 6 Nordic skiers (2 with PL, 1 with LLA, and 3 with SCI), and 14 ISH players (11 with LLA, 1 with SCI, 1 with PL, and 1 with femur agenesis). There were no differences among groups in mean age, which ranged between 34.7 ± 5.24 years old in Alpine skiers and 43.2 ± 8.35 in Nordic skiers, and mean height (range from 1.74 ± 0.05 m in Nordic skiers to 1.83 ± 0.09 m in Curlers). Body mass was higher in Curlers (83.8 ± 26.36 kg), because of a very heavy athlete (see the high standard deviation), than in the rest of the athletes (71.9 ± 11.26). Each group, with the exclusion of ISH, included WSA with the whole range of functional classes (LW10–12).

Percentage of fat mass is determined from skinfold measurements, elaborating the body density calculation with the four skinfold (biceps, triceps, subscapular, and medial suprailiac) measurements of the Durnin and Womersley equation. Eleven skinfolds (abdominal, triceps, biceps, chest, pectoral, medial calf, midaxillary, subscapular, anterior suprailiac, medial suprailiac, and thigh), however, are measured during the preparticipation screening for a better assessment of fat mass. Indeed, to our knowledge, no fat mass assessment validation for individuals with locomotor disabilities has been provided for these measurements and therefore, because only general ideas can be derived from the percentage of body mass values, a norm of best practice is to follow during the time differences in skinfold thickness. Nordic skiers, as typically found in endurance athletes that must carry their body weight during their performance, had the lowest body mass (62.6 ± 5.83 kg) and also the lowest fat mass values ($13.5 \pm 2.20\%$). Curlers, who can get benefits from a high body mass for a more stable posture when throwing the stone, had the highest values of fat mass ($27.2 \pm 6.70\%$), but again these values, which can be considered pathologic, overall derive from an obese athlete (fat mass = 34.3%). Intermediate

values were found in ISH players ($21.3 \pm 5.53\%$) and in Alpine skiers ($19.4 \pm 8.48\%$).

For an effective evaluation of both aerobic and anaerobic fitness, it is essential to plan correct stress protocols and to choose appropriate ergometers. To evaluate athletes with locomotor disabilities, ACEs, wheelchair ergometers, and treadmills are the most widely used. The ACE has been extensively used as an instrument to evaluate individuals with SCI from both a clinical and functional point of view. Its popularity derives from the following advantages: low cost, high reproducibility (regardless the type of impairment of the subject), and high efficiency due to the coordinated movement (circular alternated movement of the arms). The latter characteristic allows a fine regulation of the workload and the possibility to assess appropriate protocols for each purpose (graded aerobic exercise tests and anaerobic constant power or constant torque exercise tests). The major disadvantage of ACEs is that it is not task specific. Because the purpose of the screening evaluation is to compare athletes competing in different sport disciplines and in which locomotion is peculiar to each one (e.g., Nordic skiing mobility differs from the ISH mobility), the present reference values are obtained with ACEs for all athletes and for both (aerobic and anaerobic) general PF evaluations.

Aerobic fitness (VO_{2peak} and VT) is assessed through an integrative cardiopulmonary continuous incremental multistage exercise test carried out up to volitional exhaustion (Bernardi et al., 2010). The workload of an iso-power ACE (ER-800, Ergoline, Germany) is appropriately graded to evaluate subject's ability to tolerate increasing intensities of exercise. Pulmonary, cardiac, and metabolic responses to the exercise test are monitored through a breath-by-breath metabolic chart (Quark b^2, Cosmed, Italy). Heart responses are also beat by beat monitored through electrocardiography to assess possible manifestations of ischemia, arrhythmia, or other cardiac abnormalities.

When choosing the protocol a compromise between clinical and functional evaluations must be found, so the effort phase (excluding the warm-up) of the graded exercise test should last about 10 min modulating appropriately the duration and the workload of warm-up and of each step increment. The test consists of a 3-min warm-up phase at a constant

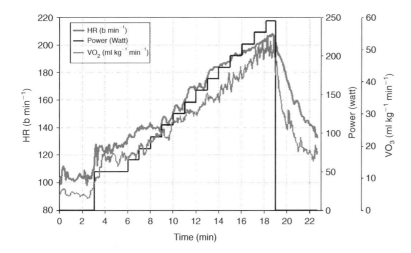

Figure 13.7 Heart rate (HR), (top line in gray) oxygen uptake (VO₂), and mechanical power of a successful Nordic sit-skier with spinal cord injury during an incremental maximal exercise test carried out with an arm cranking ergometer.

power ranging from 10 to 50 W. This phase is followed by a ramp fashion effort phase with increments of either 10 or 15 W every minute depending upon functional classification and estimated aerobic fitness of the athlete. The test is interrupted when the athlete is unable to maintain the power despite constant encouragement, or when at least two of the following criteria are attained during the exercise phase of the test: (1) a HR equivalent to 100% of their age predicted maximum (220—age, years), (2) levelling off or decline in the $\dot{V}O_2$ with increasing work rate, and (3) a respiratory exchange ratio $\geq$ 1.10. Figure 13.7 shows metabolic and cardiac responses to an ACE maximal exercise test in a successful NSS with SCI. The very high HR_{max}, VO_{2peak}, and power output values reached at the end of the test demonstrate

the very high aerobic fitness of NSS (see Bernardi et al., 2010, for a comparison with disabled athletes competing in Summer Sports). It is very interesting to note the fact that the athlete was able to reach very high HR values (over 200 beats/min) in spite of his age (35 years old). Indeed athletes with SCI may have a reduced venous return and therefore a reduced stroke volume, relying more on HR to increase their cardiac output. At each intensity level, SCI athletes display higher HR values (about 10–15 beats/min) than athletes with other locomotor disabilities (e.g., amputation or PL). When appropriately trained, athletes with SCI can reach maximal HR values higher than those expected in relation to age. Table 13.3 shows PF data in the WSAs of the four sports disciplines.

Table 13.3 Mean and standard deviations values of the physical fitness components evaluated in Italy during health and fitness preparticipation (Paralympic Games) screenings. Data of maximal aerobic power (oxygen uptake peak—VO₂ peak), maximal mechanical work carried out in an exhaustion test, and sum of the MVCs of each upper limb (see text) are expressed in relative values, normalized per kg of body mass, while explosive (all-out) power in a 10-s-long Wingate test is expressed as absolute values.

Sports	V'O₂peak (ml/kg/min)	Exhaustion test (J/kg)	Upper body strength (N/kg)	10-s-long Wingate test (W)
Curling	24.6 ± 9.36	158.0 ± 32.05	12.3 ± 0.22	269 ± 108.2
Sitting Nordic ski	47.4 ± 8.23	277.1 ± 77.08	15.2 ± 1.76	364 ± 37.1
Sitting Alpine ski	31.8 ± 6.63	205.1 ± 66.48	15.4 ± 4.03	463 ± 118.3
Ice Sledge Hockey	36.8 ± 4.75	235.5 ± 35.71	13.3 ± 4.26	422 ± 52.2

As expected NSS show the highest relative VO_{2peak} values, which correspond in absolute values to 2.89 ± 0.524 l/min. NSS relative values are significantly higher than those of the other groups. Because no adaptive effect can be expected from their sport, Curlers display the lowest VO_{2peak} relative and absolute (1.90 ± 0.355 l/min) values. These values are similar to sedentary individuals with SCI. Curlers should be encouraged to engage in aerobic exercises to increase their cardiovascular fitness. ISH players have VO_{2peak} absolute values (2.7 ± 0.38 l/min) similar to athletes competing in intermittent sports such as wheelchair basketball (Bernardi et al., 2010). Aerobic fitness is confirmed to be an important determinant of ISH performance.

With the same ACE and with the same instruments used to monitor pulmonary, cardiac, and metabolic responses as in the aerobic exercise test, we set up a constant load exercise test to assess anaerobic capacity, the greatest amount of mechanical work that can be carried out during a high-intensity exercise (intensity ranging between 130% and 170% VO_{2peak}). The athlete is requested to reach a revolution speed ranging from 70 to 90 rpm in 20 s while the power corresponds to 20 W and then, after that power is abruptly increased up to the high intensity level, to maintain the revolution speed at the imposed power as long as possible. The test is terminated when the athlete is no longer able to maintain the power (cadence drops below 70 rpm) for more than 3 s. This exhaustion exercise test has an average duration of about 70 s and is able to elicit a BL production (BL peak values after the test) significantly higher than the 30 s long all-out Wingate test, being for this reason more reliable in assessing lactic anaerobic capacity. Figure 13.8 shows the typical metabolic and cardiac responses to the exhaustion test. The VCO_2 response, which passes the VO_2 value before the end of the exercise, demonstrates the high intensity of the test.

NSS (Figure 13.9) show the highest values of maximal mechanical work at the exhaustion test. This result is an expression of the high anaerobic capacity of these athletes. Anaerobic capacity, besides maximal aerobic power, is an important PF determinant of the performance in Nordic skiing. When expressed in absolute values, maximal mechanical work of NSS

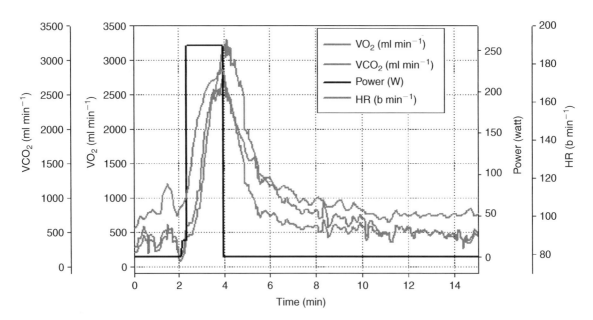

Figure 13.8 Typical oxygen uptake (VO_2), carbon dioxide production ($V'CO_2$), and heart rate (HR) responses to the exhaustion test (mechanical power as a function of time is also shown).

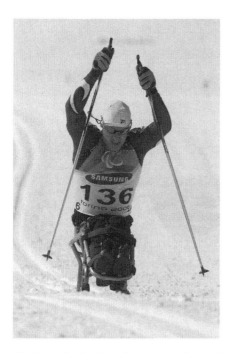

Figure 13.9 Nordic sit skiers show tremendous values of aerobic power but are also characterized by a high anaerobic capacity. Reproduced courtesy of Lieven Coudenys.

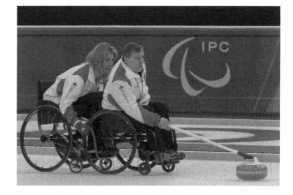

Figure 13.10 Curlers can be considered as control subjects because the sport does not modify their health related physical fitness characteristics. Reproduced courtesy of Lieven Coudenys.

(17.1 ± 5.20 kJ) is similar to that of ISH players (17.6 ± 2.93 kJ), showing the importance of this PF component in this intermittent sport especially for players who must stay for long periods of play on the ice without rest phases. Indeed ISH have significantly higher absolute values than Curlers (control group, Figure 13.10). To improve the ability to produce (for energy purposes) and sustain lactic acid, for both NSS and ISH players, we recommend interval training based on four to six repetitions of high-intensity exercise at levels similar to those of the exhaustion test. This interval training can be carried out with an ACE in the gym but training with a treadmill or on-field with a sledge would be much more effective (e.g., see the ISH section on training).

Strength and maximal explosive power are also routinely evaluated during the preparticipation screening. Strength is evaluated through isometric maximal voluntary contractions (MVCs) of each upper limb keeping, with the trunk erected, both shoulder and arm at 90° angles (MK7 dynamometer, Dal Monte, Italy). In this way not only the upper limb muscles but also the muscles connecting the

upper extremity to the vertebral column (trapezius, rhomboideus minor, rhomboideus major, latissimus dorsi, levator scapulae) and the muscles connecting the upper extremity to the anterior and lateral thoracic wall (pectoralis major, pectoralis minor, subclavius, serratus anterior) are globally evaluated. The two best values of three MVCs of each upper limb are summed to give the final result. Values measured with the same equipment in summer sports disabled athletes showed high correlations with the mean power obtained during a 30-s-long ACE Wingate test. Alpine skiers, in particular the most successful ones, show tremendous values of strength, especially when expressed as absolute values (1223 ± 235.1 N). This is definitely a major adaptation to this sport and should be specifically trained to improve performance. Nordic skiers showed relative strength values similar to Alpine skiers, these values being significantly higher than Curlers. The impact of this PF component in cross-country performance is also demonstrated. Strength training, both to improve performance and for health purposes, should be incorporated in the training programs of all WSAs.

Maximal explosive power is evaluated through a 10-s-long all-out test (Wingate test) carried out with a constant torque ACE (Excalibur, Lode, Holland). The torque in which the athlete applies the highest power is previously assessed. Alpine skiers showed the highest mean power in absolute (Table 13.3) and relative values (5.9 ± 1.81 W/kg). ISH players and Nordic skiers show similar relative values. Significantly lowers values are displayed by the Curlers when the data of these athletes, both in absolute and relative values, are compared with those of the other WSA pooled together. From the comparison among groups of these power values and taking into account the above-mentioned characteristics of the sports, we can conclude that specific training procedures to improve explosive power should be incorporated in the training schedule of ISH players. To accomplish this purpose specific on-ice drills should be carried out.

Conclusions

This chapter has shown the relevant importance of PF assessment to guide training prescription, and therefore to make the functional basis to increase performance in ISH players and in athletes with locomotor impairments competing in Curling, Alpine, and Nordic skiing. However, in these sports, success seems to be strictly related to the global amount of on-field training because athletic preparation does not support sufficiently motor skills and functional capacities which are the basis for the best performance. Preparation for Winter Games, therefore, besides off-snow and off-ice training consists of a great volume of on-field training which are often performed in mountain environment with cold temperature and low oxygen. These training procedures require appropriate adaptations (regarding duration and intensity of training) and specific awareness to allow the best sport results in the safest conditions for the athletes.

Acknowledgment

Most of the information shown in the Ice sledge hockey section of the chapter derives from a deep and illuminating research carried out by Dr. Heinz Nowoisky. A book on this topic in German language has been recently published. We acknowledge his support providing the enormous amount of data of his research that are here summarized.

We thank Dr. Silvia Carucci M.D., Dr. Paolo Emilio Adami M.D. and Dr. Livio Zerbini for their valuable assistance in processing some data of this chapter. We also thank Florian Planker, Roland Ruepp, Enzo Masiello and Winkler Werner, athletes of the Italian Paralympic team, for their experienced advises.

References

Andersen, R.E. & Montgomery, D.L. (1988). Physiology of Alpine skiing. *Sports Medicine*, **6**, 210–221.

Bernardi, M., Guerra, E., Di Giacinto, B., Di Cesare, A., Castellano, V. & Bhambhani, Y. (2010). Field evaluation of Paralympic athletes in selected sports: implications for training. *Medicine & Science in Sports & Exercise*, **42**(6),1200–1208.

Boot, C.R., Binkhorst, R.A. & Hopman, M.T. (2006) Body temperature responses in spinal cord injured individuals during exercise in the cold and heat. *International Journal of Sports Medicine*, **27**, 599–604.

Dicianno, B.E., Aguila E.D., Cooper R.A., et al. (2008). Acute mountain sickness in disability and adaptive sports: preliminary data. *Journal of Rehabilitation Research and Development*, **45**, 479.

Eisenman, P.A., Johnson, S.C., Bainbridge, C.N. & Zupan M.F. (1989). Applied physiology of cross-country skiing. *Sports Medicine*, **8**, 67–69.

Pandit, J.J., Bergstrom, E., Frankel, H.L. & Robbins, P.A. (1994). Increased hypoxic ventilatory sensitivity during exercise in man: Are neural afferents necessary? *Journal of Physiology*, **477**, 169–176.

Pokorski, M., Morikawa, T. & Honda, Y. (1995). Breathing pattern in tetraplegics during exposure to hypoxia and hypercapnia. Materia Medica Polona. *Polish Journal of Medicine and Pharmacy*, **27**, 97–100.

Veicsteinas, A., Ferretti, G., Margonato, V., Rosa, G. & Tagliabue, D. (1984). Energy cost of and energy sources for Alpine skiing in top athletes. *Journal of Applied Physiology: Respiration Environmental Exercise Physiology*, **56**, 1187–1190.

Recommended reading

American College of Sports Medicine (2009). ACSM's Guidelines for Exercise Testing and Prescription, 8th edition. Lippincott Williams & Wilkins, Baltimore, MD.

Chapter 14
Contribution of sport science to performance—wheelchair rugby

Laurie A. Malone[1], Natalia Morgulec-Adamowicz[2] and Kevin Orr[3]

[1]Department of Research & Education, Lakeshore Foundation, Birmingham, AL, USA
[2]Department of Adapted Physical Activity, The Józef Piłsudski University of Physical Education, Warsaw, Poland
[3]Canadian Wheelchair Sports Association, Ottawa, ON, Canada

Wheelchair rugby—history

Wheelchair rugby, an exciting fast-paced sport, was first developed in Canada in the 1970s as a team sport for quadriplegic athletes seeking an alternative to the popular sport of wheelchair basketball. It was originally referred to as "murderball" due to the extreme physical nature of the sport.

As the sport grew in Canada, wheelchair rugby first appeared in the United States as a demonstration event at a regional multisport competition in the late 1970s. Soon afterward, the first team was formed in the United States, followed by the first international tournament in 1982 with teams from the United States and Canada (Figure 14.1). Throughout the 1980s, other local and national tournaments began to take place in various countries. The first international wheelchair rugby tournament to include a team from outside North America, specifically Great Britain, was held in 1989. As an exhibition event, wheelchair rugby was first played at the World Wheelchair Games in 1990.

In 1993, the International Wheelchair Rugby Federation (IWRF) was founded with 15 charter member teams. The following year wheelchair rugby was officially recognized by the International Paralympic Committee as a Paralympic sport and in 1995 the first Rugby World Championships were

The Paralympic Athlete, 1st edition. Edited by Yves C. Vanlandewijck and Walter R. Thompson. Published 2011 by Blackwell Publishing Ltd.

held with eight teams competing. In 1996, wheelchair rugby was included as a demonstration sport at the Atlanta Paralympic Games, and finally was included as a full medal sport at the 2000 Sydney Paralympic Games. There are approximately 25 countries, divided into three zones, actively playing wheelchair rugby. The major international competitions in wheelchair rugby include Zone Championships (held in each odd-numbered year), the World Championships (quadrennially in even-numbered years, opposite the Summer Paralympic Games), and the Paralympic Games.

The game

Wheelchair rugby is a full contact (chair-on-chair) game played on an indoor hardwood court measuring 15 m in width by 28 m in length. The object of the game is to score more points than the opposing team; one point is awarded when a player who has possession of the ball passes two wheels over the goal line. The game is played in four 8-min stop-time quarters with additional 3-min overtime periods if necessary. Each team is allowed six time-outs, plus one extra time-out for each overtime played. The team with the greatest point total at the completion of the game is declared the winner.

In sanctioned play, athletes compete in manual wheelchairs specifically designed for wheelchair rugby according to the IWRF specifications. A regulation volleyball is used and must be bounced or

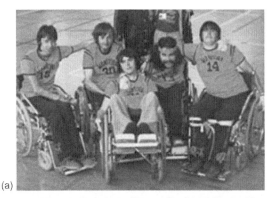

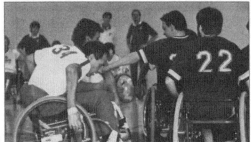

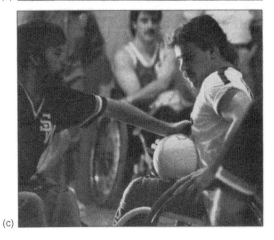

Figure 14.1 (a) First wheelchair rugby team in the world; includes the 5 players who created the game and promoted it in Canada and then the US growing to what it has now become, a worldwide Paralympic sport. The players are (from right to left): Paul LeJeune (deceased), Chris Sargeant, Duncan Campbell, Jerry Terwin, and Randy Dueck. Photo courtesy of the Canadian Wheelchair Sports Association. (b) DRIve Quad Rugby Classic on February 27, 1988. Southwest Sowhats (Canada) Mike LaRochelle (22) and Harry DeBryne attempt to block Dallas Wheelchair Sidekicks' Andy Beck (34) and Dwight Goodman. ©Paralyzed Veterans of America, Sports 'n Spokes. (c) DRIve Quad Rugby Classic on February 27, 1988. Sowhat Mike LaRochelle challenges Sidekick Dwight Goodman. ©Paralyzed Veterans of America, Sports 'n Spokes.

passed between teammates at least once every 10 s during play. The ball may be passed, thrown, batted, rolled, dribbled, or carried in any direction subject to the restrictions laid down in the rules.

Contact between wheelchairs is permitted and forms an integral part of the game. Collisions, often with great impact, are frequent as players try to stop their opponents and take control of the ball. Contact that is considered dangerous, such as hitting an opponent's chair behind the rear wheel, is not permitted and will result in a penalty. Physical contact between players is not allowed.

If a penalty is received when a team is on offense, the play results in a turnover. On defense, if a player is penalized, he/she is sent to the penalty box and is released when the opposition scores a goal or after 1 min is served.

Some actions that result in a turnover include:
• player with the ball does not dribble or pass within 10 s;
• ball is not advanced over half court within 12 s;
• ball is not inbounded within 10 s;
• team does not score within 40 s after the ball is inbounded (2008 IWRF Rule, Article 53 and Article 87: 42nd Violation);
• offensive player is in the key (a specified area in front of the goal) longer than 10 s.
A penalty is given if more than three defenders are in the key at one time, or when a player hits an opposing player's chair behind the axles causing the chair to dramatically turn (spin).

Player classification

To create a fair and equitable competition, wheelchair rugby uses a classification system based on the levels of function in the hands, arms, shoulders, and trunk, giving a wide range of persons the opportunity to play. To be eligible for wheelchair rugby, individuals must have a neurological diagnosis, which affects at least three limbs and the trunk, or a nonneurological condition that affects all four limbs and the trunk. Wheelchair rugby is a sport that was originally developed for athletes with tetraplegia due to spinal cord injury and neuromuscular conditions such as poliomyelitis, but now includes athletes with conditions such as cerebral palsy, muscular dystrophy, and various types of central and peripheral nervous system conditions. Athletes with nonneurological conditions may also be eligible to play wheelchair rugby, if they have similar impairment and activity limitation to an athlete with tetraplegia, or tetra-equivalent impairments such as arthrogryposis multiplex congenita, multiple amputations, amelia, and other similar musculoskeletal conditions.

The classification system consists of seven classes ranging from 0.5 to 3.5; the higher the class, the lesser the impact of the impairment on the wheelchair rugby performance. Each player is given a point value corresponding to their functional level. To ensure that teams field a mix of athletes of all functional levels, the classification point value of players on the court at any one time cannot exceed eight points per team. For each female player on the court, however, a team is allowed an extra 0.5 points over and above the eight points for the team.

Annual performance plan

Annual performance plans are an integral part of elite sport; however, many Paralympic teams are far behind their Olympic counterparts in the development and effective use of such plans. These plans typically outline specific goals in the areas of athlete recruitment, emerging athletes, national team athletes, athlete support services, training schedule, sport science testing, performance standards, competition opportunities (domestic and international), and coach development.

Within Paralympic sport, some sports have well-defined plans, whereas others are still working toward better development and coordination. As Paralympic sport continues to grow and becomes more and more competitive, wheelchair rugby teams will have to spend more time focusing on this very important aspect of program design and success.

Since wheelchair rugby first appeared at the Paralympic Games in 1996, the following teams have

Table 14.1 Paralympic Games and World Championship wheelchair rugby medal winners since 1996.

Year	Event	Gold	Silver	Bronze
1996	Atlanta Paralympic Games (*demonstration event*)	USA	Canada	New Zealand
1998	World Championships	USA	New Zealand	Canada
2000	Sydney Paralympic Games (*full medal event*)	USA	Australia	New Zealand
2002	World Championships	Canada	USA	Australia
2004	Athens Paralympic Games	New Zealand	Canada	USA
2006	World Championships	USA	New Zealand	Canada
2008	Beijing Paralympic Games	USA	Australia	Canada

dominated the sport: USA, Canada, Australia, and New Zealand (Table 14.1).

Development of an annual training program

One of the most important aspects of performance optimization in all elite sports is a well-structured training program. Based on the competition schedule (including national and international events), the coach should develop the annual training program in accordance with the training concept of periodization. It is important that periodization is not limited to the structure of the training program, i.e., pre-season (preparatory phase), in-season (competition phase), and off-season (transitional phase), but also applies to the methodology of developing the dominant physiological requirements of the sport (e.g., strength, endurance, and speed). While setting objectives for the training program, the coach has to consider factors such as physical preparation (e.g., strength, speed, endurance, power, flexibility, and coordination), technical preparation (offensive and defensive skills), tactical preparation (both individual and team tactics), and psychological skill development (e.g., imagery and self-talk). An inherent part of the annual training program is player evaluation and skill assessment. Systematic and consistent evaluation is needed to provide information regarding the status of each training factor in order to determine specific strengths, weaknesses, and limitations of an athlete and how best to structure their training program (Table 14.2).

Fundamental skills of wheelchair rugby

Wheelchair rugby is a contact game composed of many fundamental sport-specific skills including wheelchair maneuverability, ball handling, passing and catching, picking, blocking, and screening. On a technical level, these skills depend on strength, speed, endurance, coordination, and flexibility; however, individual athlete technique will vary depending on the level of function. Tactical skill is also important to ensure that plays are well-timed and coordinated.

Wheelchair maneuverability and propulsion technique are dependent on muscle availability and wheelchair design and setup including seating position, and type of push rims and spoke guards used. Picking the ball off the floor is a skill that must be mastered by all players on both the right and left sides of the wheelchair. Dribbling can be done one-handed, two-handed, or in front of the footrest. Passing and catching require clear communication between teammates, an awareness of each other's ability, and an understanding of skill mechanics with slight modifications based on each player's role on the court. There are many types of passes, and development of passing skill is an important consideration for all players. Individual training for specific passes, however, will depend on the position that the athlete plays during competition. Picking, blocking, and screening are other important aspects of the game, all used to create an advantage for the team. A "pick" is a maneuver in which a player uses their chair to stop an opponent's chair. Typically, a low pointer will use their chair to "grab" the opponent's chair,

Table 14.2 Structure of an annual training program.

Training phases	
Pre-season/preparatory phase	• Develop a high level of physical conditioning • As this phase progresses, training becomes more specific and represents a transitional shift toward the competitive season with focus on sport-specific exercises and movements (i.e., agility, coordination, endurance, flexibility, and speed) • Skill mastery; develop, improve, and perfect technique • Develop teamwork among players; synchronize plays and tactical moves • Develop psychological skills (i.e., imagery, self-talk)
In-season/competitive phase	• Continue perfecting technique to enable performance at the highest level • Continue improvement of sport-specific and psychological skills • Technical (offensive and defensive skills) and tactical (individual and team) development must be at the peak • Maintain physical conditioning
Off-season/transitional phase	• Recovery • Evaluation of prior season and results • Active rest, cross-training

otherwise known as holding a pick. A block, set with the chair, is used to limit or stop the actions or movements of an opposing player, forcing them to change direction or travel off their desired path. A play in which teammates form a protective barrier for the ball carrier to advance the ball is called a screen. Picks, blocks, and screens are tools that can be used on offense and defense.

Equipment selection and maintenance

Wheelchair rugby is played in a manual wheelchair, custom-designed for the sport and adjusted to suit the individual player's comfort and safety needs. The wheelchair setup is extremely important and should be specific to the individual athlete. Following a proper setup the player should fit snugly into the chair.

The wheelchair is considered to be a part of the player. Each player is responsible for ensuring that his/her wheelchair meets all specifications for the duration of the game. If a wheelchair does not meet these specifications, it cannot be used until brought into compliance. The rules include detailed specifications for the wheelchair and key design features (e.g., wheelchair height and length, diameter of wheels, and cushion thickness). All wheelchairs must be equipped with spoke protectors and an anti-tip device at the back. In addition, the wheels are attached at an angle (camber) for greater stability.

There are two types of chairs, each designed for the role the individual player on the court. The offensive chair, set up with wings between the front bumper and the rear wheels and spoke guards flush with the push rim, is designed to prevent being easily picked or held by an opponent (Figure 14.2). A defensive chair sits low with lots of camber and is designed for blocking and picking (Figure 14.3). The defensive chair typically has a long front end and open space between the rear wheel and the front of the chair to maximize the ability to hit and hold an opponent. Typically, higher point players (2.0–3.5) will play in an offensive chair and lower point players (0.5–1.5) will play in a defensive chair (Figures 14.4 and 14.5).

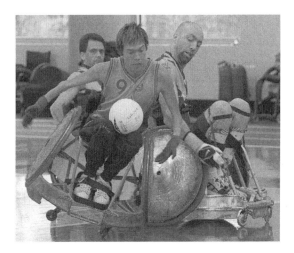

Figure 14.2 An offensive chair, set up with wings between the front bumper and the rear wheels and spoke guards flush with the push rim, is designed to prevent being easily picked or held by the opposition. Sweden player Stefan Jansson on left, Lakeshore Demolition player Bryan Kirkland on right. Photo courtesy of Lakeshore Foundation. Photographer Brian Love.

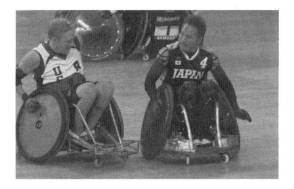

Figure 14.3 A defensive chair typically has a long front end and open space between the rear wheel and the front of the chair to maximize the ability to hit and hold an opponent. USA defensive player (Scott Hogsett) on left getting in position to "hold" Japan offensive player (Shinichi Shimakawa). Photo courtesy of Kelly Gumbert.

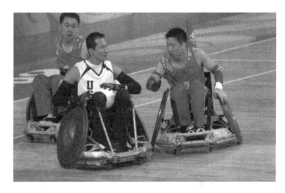

Figure 14.4 Offensive players Will Groulx (USA) and Jun Chen (China) go head to head at the Beijing Paralympic Games. Photo courtesy of Kelly Gumbert.

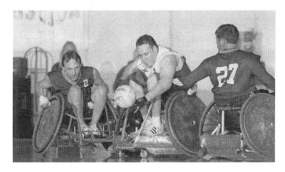

Figure 14.5 Low point player Eddie Crouch (on left) in defensive chair holding opponent; high point players Ross Morrison (middle) and Joel Wilmoth in offensive chairs vying for the ball. ©Paralyzed Veterans of America, Sports 'n Spokes, photograph by Mark Cowan.

Wheelchair rugby—scientific studies

There is limited published scientific literature regarding wheelchair rugby; however, recently this topic has become popular at scientific conferences. Many unpublished studies have examined topics ranging from classification procedures and principles to skills testing by class. To date, only a few published studies have attempted to analyze actual performance of wheelchair rugby players. (Table 14.3).

It has to be noted that the results of these studies often have been inconsistent. This is typically explained by problems with the samples used, which are small and combine persons with complete and incomplete quadriplegia. The variations in results are also caused by the diversity of testing equipment (e.g., wheelchair ergometer, arm crank ergometer or wheelchair treadmill) and measurement protocols (e.g., resistance or duration) used. However, the results of such studies may still provide insight regarding the parameters important for wheelchair rugby performance and the methods to be used in optimization of athlete performance.

The combination of training factors (e.g., physical, technical, and psychological) ultimately determine the performance of wheelchair rugby athletes and

Table 14.3 Research related to athlete performance in wheelchair rugby (WCR).

References	Type of performance	Sample size (n)	Results
Hopman et al. (1996)	Aerobic	8	No significant change of physiological response to maximal arm crank effort was observed in Dutch WCR athletes after 6 months training (VO_2 peak = 1.03 ± 0.42 l/min).
Morgulec et al. (2006)	Aerobic	14	One year training showed improvement of aerobic performance on a wheelchair treadmill in Polish WCR athletes (Pre: VO_2 peak = 1.41 ± 0.35 l/min, Post: VO_2 peak = 1.97 ± 0.43 l/min).
Abel et al. (2008)	Aerobic	12	Energy expenditure in German WCR athletes was 63.5 ± 12.9 kcal/h at rest, and 248.5 ± 69.4 kcal/h during training as measured by a portable metabolic system.
Barfield et al. (2010)	Aerobic	9	WCR on-court training enables some athletes to achieve a training intensity associated with improved cardiorespiratory fitness.
Morgulec et al. (2005)	Anaerobic	19	A comparison of active Polish WCR athletes and sedentary individuals with quadriplegia on Wingate anaerobic performance found significantly higher mean power (112.76 ± 30.19 W, 74.20 ± 54.37 W respectively), relative mean power (1.57 ± 0.40 W/kg, 1.06 ± 0.71 W/kg respectively), fatigue index and peak lactate accumulation in the active group. However, no significant differences were found between the active and sedentary individuals in peak power (149.95 ± 55.10, 112.00 ± 81.75 W, respectively) or relative peak power (2.08 ± 0.72, 1.60 ± 1.09, respectively).
Goosey-Tolfrey et al. (2006)	Aerobic and anaerobic	4	Elite British WCR athletes with quadriplegia had relatively high arm crank aerobic (VO_2 peak = 0.89 ± 0.06 l/min) and anaerobic 5-sec sprint test (PP = 228 ± 67.81 W, rPP = 3.08 ± 0.93 W/kg) performance.
Taylor et al. (2010)	Respiratory mechanics	7	Highly trained WCR players with cervical spinal cord injury do not develop exercise-induced diaphragmatic fatigue and rarely reach mechanical ventilatory constraint.
Yilla and Sherrill (1998)	Sport-specific skills	65	The *Beck Battery of Quad Rugby Skill tests* (maneuverability with the ball, pass for accuracy, picking, sprinting, and pass for distance) is valid and reliable for male WCR athletes, aged 18–51.
Furmaniuk et al. (2010)	Functional abilities	40	WCR training may maintain and improve functional abilities in persons with incomplete tetraplegia.
Mason et al. (2009)	Wheelchair maneuverability	10	Gloves that have been modified for the specific demands of wheelchair rugby are more effective for aspects of mobility performance than other glove types.

References	Type of performance	Sample size (n)	Results
Sporner et al. (2009)	Game dynamics	18	WCR athletes at the National Veterans Wheelchair Games on average traveled 2364.78 ± 956.35 m at 1.33 ± 0.25 m/s with 242.61 ± 80.31 stops and starts in 29.98 ± 11.79 min of play per game. Information was captured by a data logger attached to the wheel of each athlete's wheelchair.
Sarro et al. (2010)	Game dynamics	8	During the final match of a WCR tournament players covered 2294.7 ± 391.5 m in the first half and 2245.4 ± 431.5 m in the second half. The average velocity was 14.5% greater in the first (1.22 ± 0.21 m/s) than in the second half (1.05 ± 0.20 m/s). Data were captured using 2 overhead cameras and image processing techniques.
Molik et al. (2008)	Game efficiency	105	Offensive game efficiency as measured by a videotape observation technique was lower in class 0.5 elite WCR players as compared to all higher class players. No differences were found in game efficiency between classes 2.5–3.5.

GES-game efficiency sheet; IWRF-International Wheelchair Rugby Federation; MP-mean power; rMP-relative mean power; PP-peak power; rPP-relative peak power; VO_2 peak-peak oxygen uptake.

influence team success. Thus, recently sport scientists working with wheelchair rugby teams have focused on the monitoring and assessment of sport-specific skills, physical fitness, game efficiency, and time–motion game analysis. With regard to skill assessment in rugby, data between programs is difficult to compare. Typically the majority of skills tests used have not been assessed for reliability and validity. In addition, different testing protocols and instruments are used, so skill performance norms/standards have not been determined.

Rugby skills assessment

To assess an athlete's performance level as part of the training program, a variety of skills should be assessed on a regular basis including passing, sprint speed, agility, and endurance.

Sport-specific skills testing should be conducted at various points throughout the season—at the beginning of the competitive season, halfway through the season, and when the athletes are performing at their peak. Such testing is beneficial for all players from novice to expert-level athletes. The skills assessment can and should be used to monitor progress, and can be used for comparison to other athletes with a similar classification.

As part of the assessment process, the coaching staff should also rate the athletes on important intangible skills that cannot be "measured" quantitatively.

These subjective skills include things such as communication, attitude, commitment, leadership, contribution to team chemistry, coachability, desire, and determination.

Sport-specific skills testing should be conducted at various points throughout the season—at the beginning of the competitive season, halfway through the season, and when the athletes are performing at their peak. Such testing is beneficial for all players from novice to expert-level athletes. The skills assessment can and should be used to monitor progress, and can be used for comparison to other athletes with a similar classification.

Basic skills tests

Passing tests typically include throws from different positions and distances to a target. Tests to assess speed and acceleration will include sprints from different distances. Although a standard stopwatch is often used for timing, more accurate and precise measures can be obtained with timing lights or a laser camera. Speed can also be combined with agility by adding cones to create a slalom-type course with various weaving maneuvers. It is also important to include tests with quick changes in direction (e.g., forward–backward, left–right). With any of these tests, the ball can be added with requirements to dribble according to the game rules.

The *Beck Battery of Quad Rugby Skill*, the only published series of skills tests deemed valid and reliable, is one option to assess sport-specific skill performance in wheelchair rugby athletes

(Yilla & Sherrill, 1998). Athletes use their own rugby competition chair during testing, and it is best to repeat the tests at the same location to eliminate any influence of different floor surfaces. The assessment battery includes five tests:

1. Maneuverability with the ball—maneuver chair through a course of gates while bouncing the ball at least once every 10 s. The score is the total number of gates completed in 30 s; two trials.

2. Pass for accuracy—ball thrown at target with point value designated by portion of target hit. The score is the total point value for two trials; three attempts each trial.

3. Picking—measures the skill of setting two picks on each chair in a course. The score is the time taken to complete the 18-m course; two trials.

4. Sprinting—measures the skill of sprinting, and the score is the time taken to complete the 20-m sprint; two trials.

5. Pass for distance—measures the skill of passing for distance, and the score is the total point value for two trials; three attempts each trial.

Before commencing the *Beck Battery of Quad Rugby Skill tests*, athletes have a 10-min structured group warm-up. Every athlete should complete two trials of all tests with a 2-min rest minimum between trials. The total score for each test is the average from two trials.

Aerobic and anaerobic performance

Wheelchair rugby combines short intense bouts of exercise over an extended playing time; thus, it requires aerobic as well as anaerobic capacity.

Aerobic performance: VO$_2$ peak test on an arm crank ergometer

To assess aerobic capacity (endurance) of wheelchair rugby athletes, peak oxygen uptake (VO$_2$ peak) is measured. For peak testing, athletes should arrive at the laboratory in 30-min intervals. Participants are asked to void their bladder prior to testing, and the lab technician measures blood pressure to ensure autonomic dysreflexia is not exhibited. A heart rate (HR) monitor transmitter is positioned around each athlete's chest while the receiver is strapped to the athlete's chair. Electrodes on the HR monitor are moistened to ensure the HR signal

is transmitted appropriately despite the absence of sweating. Athletes, seated in their preferred wheelchair, are positioned in front of the arm ergometer with the ergometer axle adjusted to be parallel to the participant's shoulder joints and at a distance to allow slight elbow flexion (i.e., 5–10 deg) during the shoulder extension phase of rotation. The mask and nose clip are positioned securely on the face, ensuring that no expired air can escape.

The peak exercise protocol is based on asynchronous arm ergometry models previously reported in the literature (Goosey-Tolfrey et al., 2006). Each athlete completes a 5-min warm-up period at 60 rpm on a self-selected workload of 10–30 W. Two minutes of intermittent exercise then follow to prepare the athlete for testing (cycles of 30 sec rest, 30 sec exercise). After the warm-up and test preparation, stage increases occur continuously every 2 min. Initial watt resistance is set at a rating of perceived exertion (RPE) that approximates 10–12 on the RPE scale (approximately 60% peak power output). Workload is increased by 5 W for participants with a classification below 2.0, and is increased by 10 W for athletes with a classification of 2.0 or above. Oxygen consumption, HR and RPE are recorded in the final 5 s of each stage. The test is terminated when no further increase is detected in HR or VO$_2$ after an increase in workload, or when the participant reports volitional fatigue. Upon completion of the VO$_2$ peak test, participants are asked to cool down for a self-determined amount of time at 10 W, followed by a post-test blood pressure check. This second blood pressure measurement is taken approximately 3–5 min after cooldown, and is evaluated to ensure participants are not exhibiting hypotension following exercise (Claydon et al., 2006; Dela et al., 2003).

Information from peak VO$_2$ tests can be used to establish workout training intensities, prescribe exercises, and can be used in conjunction with field tests (sport-specific measures) to better address the demands of the sport. In one study (Barfield et al., 2010), data were analyzed to determine the number of continuous minutes that rugby players spent above 70% HR reserve under various rugby training activities. The percent of time spent at or above 70% HR reserve varied across athletes and conditions. Continuous pushing as a warm-up drill at the beginning of practice was the least variable training condition among the athletes averaging greater than 73% of time above the target HR. Scrimmage training was highly variable across athletes with a range of 0–98% of time above the criterion. These results indicate that wheelchair rugby training enables some players to reach a training intensity associated with improved cardiorespiratory fitness and that the activity type during a training session dictates the extent to which individuals sustain such a threshold.

Aerobic performance: VO$_2$ peak test on a motor-driven treadmill

Another method to measure aerobic capacity is performance of a maximal exercise test on an oversized motor-driven treadmill (Figure 14.6), connected online to a computer, with specialized software used to monitor and collect performance data. Peak oxygen uptake is determined using a continuous incremental test protocol to voluntary fatigue. Ventilation (VE) and VO$_2$ peak are measured via open-circuit spirometry. Peak oxygen consumption is defined as the highest oxygen consumption achieved by an athlete during the maximal exercise test, and is expressed as an absolute value in liters per minute. The relative peak oxygen consumption (rVO$_2$ peak) with respect to body mass is expressed as milliliters of oxygen per kilogram of body weight per minute. Ventilation and gas exchange are measured breath-by-breath, and data are averaged over each 10 s period. Athletes perform the maximal exercise test on a motor-driven treadmill with their rugby wheelchairs and gloves.

The test protocol consists of a 5-min warm-up at a speed of 2 km/h. Immediately following the warm-up, the continuous incremental test begins with the speed set at 4 km/h for all athletes. After 3 min and every 3 min thereafter, the speed is increased by 2 km/h to voluntary athlete fatigue. Throughout the test, participants are verbally encouraged to give a maximal effort. It has to be noted that, during this protocol, some 0.5 athletes may reach a maximum velocity before they achieve VO$_2$ peak. In such cases, individualized modification of the protocol (e.g., changing the starting velocity and increments) should be considered.

Anaerobic performance: Wingate Test on an arm crank ergometer

The Wingate Anaerobic Test (WAnT) has been accepted in laboratories around the world for the assessment of muscle power, muscle endurance, and fatigability. Conceptually, the testing of anaerobic performance of persons with neuromuscular disease is based on principles similar to those used in able-bodied populations. An arm ergometer is often used to evaluate anaerobic performance. This method seems to be more available in many laboratories, because of the lower cost and portability of the device. Jacobs et al. (2004) established reliability and validity of arm cranking for the measurement of anaerobic performance in persons with quadriplegia.

For a Wingate test, the athlete sits in his/her own braked daily use wheelchair held by two research team assistants (Figure 14.7). The height of the arm

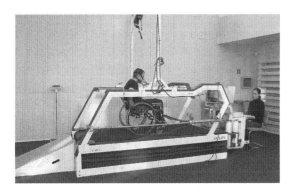

Figure 14.6 One method to measure aerobic capacity is performance of a maximal exercise test on an oversized motor-driven treadmill. (Photo courtesy of Mariola Godlewska)

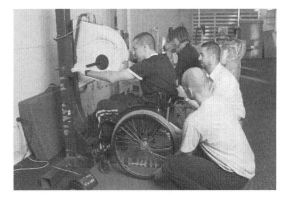

Figure 14.7 For a Wingate test, the athlete sits in his/her own braked daily use wheelchair held by two research team assistants. (Photo courtesy of Mariola Godlewska)

ergometer axis should be positioned at a height parallel with the athlete's shoulder joints. The horizontal distance from the arm ergometer allows for a slight flexion at the elbow at the furthest point of the cranking movement. For participants with severe impairment of hand function, an elastic bandage can be used to fix the hands to the handlebars. The test protocol consists of a 2-min warm-up—cranking at 60 revolutions per minute (rpm) without resistance. The Wingate test resistance equates to 1–3.5% of body mass. Optimization of the braking force is based on Jacobs et al.'s (2004) recommendations of resistance loading during arm WAnT in individuals with quadriplegia (C5: 1–1.5%, C6: 1.5–2%, C7: 2.5–3.5%). The participant cranks as fast as possible with measuring started as soon as 25 rpm is registered by the system. The counting of revolutions lasts exactly 30 s. Verbal encouragement is given throughout the test. Usually, four indices are measured during the WAnT: peak power output (PP) defined as the highest 5-s power output, mean power output (MP)—the average power sustained throughout the 30-s period, the lowest power output (LP)—the lowest 5-s power output, and time to achieve PP (tPP). The WAnT Software Package also calculates the fatigue index (FI) defined as the percentage of decline in power output (FI = PP − LP/PP × 100), and peak power output (rPP) and mean power output relative to body mass (rPP, rMP respectively).

Tests of game efficiency

To examine offensive game efficiency in wheelchair rugby, a game efficiency sheet (GES) was developed by Molik et al. (2008). Games are recorded by video cameras and later analyzed by experienced observers (wheelchair rugby coaches, classification officials, and/or referees), who register results on a GES. Playing time is calculated for players in each game. Athletes who participate for more than 8 min during the game (typically championship games) are included in the analyses. Information obtained from the GES provides an opportunity to analyze the individual and team offensive efficiency in wheelchair rugby. The following 11-game efficiency parameters are documented on the GES:

- sum of all points scored
- points scored after receiving a pass into the key area

- points scored after an athlete drove into the key area
- assists
- turnovers/losses of the ball
- steals/interceptions
- balls caught
- balls passed
- personal fouls
- percentage of balls caught
- percentage of passes caught by teammates

Each parameter of GES was tested for interobserver reliability. Due to low reliability values ($r < 0.90$), three parameters were excluded from the final analyses: points scored after a fast attack (FA), blocks (BL), and screens made in key area (SC). High levels of reliability ($r = 0.9 - 1.0$) for the remaining 11 parameters were identified.

An examination of the validity of the GES was not undertaken as the GES measures the tangible behaviors of athletes during the game analogous to time sprinting, shot scored, or rebound made. If in subsequent investigations, these measures are manipulated (i.e., differentially weighted as a result of a factor analysis), then there would be cause to perform a validity study.

Time–motion analysis

An understanding of game dynamics is essential to optimize development of effective coaching strategies and training programs for wheelchair rugby. For a team to gain the competitive edge required for success, there is a need to fully understand the game dynamics and player requirements involved. The first phase of this requires determining player trajectories, distances, and velocity traveled in competitive wheelchair rugby games.

For example, information regarding distance covered according to player position can be used to better plan subsequent training sessions or for evaluating players' performance during competitions. Recently, more sophisticated kinematic analysis systems have been developed with automatic tracking systems based on image processing techniques that allow for the simultaneous evaluation of all players during a game (Figure 14.8). Such a system models the player as a simple dot on the field plane and measures its position as a function of time with an improved temporal and spatial resolution, when compared to methods based on visual estimate (Figure 14.8). Prior to a game, the distances between calibration points on the court are measured, and these positions are used to generate the calibration parameters for the cameras. These parameters and the position of the players in the video sequences are used to reconstruct the 2D coordinates of each player using the direct linear transformation (DLT) method.

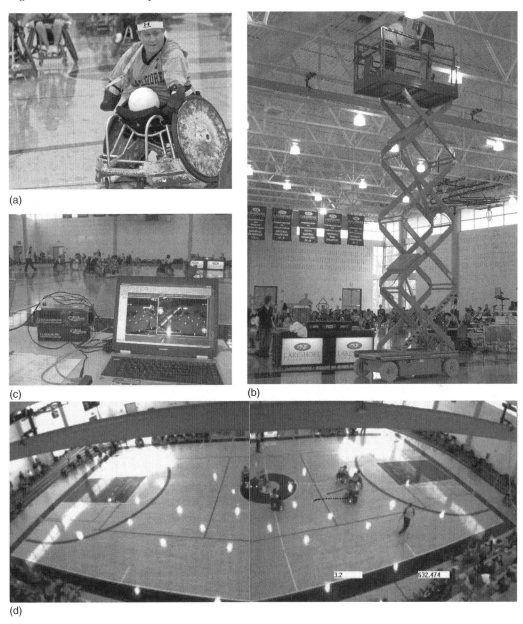

(a)

(c)

(b)

(d)

Figure 14.8 A sophisticated kinematic analysis system developed with automatic tracking based on image processing techniques allows for evaluation of all players during a game. (a) Lakeshore Demolition player Bob Lujano. Photo courtesy of Lakeshore Foundation, photographer Brian Love. Parts (b) and (c) Cameras mounted on ceiling, images sent to courtside computer. Photos courtesy of Laurie Malone. Part (d) Processed camera images showing player trajectory trails (representing player position in previous frames) during a game. Photo courtesy of Ricardo M. L. Barros. Parts (e) and (f) Trajectories of each player on Team A and Team B showing distance traveled during one quarter of play. (Figures modified from Sarro, Karine J., Misuta, Milton S., Burkett, Brendan, Malone, Laurie A. and Barros, Ricardo M. L.(2010) 'Tracking of wheelchair rugby players in the 2008 Demolition Derby final', Journal of Sports Sciences, 28: 2, 193–200).

Player Profiles – Team A

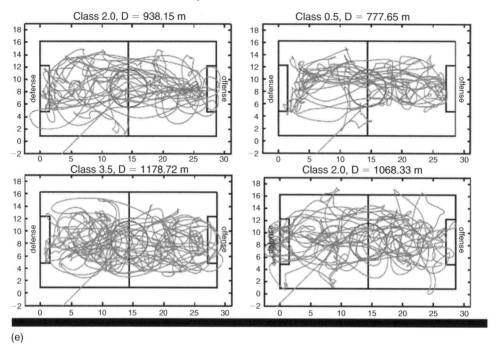

(e)

Player Profiles – Team B

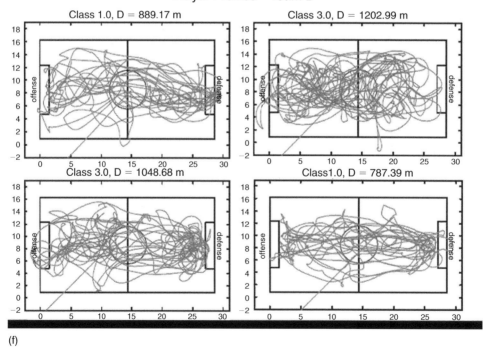

(f)

Figure 14.8 (Continued)

Video data are collected during a wheelchair rugby match using at least two high-speed cameras hung above the court. The video image is captured, measured, and visualized using a purpose-built interface; data treatment and calculations are done using Matlab® software. For each player, the following can be computed: (a) player trajectory on the court, (b) accumulated distance covered as a function of time, (c) total distance covered, (d) average velocity, and (e) distance covered during working game clock versus stopped game clock.

The method does not interfere in any way with player performance and allows analysis in real-time competitive conditions. This imaging technique is based on the simultaneous 2D kinematic analysis of the movement of all players. Relevant variables are extracted from the results of such analyses including total and partial (e.g., 1st quarter vs. 4th quarter) distances covered, velocity, and regions on the court more frequently visited by players.

Recommendations for future research

Although limited scientific data are available regarding wheelchair rugby, there is no doubt that a comprehensive sport science program is necessary for performance optimization of wheelchair rugby athletes. Sport science programs in wheelchair rugby should be more complex and include elements of nutrition, mental preparation, and injury prevention. An effective sport science program will require cooperation between experts from various disciplines (e.g., physiology, biomechanics, psychology, and nutrition) and the entire team staff, coaches, and athletes. Of great importance is the training of more sport scientists in the field of disability sport.

Given that wheelchair rugby has had a relatively short development compared to other wheelchair sports, there are many research questions that must be addressed in the future. The list given below includes just a few research ideas that could be of interest to scientific investigators:
- Energy cost of wheelchair rugby during competition.
- Effective and feasible (practical) cooling strategies during wheelchair rugby competition (thermoregulation).

- Understanding of game dynamics by player class, skilled vs. unskilled teams.
- What are the exercise capacities of wheelchair rugby athletes using different types of exercise equipment (arm ergometer, wheelchair ergometer, and wheelchair treadmill) and protocols?
- What are the valid and reliable field-based measures of aerobic and anaerobic performance in wheelchair rugby athletes?
- What are the optimal loading patterns in wheelchair rugby training during preparatory, competitive, and transition phases?
- What are the nutrition recommendations for wheelchair rugby athletes prior to, during, and in recovery from exercise?
- How to develop an evidence-based sport-specific classification system in wheelchair rugby?
- How to measure the defensive game parameters in wheelchair rugby to provide a more comprehensive, objective, and overall measure of game efficiency, especially in the context of changes in rules?
- What individual and team tactical strategies are the most successful with regard to player class?
- What type of sport injuries are common in wheelchair rugby and what methods of injury prevention are recommended?
- How psychological and mental training skills can be applied in wheelchair rugby?

A coach's perspective

Development of top-level wheelchair rugby athletes (Figure 14.9) is very similar to developing athletes in any sport. One difference between able-bodied athletes and neurologically impaired athletes is physiological adaptation to disability before sport. Athletes need to develop an aerobic base, core strength, and develop compensation for the lack of innervated muscles.

A key characteristic of structured training is that it is implemented through a comprehensive program, providing all the materials needed to plan, prepare, and conduct training efficiently. Training from the onset needs to include strength training, nutrition planning, and good aerobic and anaerobic training. The training should proceed with a sequence of exercises that progressively increase in difficulty.

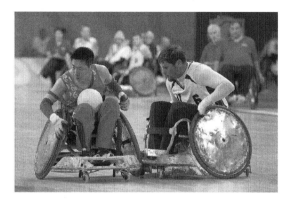

Figure 14.9 Athletes competing in wheelchair rugby. Reproduced courtesy of Lieven Coudenys.

Physiologically, the top players exhibit good aerobic conditioning, anaerobic power, and a high strength to body weight ratio. Athletes need to have a solid aerobic foundation when playing multiple games throughout a tournament. Players must also have excellent wheelchair maneuverability skills and eye–hand coordination. Good nutrition is paramount to maintaining energy and performance. A high carbohydrate diet during tournaments and proper hydration can assist well-trained athletes to sustain their energy. Top rugby athletes are typically taller athletes with long levers to efficiently propel their chairs. In addition, top athletes must have strong mental fortitude and a very strong work ethic, always trying to improve their skill level. Most top rugby athletes typically show strong drive and willingness to challenge themselves beyond the norm.

The contribution of sport science to rugby performance has resulted in improved training programs and performance on the court. In addition, the knowledge gained from the study of wheelchair rugby players can be used to improve the overall quality of lives for individuals with similar disabilities not engaged in sport. Furthermore, a better understanding of the physiological adaptation to quadriplegia, upper extremity strength and mechanics, and psychological expectations in individuals with more severe disabilities will be achieved.

Through the use of video analysis, physiological testing, and biomechanical analysis, science has greatly factored into the high performance of some international teams. Video analysis software used to evaluate game play and document events in the game allow coaches to evaluate performance of individuals and the team. By tagging certain events, this analysis provides a more efficient way to break down game film. The physiological tests that are currently being used to improve performance include thermoregulation to maximize cooling in athletes who have their systems compromised; VO_2 peak tests, HR evaluation, and blood pressure testing are all measures that continue to be explored. Some teams have also worked closely with strength and conditioning specialists to periodize workouts to peak performance and cycle training to maximize each athletes full potential.

Other areas of science that have proven valuable in wheelchair rugby have been the use of sports psychology services. The athletes work directly with the sports psychologist to work on individual mental skills and the psychologist works with the team to address team dynamics. The last area of science that is still evolving is mechanical engineering and improving the strength to weight ratio of the playing chair while reducing maintenance.

The sport of wheelchair rugby has evolved over the past 20 years since becoming a full medal sport in the Paralympic Games. Initially established as a sport to include athletes with greater physical impairment, the sport has evolved to encourage high level physical training and skill development in these individuals. Attitudes have certainly changed regarding the amount of physical load that can be placed on the quadriplegic athlete (Figure 14.10). Initial concerns that the compromised systems of athletes with cervical spinal injuries would not allow them to fully engage in athletics have been refuted.

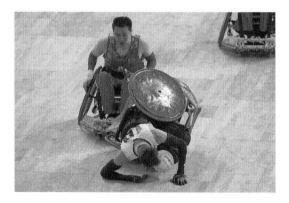

Figure 14.10 Injury patterns have declined since the introduction of sports science investigations. Reproduced courtesy of Lieven Coudenys.

References

Abel, T., Platen, P., Rojas Vega, S., Schneider, S. & Strüder, H.K. (2008). Energy expenditure in ball games for wheelchair users. *Spinal Cord*, 46, 785–790.

Barfield, J.P., Malone, L.A., Arbo, C. & Jung, A.P. (2010). Exercise intensity during wheelchair rugby training. *Journal of Sports Sciences*, 28(4), 389–398.

Claydon, V.E., Hol, A.T., Eng, J.J. & Krassioukov, A.V. (2006). Cardiovascular responses and postexercise hypotension after arm cycling exercise in subjects with spinal cord injury. *Archives of Physical Medicine and Rehabilitation*, 87(8), 1106–1114.

Dela, F., Mohr, T., Jensen, C.M., et al. (2003). Cardiovascular control during exercise: insights from spinal cord-injured humans. *Circulation*, 107(16), 2127–2133.

Furmaniuk, L., Cywinska-Wasilewska, G. & Kaczmarek, D. (2010). Influence of long-term wheelchair rugby training on the functional abilities in persons with tetraplegia over a two-year post-spinal cord injury. *J Rehabil Med*, 42(7), 688–90.

Goosey-Tolfrey, V., Castle, P. & Webborn, N. (2006). Aerobic capacity and peak power output of elite quadriplegic games players. *British Journal of Sports Medicine*, 40(8), 684–687.

Hopman, M.T., Dallmeijer, A.J., Snoek, G. & Van der Woude, L.H. (1996). The effect of training on cardiovascular responses to arm exercise in individuals with tetraplegia. *European Journal of Applied Physiology*, 74(1–2), 172–179.

Jacobs, P.L., Johnson, B.M., Mahoney, E.T., Carter, A.B. & Somarriba, G.S. (2004). Effect of variable loading in the determination of upper limb anaerobic power in persons with tetraplegia. *Journal of Rehabilitation Research and Development*, 41(1), 9–14.

Mason, B.S., van der Woude, L.H. & Goosey-Tolfrey, V.L. (2009). Influence of glove type on mobility performance for wheelchair rugby players. *American Journal of Physical Medicine and Rehabilitation*, 88(7), 559–570.

Molik, B., Lubelska, E., Kosmol, A., Bogdan, M., Yilla, A. & Hyla, E. (2008). An examination of the International Wheelchair Rugby Federation Classification system utilizing parameters of offensive game efficiency. *Adapted Physical Activity Quarterly*, 25(4), 335–351.

Morgulec, N., Kosmol, A., Vanlandewijck, Y. & Hübner-Woźniak, E. (2005). Anaerobic performance of active and sedentary male individuals with quadriplegia. *Adapted Physical Activity Quarterly*, 22(3), 253–264.

Morgulec, N., Kosmol, A., Molik, B., Hubner-Wozniak, E. & Rutkowska, I. (2006). The effect of training on aerobic performance in wheelchair rugby players. *Research Yearbook—Studies in Physical Education and Sport*, 12(2), 195–198.

Sarro, K.J., Misuta, M.S., Burkett, B., Malone, L.A. & Barros, R.M.L. (2010). Tracking of wheelchair rugby players in the 2008 Demolition Derby final. *Journal of Sports Sciences* 28(2), 193–200.

Sporner, M.L., Grindle, G.G., Kelleher, A., Teodorski, E.E., Cooper, R. & Cooper, A.R. (2009). Quantification of activity during wheelchair basketball and rugby at the National Veterans Wheelchair Games: a pilot study. *Prosthetics and Orthotics International*, 33(3), 210–217.

Taylor, B.J., West, C.R. & Romer, L.M. (2010). No effect of arm-crank exercise on diaphragmatic fatigue or ventilatory constraint in Paralympic athletes with cervical spinal cord injury. *J Appl Physiol*, 109(2), 358–66.

Yilla, A.B. & Sherrill, C. (1998). Validating the Beck Battery of quad rugby skill tests. *Adapted Physical Activity Quarterly*, 15(2), 155–167.

Recommended readings

Molik, B., Lubelska, E., Kosmol, A., Bogdan, M., Yilla, A. & Hyla, E. (2008). An examination of the International Wheelchair Rugby Federation Classification system utilizing parameters of offensive game efficiency. *Adapted Physical Activity Quarterly*, 25(4), 335–351.

Morgulec-Adamowicz, N., Kosmol, A., Molik, B., Yilla, A.B. & Laskin, J.A. (in press). Comparative study of aerobic, anaerobic and skill performance to classification in wheelchair rugby athletes. *Research Quarterly for Exercise and Sport*.

Wheelchair rugby was featured in the Oscar-nominated 2005 documentary *Murderball*. It was directed by Henry Alex Rubin and Dana Adam Shapiro, produced by Jeffrey Mandel and Shapiro, and distributed by ThinkFilm. It was nominated for Best Documentary Feature for the 78th Academy Awards.

Yilla, A. & Morgulec, N. (2002). Preliminary analysis of the performance of polish wheelchair rugby athletes. *Physical Education and Sport*, XLVI(Suppl. 1), 506–507.

Chapter 15
Contribution of sport science to performance—swimming

Brendan Burkett

School of Health and Sport Sciences, University of the Sunshine Coast, Maroochydore DC, QLD, Australia

Paralympic swimming—history

Paralympic sports evolved from rehabilitation programs in the 1940s, and as such were built on medical science knowledge with an application to exercise. These programs initially focused on spinal-cord-injured athletes, and the competitive sports program became an extension of the rehabilitation program. Many of the pioneers in disability sports were medical doctors, particularly as the athlete with a disability programs grew out of the rehabilitation institutions. The rehabilitation practitioners who developed these initial programs were in fact pioneers of the modern-day exercise scientist.

The evolution of rehabilitation programs for swimming has resulted in the modern-day Paralympic swimming program. Compared to able-bodied or Olympic swimming, Paralympic swimming has a shorter history of competition, with the first Olympic Games held in 1896, and the first Paralympic Games in 1960. At the 1988 Seoul Olympic Games, the first international swimming sports science project was conducted. This sports science project analyzed the swimming race and measured determinant factors such as start time, stroke rate, stroke length, distance per stroke (DPS), turn time, finish time, and the swimming velocity within each of the 25-m segments.

The Paralympic Athlete, 1st edition. Edited by Yves C. Vanlandewijck and Walter R. Thompson. Published 2011 by Blackwell Publishing Ltd.

As with Olympic sports, the Paralympic Games have experienced an increase in the number of official sport scientists as part of each country's Paralympic team. From these valuable data, the coach and athlete are able to evaluate swimming performance and determine how to enhance this swimming performance for future events, and/or to identify which components to work on in their training, such as stroke count, swim pace, race strategy, aerobic fitness, and maximum speed work.

At the 1992 Barcelona Paralympic Games, the first international Paralympic swimming race analysis was conducted. This swimming race analysis continued at the 1996 Atlanta Olympic and Paralympic Games (although different research teams were involved), and at the 2000 Sydney Olympic and Paralympic Games exactly and the same analysis was conducted for Olympic and Paralympic swimmers. Unfortunately, there was no international swimming analysis conducted at the 2004 Athens Olympic and Paralympic Games, or the 2008 Beijing Olympic and Paralympic Games. This was considered a major loss to furthering Olympic and Paralympic sporting performance. Despite the lack of a coordinated international program, the need for this sport science information was demonstrated as in the 2004 Athens and 2008 Beijing Games, several countries conducted their own individual sports science analysis. The growth of sport science within the Games is also reflected in the organization of the International Paralympic Committee (IPC), with the IPC Sport Science, Research and Education Committee installed in 1994. This committee coordinates the applications for sport science research projects that are now being conducted at all IPC-sanctioned events, including the Paralympic Games. As with the majority of Paralympic sports, the coaches, athletes, and scientists take the knowledge and experience from Olympic performances and then apply (sometimes with modification) to the Paralympic sport. For example, when designing the training program for a Paralympic swimmer, the coach and sport scientist would use the Olympic swimmer's training regime as the starting point. As with any sport science analysis, the adaptation process of the athlete must be carefully monitored; this knowledge will enable the strategy for performance enhancement to be developed. Sport science has played a major role in accurately and reliably monitoring the performance of the athlete. From these valuable scientific data, the coach can be equipped to make informed decisions on the Paralympic swimmer's training program.

Swimming classification

To provide a fair and equal playing field, the competition for athletes with a disability incorporates a classification system. For swimming, the current functional classification system (which is based on the athlete's function rather than the inaugural classification system which was based on the medical disability of the athlete) has been used since the 1992 Barcelona Paralympic Games. Based on sport science feedback, this classification system is constantly evolving with some modifications taking place every 2 years, coinciding with the IPC General Assembly.

Competition for persons with locomotor disabilities is organized under a functional classification system in which swimmers with various disabilities compete against one another in one of ten S-classes (for freestyle, backstroke, and butterfly), and SB-classes (for breaststroke). The separate classes are to accommodate the distinct arm-dominant freestyle, backstroke, and butterfly strokes, when compared to the leg-dominant breaststroke. Swimming is one of the few sports that combine the conditions of limb loss, cerebral palsy (coordination and movement restrictions), spinal cord injury (weakness or paralysis involving any combination of limbs), and other disabilities (such as dwarfism,

major joint restriction conditions) within, as well as across classes. In the functional classification system, function decreases from class S10 downward. Swimmers with visual impairment are divided into three classes: S11, S12, and S13. Where a person with normal vision could read newsprint at a distance of 100 cm, an S13 swimmer needs to be at 10 cm, an S12 at 4 cm, and an S11 could not read this at all. S11 swimmers are also required to wear blackened goggles, and to ensure safety they use tappers during competition. The tappers, positioned on the pool deck at each end of the pool, notify the swimmer that he/she is approaching the wall with a gentle tap using a long rod with a soft bulbous end. The international swimming community also includes swimming classes for athletes with an intellectual disability (S14) and hearing impairment (S15). These athletes presently compete outside the Paralympic Games.

Fundamental sport science parameters in swimming

The contributions to swimming from sport science knowledge have been derived from the traditional disciplines of exercise physiology, biomechanics, and motor control. As swimming requires the complex integration of these parameters, the following subsections have avoided the traditional "discipline silos," and are structured rather around swimming-specific variables. Swimming performance is typically defined by the fundamental parameters of velocity, stroke rate, stroke length and stroke index, active drag, power output, and propelling efficiency, as well as by hand kinematics and kinetics during underwater phases. Swimming performance has also been examined from the standpoint of energetic characteristics, including lactate production and degradation, oxygen consumption, and heart rate variability. The cyclic action of swimming is characterized by the alternation of propulsive and resistive impulses, and the goal for the swimmer is naturally to increase propulsion and reduce resistance while moving in the dense medium of water (Figure 15.1).

Swimmers with a locomotor disability competing at the Paralympic level have been found to exhibit

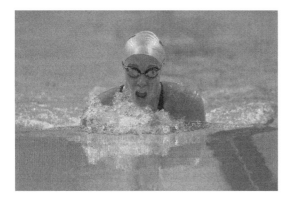

Figure 15.1 Swimming athlete competing at the Paralympic Games. Reproduced courtesy of Lieven Coudenys.

some similar patterns of stroke rate and race velocity patterns, while other components such as start, turn, and finish times differ, when compared to the higher swimming velocity of Olympic swimmers.

Stroke rate, stroke length, and velocity

The stroke rate in swimming is defined as the number of strokes per unit of time (stroke/min), and is measured using a base-three (or similar) stopwatch, which is a common watch used by swim coaches. The stroke length is the distance the body travels during one arm stroke (from the entry in the water of the hand at the first cycle to the entry in the water of the hand at the second cycle), and is measured in meters per stroke. The velocity, which is the product of stroke rate and stroke length, can also be measured from first principles as the distance traveled divided by the time. Elite swimmers and coaches are able to determine the best ratio between stroke rate and stroke length for the specific distance they are swimming. Furthermore, an elite swimmer can manipulate the stroke rate, and/ or the stroke length, without causing detriment to the other variable. This new swimming profile can result in a faster swimming velocity and reduced energy expenditure. It should be noted that it takes a considerable amount of knowledge and skill to obtain this swimming profile. The velocity profile within a 100-m swimming race generally (this will vary between each individual swimmer) decreases

by around 3.5% per 25-m section of the race, with a slightly higher decrease of 5.9% following the turn. To achieve a certain velocity, the swimmer adopts an individual ratio between stroke rate and stroke length. The stroke rate generally decreases by 6% at the beginning of the race and then by 1.5% over the remaining sections. The stroke length first increases by ~2%, followed by an ~3% decrease for the remaining 25 m. This relationship between rate and length can be manipulated by the sport scientist and coach.

Inter-arm coordination and stroke index

Inter-arm coordination is the timing between the left and right arm of the swimmer, and is naturally only apparent in the bilateral strokes of freestyle and backstroke. The inter-arm coordination is commonly defined as a catch-up stroke, or a superposition stroke; and is a function of velocity, stroke length, stroke rate, stroke index, and most importantly the swimmer's preferred swimming style. Of these external variables, the velocity of the swimmer has been found to have the greatest impact on the inter-arm coordination profile. Typically, the inter-arm coordination switches from a catch-up to a superposition mode at a velocity of ~1.8 m/s and/ or at a stroke rate of 50 strokes/min. In contrast, the stroke length is either similar or shorter. Stroke length has been found to increase from the 50-m to the 200-m race, and decrease from the 200-m to the 1500-m race. The cause of this change was thought to be the fact that swimmers develop greater propulsive power per stroke in the 200-m race. As swimming velocity increases from the 200-m to the 100-m event, the stroke rate also increases. The inter-arm coordination typically changes from a catch-up mode, at long- and mid-distance pace, to a superposition coordination mode when sprinting. Expert swimmers have been able to generate a greater maximal stroke length and, more importantly, can maintain this longer stroke length as the stroke rate increased, culminating in a faster swim. For a given race pace, the swimming velocity was found to positively correlate to stroke length, this last parameter being the most discriminate variable. From this new scientific knowledge, a new stroke index was developed, which was defined as the product of stroke length and swimming velocity. As the swimming performance increases, so does the stroke index.

Aerobic capacity and recovery

To design the training session, the Paralympic athlete and coach often seek advice from the exercise physiologist to determine the appropriate intensity and duration for training. The most common measures are heart rate and blood lactate. The measurement of lactate production after racing events and during recovery is a common practice within swimming programs, as this variable can be related to swimming performance. The predominant energy system used in swimming during sprinting events is the anaerobic system. This is due to the short duration of these swimming events and the muscle fiber types principally used. The incremental swimming training regime and recovery strategies are a direct contrast as they primarily use aerobic metabolism, which assists in the removal of lactate from the muscle tissue and vascular system.

The anaerobic system in the human body functions without oxygen, and a major limitation of this system is the production and accumulation of lactic acid in the muscles and body fluids. Simply put, the primary cause of lactate production and accumulation is when there is a discrepancy between the demand and the availability of energy from the aerobic processes of exercise. A useful tool during testing of an athlete's lactate levels is a rating of perceived exertion (RPE) scale because it allows coaches and swimmers to determine the perceived intensity at which they are exercising. The RPE is a subjective rating of exertion and fatigue, which corresponds to a number on the scale. The represented number can correspond to a percentage of maximal heart rate, maximal oxygen consumption (VO_2 max), or heart rate reserve, and indicates a classification of intensity. Within the rating scale, the lowest number corresponds to a very light intensity, and as the intensity increases, the numerical value also raises to a maximum.

Established relationships currently exist between heart rate, blood lactate and the training intensity, or training zone. Using this knowledge, the coach and athlete have a scientific measure that

their training will result in the desired performance outcome. A commonly accepted sport science measure to quantify aerobic capacity in swimmers is to use an incremental test set of 7 times 200-m swims on a descending time of 5 s quicker. A blood sample is taken and lactate level measured after each 200-m swim. This swim will enable the relationship between lactate, swimming speed, and lactate tolerance (ability to remove lactate from the working systems at specific intensities) to be quantified. Of the limited studies that have been conducted on the effect of exercise on a person with a disability, there exists a wide range of variability in the suggested recommendations for exercise. There are also limitations in following the current methods of analysis. For example, to determine oxygen uptake (VO_2) with an Olympic athlete, the most common method is to measure the VO_2 as the subject runs on a treadmill, or cycles on a cycle ergometer. A spinal-cord-injured athlete, or any athlete who does not have the function of their lower limbs (amputee, cerebral palsy, and les autres), will not be able to pedal the cycle ergometer. Some research studies have then modified the oxygen uptake test and have the athlete use a hand crank. The reliability of this method of assessment needs further investigation. In addition, for those confined to a wheelchair and will not fit on a conventional treadmill, it will require a specifically built wide treadmill that can safely accommodate the wheelchair. While research into disabled swimmers recovery is limited, athletes have been encouraged to develop individual recovery management plans because their recovery approach is not the same due to the nature of their disabilities. The purpose of the personalized recovery plan is to allow a swimmer to recover more appropriately. Training and recovery devices such as a pool buoy are also in use to improve lower-limb buoyancy, which may prove beneficial in improving upper-limb stroking technique. The use of these devices could assist in the reduction of lactate production in disabled swimmers, as the swimmer is being artificially assisted in flotation, hence there is a decrease in drag.

An analysis of the aerobic capacity of swimmers in 400-m race at the 2000 Sydney Paralympic Games found that the sample of visually impaired swimmers had a lower aerobic capacity level when compared to the Olympic swimmers. The average aerobic capacity of the small group ($n = 8$) of visually impaired swimmers, measured with an arm crank, was 41.17 ml/kg/min. In comparison to other studies, wheelchair athletes regularly obtain VO_2 peak values above 50 ml/kg/min, and able-bodied swimmers have reported values of over 65 ml/kg/min. Even considering a possible difference between arm cranking and swimming, values of 20% of these visually disabled swimmers do not approach the peak VO_2 levels of elite able-bodied athletes.

Metabolism and thermal adjustment

A branch of exercise physiology is bioenergetics and metabolism, and this topic is discussed in detail in Chapter 3. The net result of energy intake and expenditure and the development of legal ergogenic nutritional aids (supplements that are legal but could enhance the performance of the athlete) are of particular interest to the Paralympic athlete and coach. With the difference between gold and silver, or bronze and fourth, being as small as 0.35%, or 0.01 s, anything that can make a difference to athletic performance is eagerly sought by the Olympic and Paralympic athlete.

Thermal adjustment is also a very important component of exercise, particularly as the chemical reaction of converting energy intake into muscular activity produces a by-product of heat. The preparation and possible adaptation to the hot and humid environments of the past Athens and Beijing Paralympic Games were major issues for Olympic and Paralympic athletes. As with other applications, the initial sport science knowledge develops "generic" guidelines and principles. From this starting point, the Paralympic coach and sport scientist will either adopt the same guidelines or modify this approach to address the unique characteristics of the athlete with a disability. With reference to heat adaptation, the able-bodied athletes dissipate their heat through their limbs and available surface area.

Despite competing in an aquatic environment, the ability to accommodate thermal regulation for the Paralympic swimmer is challenging. For example, the athlete with a spinal cord injury tends to have a reduced lower-limb surface area due to the associated muscular atrophy; a similar scenario exists for the amputee who has lost part or all of a limb. This different surface area will naturally influence thermal regulation. Furthermore, the modified neuromuscular system for some athletes with cerebral palsy has resulted in heightening their sensitivity to hot and cold climates.

Mood state and visualization

As with Olympic athletes, the Paralympian is confronted with the similar issues of the psychological effects of exercise, the problem of exercise adherence, motivation, and the anxiety experienced pre-competition as well as in the middle of the major event. The established process of proactively controlling the athlete's mood state, visualization, and pre-competition thought process is of particular importance to the outcome of the sporting performance. In most cases, the Paralympic athlete can apply similar visualization processes as the Olympic athlete, but for some disabilities this is not possible. In using visualization techniques, the athlete will often watch a video of a past performance, usually their best performance, so as to "visualize" the perfect race. For the athlete with a visual impairment or blindness, this is not possible, so they need to resort to other techniques such as hearing or to rely on their confidence in the predefined race strategy. For swimmers with cerebral palsy, there are a very small number of athletes who may also have an intellectual disability. This could restrict their ability to use the power of the mind to modify the mood state, concentrate, or follow the race plan. Likewise, when using muscle relaxation techniques to bring the athlete into the desired mood state, the common procedure of systematically contracting and relaxing muscle groups within the body to create an overall level of relaxation may need to be modified for the athlete with an amputation. This loss of limb or in the case of the athlete with a spinal cord injury, there may be limited or no ability to systematically contract and relax. The athlete who has an intellectual disability may have a different response mechanism to the "burn out or staleness" that is common in athlete following long periods of training and competition. Sport science has contributed to developing novel mechanism to address these issues, such as incorporating other sensor cues of smell and a more detailed description of the environment or mood state; these are discussed in more detail in Chapters 7 and 11.

Disability-specific swimming profile

As there are specific and unique biological requirements associated with particular physical disabilities, an overview of the classification of disability
in Paralympic competition will lend clarity to the
subsequent discussion. The original classification
system was based on a medical model and athletes
competed within five classes of disability: athletes
with an amputation, defined as having at least one
major joint in a limb missing (i.e., elbow, wrist,
knee, and ankle); athletes with cerebral palsy,
defined as having the cerebellar area of the brain
affected, which, through palsy, affects the control
of movement; athletes with a spinal cord injury or
other condition that causes at least a 10% loss of
function in the lower limbs (e.g., traumatic paraplegia or quadriplegia); athletes with a visual impairment (i.e., perception of light or hand movement
to a visual acuity between 2/60 and 6/60 and/or a
visual field of $>5°$ and $<20°$); and athletes classified as "Les autres", a French phrase meaning the
"others"; this group comprises athletes who do not
fit within one of the other disability groups, but
nevertheless have a permanent physical disability
(e.g., one femur shorter than the other, resulting in
a significant difference in leg length). The athletes
have a permanent physical disability, but they do
not technically meet the criteria of amputation or
spinal cord, so they are part of the les autres group.
The following section describes some of the specific requirements for swimming for each of these
disability groups.

Swimmers with an amputation

The swimmer with an upper-limb amputation
(Figure 15.2) tends to have an increased stroke
rate and shorter stroke length, when compared to
a fully functional upper-limb swimmer. Naturally,
the swimmer with an upper-limb amputation will
rely more on their ability to kick as this will directly
translate into their swimming performance. Despite
the loss of the upper limb, maintaining musculoskeletal symmetry is paramount, and the swimmer
should be encouraged to use an adapted hand pad-
dle to provide necessary resistance to the amputated
limb during training. This load will then facilitate

hypertrophy around the remaining musculature
and aim toward developing musculoskeletal symmetry for the athlete. Based on the biomechanics of body roll and developing swimming forces,
if unsure, the swimmer should breathe on their
amputated side as this will enable the intact limb to
remain longer underwater and, therefore, generate
propulsive force. From sport science observations,
the majority of swimmers follow this profile; however, if the swimmer feels more comfortable breathing to the other side, this should determine the side
of breathing.

The swimmer with a lower-limb amputation
should be able to maintain a similar stroke rate and
stroke length profile as the able-bodied swimmer.
However, the timing and type of kick may vary.
Swimmers with a lower-limb amputation tend to utilize a "crossover" kick, i.e., to kick down on one side
in time with the alternate arm stroke, and then to
crossover and kick on the other side to counter that
arm stroke. Some swimmers have utilized the typical one side only kicking, but this tends to inhibit
their longitudinal body roll in the water. The kick
rate of the swimmer with lower-limb amputation is
naturally slower than that of a two-legged swimmer.
There is also a higher than normal issue with shoulder injury for the lower-limb amputee. This is attributed to the increased load on the shoulder on the
opposite side to the leg amputation, as this shoulder
needs to "skull the water" to maintain balance in
the water as well as generating underwater force. As
with the swimmer with an upper-limb amputation,

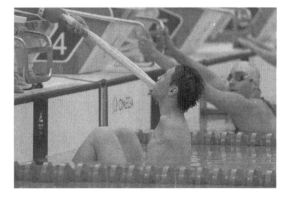

Figure 15.2 Swimmer with upper-limb amputation
at the start of a race. Reproduced courtesy of Lieven
Coudenys.

the lower-limb amputee should also be encouraged to use a modified fin during training to provide the required overload for their residual stump and subsequently develop musculoskeletal symmetry.

Swimmers with cerebral palsy

The swimmer with cerebral palsy generally has two distinct profiles, which relate directly to the level of severity of the disability. For the swimmer with mild cerebral palsy, their swimming stroke will initially be very similar to an able-bodied athlete. That is the stroke rate, stroke length, and overall technique will be consistent, but over a short period of time of around 30 s, the technique will deteriorate due to the disability. This phenomenon of a decrease in technique is common in athletes with cerebral palsy, and is often related to the level of fitness. For the swimmer with mild cerebral palsy, the level of fitness is not the critical factor in the change of technique; rather it is the consequence of the disability. From sport science analysis, the mechanism to address this issue is to establish a lower-intensity race strategy in the earlier stages of the race as this will enable the athlete to counter the effects of fatigue in the later stages of the race. For swimmers with a more severe level of cerebral palsy, the ability to control their technique can become a challenge and, therefore, a focus on following a traditional swimming technique should be reduced. Rather, the athlete and coach need to identify a stroke profile that the athlete can maintain and explore the propulsion and resistance profile further. Temperature regulation is a key issue for swimmers with cerebral palsy, particularly in cold water less than 26°C. Sport science analysis has found strategies such as increasing the use of dryland warm-up so that the time spent in the water can be maximized for the main set swimming. A similar process for a greater dryland warm-down, in which the swimmer may conduct their warm-down out of the water, can also be adopted to address this issue. Finally, some swimmers with cerebral palsy may be more emotional in a stressful situation, such as competing at the World Championships or Paralympic Games. This is a function of the athlete's disability, and knowledge of this can alert the coach and support staff prior to this possible issue becoming a problem.

Swimmers with a spinal cord injury

Swimmers with a spinal cord injury have two key factors to consider: first, avoiding overloading the shoulders of the swimmer as the athlete relies on the shoulder to propel their wheelchair (with a possible shoulder injury, daily mobility will subsequently be impaired). This issue can be addressed by carefully monitoring the athlete's range of movement internally and externally using a regular sport science screening measure, as discussed in sports medicine (Chapter 4). This will enable valuable feedback on the intensity levels of both the in-water and dryland training regimes. Correct sport science assessment can avoid potential shoulder injury issues; unfortunately, the second issue can be more challenging to address. As the swimmer spends the majority of the day in a wheelchair, and when coupled with the low stimulation to the lower limbs, the athletes can develop a "fixed" contracture at the hips. That is, the hip joint will maintain the approximate 90 sitting flexed position, regardless if the athlete is sitting upright in a chair or lying prone or supine in the water. In the prone freestyle, breaststroke, and butterfly strokes, this fixed hip contracture will create an excessive frontal drag profile and significantly affect the swimmer. In the supine backstroke position, the upright fixed hip position will exaggerate body roll and further challenge the limited (or lack of) abdominal control. Sport science has assisted this issue by having the swimmer utilizing a "pull buoy" when swimming in the prone position (Figure 15.3). The floatation of the buoy in the water actively encourages extension of the hip joint. This alone will not resolve the situation, and the athlete in a wheelchair, regardless of the sport in which they participate, should daily extend the hip joint to avoid a more permanent fixed contracture.

Swimmers with visual impairment or blindness

Broadly speaking, there are no physical differences between an Olympic swimmer and a swimmer with a visual impairment or blindness. However, the lack of vision can affect the opportunities to take part in training and competition, the ability to learn proper swimming technique, and the potential to monitor

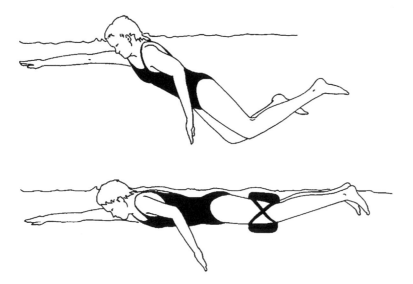

Figure 15.3 Image of swimmer with pool buoy.

one's race speed patterns through visual feedback. Disabilities, such as visual impairment or blindness, have not been found to influence the race strategy in a 100-m race when compared to Olympic swimmers (Burkett & Mellifont, 2008). When comparing the Olympic swimmer and the swimmer with a visual impairment at the 2000 Sydney Games, within the four clean swimming sections of the 100-m event, there were no significant differences in stroke rate between the Olympic or Paralympic swimmers. Despite the difference in average swimming velocity, as the stroke rate was not normalized for time, this suggests that a very similar race strategy is adopted by both the Olympic and Paralympic swimmers. This result of similar race patterns between Olympic and Paralympic swimmers have been found in other studies. This sport science knowledge demonstrates that the visually impaired swimmers studied did not require the ability to "see" the opposition swimmer to perform; rather they employed a suitable race strategy.

Swimming race analysis

Competition or swimming race analysis has become a regular feature at most international swimming events with official video recordings conducted above water during the Olympic Games since 1988. In an Olympic year, potential Olympic medal swimmers need to improve their swimming performance by ~1% within competitions, and 1% within the year leading up to the Olympics. Additional enhancements of ~0.4% between competitions have been found to substantially increase a swimmer's chance of a medal. Variables that are commonly measured include start, turn, and finish times, as well as 25- and 50-m lap split times. Using time data and segment distances, mid-pool swimming speed at various points in a race can be calculated. Additional performance indicators include the swimmer's arm strokes/minute, or stroke rate, and the distance covered per arm stroke, or stroke length. The swimmer's race pattern is defined by the within-race changes in stroking parameters and resultant changes in swimming speed.

Swimming race analysis for functional swimmers (S1–S10)

From sport science analysis of the 100-m freestyle finalists at the 2000 Sydney Paralympic Games, it was found that races were won or lost by better maintaining velocity in the second half of each 50-m race lap and that differences in velocity between swimmers were more related to stroke length than stroke rate (Daly et al., 2003). This knowledge is essential to guide the training strategies for the Paralympic swimming coach. Furthermore, within-race velocity changes were more related to changes in stroke rate, and stroke rate changes were also responsible for velocity changes between qualifying heats and finals in the first part of races. Stroke length was responsible for better velocity maintenance at the end of races. In a more recent study, 724 official finals times were analyzed for 120 male and 122 female Paralympic swimmers in the 100-m freestyle event at 15 national and international competitions between 2004 and 2006 (Fulton et al., 2009). Separate analyses were performed for males and females in each of three Paralympic subgroups: S2–S4, S5–S7, S8–S10 (most through least physically impaired). Swimming performance progressed by ~0.5% x y^{-1} for males and females. Typical variation in mean performance time between competitions was ~1% after adjustment for the ability of the athletes in each competition, and the Paralympic Games was the fastest competition. Thus, taking into account variability, progression, and level of competition, Paralympic swimmers who want a substantial increase in their medal prospects should aim for an annual improvement of at least 1–2%, which is higher than the current 1% for Olympic swimmers.

Other studies to compare the stroking parameters of Paralympic swimmers have been conducted over a 4-year period of 2002–2006, analyzing 13 competitions including the Paralympic Games, World Championships, and several national championships. In total, 442 races of 100-m heat (225 performances) and finals (217 performances) were profiled. On average, start time correlated the highest with race time, showing near-perfect correlations for classes S7 ($r = 0.90$), S8 ($r = 0.97$), and S10 ($r = 0.90$). Turn time correlations were very high and consistent for all classes ($r = 0.78$–0.89), and finish time was consistently the lowest of the three race times for all classes showing moderate to high correlations ($r = 0.30$ for class S8 to $r = 0.67$ for class S10). This is somewhat in contrast to the findings for 1996 Atlanta Paralympic heat swims where start time was not found to be as important ($r = 0.6$ and lower for classes S7 and above), indicating an evolution in the race profile of Paralympic swimmers. When comparing the final race time with the stroke parameters for the different Paralympic classes, several relationships were found, such as small correlations for stroke rate in the class S7 and S10 swimmers ($r = -0.05$ to -0.27), indicating that stroke rate may not be as important as stroke length for these swimmers. Stroke rate correlations for classes S8 and S9 were moderate ($r = -0.51$ to -0.78), indicating that high stroke rate may be optimal for these classes. Classes S8 and S9 showed very small correlations for stroke length ($r < -0.13$). As expected, a high velocity in any 25-m segment of a 100-m swimming performance is beneficial for optimal final time, with a correlation analysis showing strong relationships between 25-m segment times and velocity to final race time in all events. Sport science analysis has found that different classes of swimmers do not possess the same skill level for start, turn, and finish time, suggesting that different strategies are evident between Paralympic swimming classes. Recognizing differences in strategies between classes is important and may be the key to optimizing performance for Paralympic swimming. The majority of results for stroke parameters between the classes suggest that, in accordance with research in able-bodied swimming, focusing on stroke length is important for achieving optimal race time. These results suggest that swimmers should concentrate on using a long stroke and taking fewer strokes per lap for 100-m events to achieve optimal race time.

S9 race analysis case study—an application of sport science knowledge

Several longitudinal studies have tracked the performance of individual swimmers from their inaugural international competition as a 14-year-old, through to their Paralympic and world record performances 4 years later. This progression can provide an insight into the differences in skill level and subsequent motor skills in swimming. As seen in Table 15.1, the individual swimmer's performance improved 10% from the final appearance performance at the 2002 World Championships, to the medal performance at the 2004 Paralympic Games, and an additional 2.6% to set the world record performance at the 2006 World Championships. More importantly, these data identify the details that contribute to this, such as stroke rate and length, segmental velocity, start and turn times. The key areas of improvement

Table 15.1 S9 race analysis case study: evolution of performance and race parameters (2002–2006).

Worlds final (2002)	Canada final (2003)	Grand Prix (2004)	Athens heat (2004)	Athens final (2004)	Commonwealth Games (2006)	Worlds final (2006)
Key times						
Total time	1:03.97	1:02.78	0:59.64	0:58.77	0:58.15	0:57.41	0:56.67
Start time (s)	7.81	7.85	7.31	6.70	7.17	6.86	6.89
25 m time (s)	13.94	13.88	13.29	12.60	12.67	12.58	12.57
Finish time (s)	3.42	3.37	3.01	3.48	3.28	3.24	3.11
Start, turns, finish (s)	17.14	17.06	16.00	15.94	15.89	15.40	15.08
Free-swim time (s)	46.83	45.72	43.64	42.83	42.26	42.01	41.59
Splits						
50 m	0:30.50	0:30.54	0:29.20	0:28.53	0:28.34	0:28.21	0:27.87
100 m	1:03.78	1:02.63	0:59.64	0:58.77	0:58.15	0:57.41	0:56.67
50 m times						
1st 50 m	30.51	30.54	29.20	28.53	28.34	28.21	27.87
2nd 50 m	33.28	32.09	30.44	30.24	29.81	29.20	28.80
Turns						
Turn 1 (s)	5.91	5.84	5.68	5.76	5.44	5.30	5.08
Stroke count						
Lap 1	56	58	52	48	52	50	52
Lap 2	64	64	58	56	60	54	56
Averages						
Average velocity (m/s)	1.49	1.53	1.60	1.63	1.65	1.65	1.68
Average stroke rate (strokes/min)	63.8	65.5	62.7	60.6	64.9	61.4	64.6
Average DPS (m)	1.43	1.42	1.54	1.63	1.54	1.61	1.57

Note: Turn time measured as 5 m from wall.

for this swimmer were to improve turn and finish times, and to evenly pace the race, knowing that high and stable values of the stroking parameters reveal high motor skills.

Swim race analysis for swimmers with a visual impairment

The race analysis for swimmers with a visual impairment has been compared with Olympic counterparts, and there were almost no differences among these Paralympic and Olympic swimmers in the percentage of time in any one race section. In absolute terms, the Olympic swimmers were significantly faster and class S11 swimmers were slower, when comparing the 100-m freestyle event. The race speed and stroking patterns used were, nevertheless, quite similar to each other and were comparable to those found in swimmers with locomotor impairment. There were no absolute differences among groups in stroke rate, only in stroke length. The S11 swimmers demonstrated a significantly slower stroke rate, mid-pool swim speed, and race time than the other groups. The men's classes, however, were not clearly distinct from each other based on the swimming variables measured, as no significant differences were found between S12 and S13 in either event. In women, an increase in class (more sight) was associated with an increase in stroke index (swimming speed × stroke length), decrease in race time, and faster mid-pool swim speed.

While the classes S13 and S12 do not vary from one another in swimming performance, there is an obvious difference as compared to Olympic finalists as well as to S11 swimmers in both gender groups. Many visually impaired swimmers train nearly as much as Olympic swimmers and some take part in able-bodied training programs and competition. Swimmers in the S11 class might have less experience as they are least likely to train and compete with colleagues with ample vision. This sport science analysis discovered some interesting findings, such as the absolute number of strokes needed to swim a 100-m race changes by only about 3% between a heat and final race and by less than 2% between laps one and two of a two lap 100-m freestyle race. This translates into a difference of less than one half arm cycle per 50-m pool lap. So when a swimmer increases stroke rate with a resulting increase in speed, the same real number of arm cycles are used to cover the race distance because of the decreased race time.

Within the visually impaired male swimmers, there was no significant difference in stroke length across the three classes, although there was a general decrease with decreasing vision. This was significantly different from Olympic swimmers. Within the visually impaired female classes, the S12 and S13 swimmers produced the same stroke length, which was significantly longer than the S11 female class. Despite the degree of visual impairment, the majority of the performance indicators showed a similar race pattern used over the 100-m event by the Olympic and Paralympic swimmers. A most interesting feature was that swimmers with greatest degree of visual impairment (S11) adopted race start and finish times similar to the other groups. "Seeing" the opposing swimmer or the pool surroundings may not be as important as experience (movement rhythm, feeling of the water, and perceived exertion) in employing a suitable race pattern. The results indicate that the essential difference between Olympic and Paralympic swimmers with a visual impairment appear to be in physical aptitude and that there are little or no differences in the performance of classes S12 and S13.

Seeing only a little bit is enough to swim the race in an optimal manner.

Swimming start and turn

The swimmer's start is an important component of the complete swimming race as it is the section of the race where the swimmer is traveling at the fastest velocity. Typical average velocities for elite male swimmers over the first 15 m of the race are around 3 m/s, while free swim velocities are in the order of 1.8–2 m/s for elite freestylers. It is therefore imperative that the swimmer maximizes velocity at the start and continues this velocity for as long as possible. Analyses of the entire swimming race have found that the start contributes to around 10% and 5%, respectively, of the total swimming race for the 50- and 100-m events. This percentage of contribution naturally declines in the longer events. Despite the reduction in the percentage contribution in the longer events, parts of the components of the swimmer's start, such as the underwater phase and breakout stroke, are repeated with every turn the swimmer makes. Thus, any improvements in the underwater components of the swimmer's start can also apply throughout each swimming turn. Technical modifications to the swim start have been found to reduce the swimming race time by 0.10 s, and when races have been won and lost by a tenth of this margin, an effective start is critical. The swim start is defined as the distance to the 15-m mark in the race which coincides with the break start rope (the rope that goes across the pool at the 15-m mark and is dropped in case there is a break in the race and the swimmers keep swimming) and is the maximum distance a swimmer can travel underwater, as per the Federation Internationale de Natation (FINA) rules. The swim start can be divided into a number of subsections including time components (block, flight, underwater, and free swim) as well as distance components (entry, underwater, and free swim). In a study of the 200-m starts to 15 m at the 2000 Sydney Olympic Games, 95% of the variance in start time was attributed to the underwater phase, and a greater entry distance had little relationship with the start time ($r = 0.046$).

Swim start race analysis for functional swimmers (S1–S10)

Sport science research has compared the swim start of Olympic and Paralympic swimmers over a number of national elite swim training camps. The specific disability of the Paralympic swimmers enabled the researchers to monitor the influence of some of the variables that contributed to the swimmer's start. For example, the influence of block time is apparent when analyzing the swimmer with cerebral palsy, as their inhibited neural muscle recruitment results in an inefficient kinetic link required to generate a fast block time. When comparing the start time to 15 m, there was a significant difference between the Olympic and Paralympic classes, with the start time progressively increasing as the Paralympic class decreased.

Further analysis of the different components of the start highlights no significant differences in the majority of the variables between the S10 and S9 classes, despite these classes having a significant difference in swim time to both the Olympic and S8 class. This sport science knowledge identifies that a similar mechanism has been developed by the elite S10 and S9 swimmers. The only variable that distinguishes these two classes was the underwater velocity. From reviewing the underwater video footage, the S9 swimmers were not able to hold their streamline as effectively as the S10 swimmers. This could be attributed to the greater level of disability (such as a greater leg amputation), which naturally affects the swimmer's balance. The end result was that the S9 swimmers oscillate more as they correct their balance, resulting in a less effective streamline position. The S10 swimmers were able to develop an underwater velocity comparable to the Olympic swimmers, which was also significantly faster than the S9 and S8 swimmers.

The ability of the S10 swimmers to match the Olympic swimmers in the underwater velocity would relate to the minimal disability of these swimmers. For example, arm amputees within the S10 class were missing an arm below the elbow, and the loss of this limb generally only affects the arm stroke of the swimmer—the ability to hold streamline within the underwater phase of the start is not significantly impaired by the loss of the lower arm. From the analysis of the underwater video footage, as the Paralympic class of the swimmer decreased, the swimmers tended to have a wider underwater streamline profile, which naturally creates an increased resistance that consequently reduces the underwater velocity. Depending on the individual disability, an improved streamline could be attained with a focus on this technique. The swimmers with cerebral palsy may also require other specific changes such as interlocking their hands to avoid the arms drifting apart underwater. This would need to be assessed on an individual basis. From the underwater footage, the transition from the underwater phase to stroke preparation phase was generally appropriate as the swimmers maintained their streamline body position and started their first underwater arm stroke just prior to breaking the surface of the water. Kicking was maintained throughout the underwater to surface transition.

By only considering the class, and not the disability, some key features of the athletic performance are hidden. For example, sport science research has found a significant difference in the absolute start time between the Olympic and the three Paralympic classes (S10, S9, and S8), yet no significant difference was observed in start time between the three disability groups studied—arm amputee, leg amputee, and cerebral palsy. In addition, the block time of the S10 and S9, as well as the arm and leg amputees, was similar, while the cerebral palsy and S8 swimmers had a significantly slower block time, when compared to all other swim groups. This result highlights the finding that the impaired neuromuscular motor pattern in people with cerebral palsy affects the execution of movement patterns and causes delayed planning of movement.

The flight phase is naturally dependent on what the swimmer does on the block, and there are essentially two swim start styles, grab and track. Past studies have found differences between these starts, and using this sport science knowledge, the coach and athlete can objectively determine the most appropriate type of swim start. A key requirement when making any intervention on the swim start is the need to provide suitable practice following any changes in technique. Once a suitable adjustment time period has occurred, the final decision on which technique to adopt can be made. The distance variables of entry, underwater, and free swim distance all followed a similar pattern with a significant difference between the Olympic swimmers and all Paralympic classes. When comparing the Olympic swimmers with swimmers with an arm amputation, both groups generated the same entry distance. If the Olympic swimmers are used as a benchmark for ultimate performance, then this result indicates that the arm amputee swimmers, whose greatest strength is their legs, may have modified their start to maximize the entry distance to capitalize on this leg strength. For the flight and underwater distance variables, the Olympic swimmer records the longest, the S10 and S9 records a similar distance, and the S8 cohort records significantly shorter distances. Olympic swimmers traveled an underwater distance that was almost double that of the S8 swimmers relates to the difficulty the S8 swimmers have holding a streamline position due to their neuromuscular and/or major limb loss of function. This feature was noted when observing the underwater footage of the swimmers. When comparing the specific disabilities, the swimmers with a leg amputation and cerebral palsy, both had shorter underwater distances, although they were not significantly different. Both of these groups of swimmers would have a reduced kicking capability, due to the loss of a leg, or involuntary muscle spasms, which would interfere with a coordinated leg kicking action. The end result being the above water free swimming phase is more efficient when compared to the kicking dominant underwater phase.

The sport science tool of video analysis, and in particular underwater footage, enabled the underwater distance to be assessed. This sport science tool is regularly used to determine the appropriate transition from underwater to the surface for the swimmer. Factors that need to be considered in this process include the individual swimmer's underwater streamlining and kicking efficiency compared to their free swimming ability. Determining the appropriate underwater distance is a fundamental parameter for the start and turn of the swimmer. Due to the diversity in the physical ability of the Paralympic swimmers, the underwater distance traveled will depend on the strengths and weakness of the individual swimmer, although a key requirement for all groups was the smooth transition from underwater to free swimming. Studies have found a difference in the absolute distance the swimmers traveled underwater. In relative terms, there was no difference between the three Paralympic swimming

classes, although the entire group of Paralympic swimmers spent significantly less time underwater. This similar proportion of time and/or distance spent in each phase, regardless of Paralympic class, indicates that the swimmers follow a similar pattern of swim start technique.

The S10 swimmers were able to produce a similar underwater velocity as the Olympic swimmers, with the S9 and S8 swimmers both generating a significantly slower underwater velocity. The relationships changed during free swimming, with the S10 and S9 swimmers generating similar profiles that were significantly different to both the Olympic and S8 swimmers. This finding highlights that the minimal disability swimmers (S10) were able to generate good underwater velocity, but were not able to transfer this into free swimming, which probably related to their similar ability to place and hold their body in a streamline position and then to utilize two fully functional legs to drive to the surface for the breakout stroke. This skill of obtaining a streamlined body position and kicking until the swimmer slows to near race pace has been identified as a characteristic of competitive swim starts. The underwater to free swim velocity transition provides some interesting relationships, with the S9 and S8 swimmers transiting from underwater to free swimming with the least amount of drop-off in velocity. This indicates that these swimmers have determined the appropriate time and distance within their start to transit from underwater to free swimming, a critical feature identified in other studies. As previously mentioned, the free swim velocity is a function of the preceding underwater velocity; therefore, the minimum loss during the underwater to free swimming transition is critical. The aim for the swimmers was a seamless underwater to free swimming velocity transition.

Swim start race analysis for swimmers with a visual impairment (S11–S13)

Sport science assessment has found that swimmers with a visual impairment have a similar starting and turning skill, when compared to their sighted colleagues. A similar result was found for finish time variable, with studies finding no significant differences in the finish section race strategy between the

Olympic and Paralympic swimmers. This suggests that despite the lack or complete loss of vision, Paralympic swimmers still "raced" the finish section, further implying that swimmers generally follow a specific race plan over the 100 m and are less influenced by "seeing" the competitors beside them.

The S11 swimmers had a significantly longer percentage of time allocated to the turn. This greater allocation for the turn section of the race could be expected as the S11 swimmers, having no sight, may approach and maneuver at the wall more cautiously. In contrast, the classes S12 and S13 have enough depth perception to see the large black cross on the pool end walls and perform a freestyle turn. This involves a somersault with a twist so that the legs hit the wall in a correct position to push off smoothly while not actually touching the wall with the hand. The S11 swimmers have the additional aid of the tapper and will therefore need more training (experience), but nevertheless are able to complete the task required. There has been some discussion that underwater vision can be improved with studies showing that South Asian children who dive without goggles for their own food and livelihood have much better focus underwater than European children. Their eyes had adapted themselves, but these studies could not determine if this was due to evolution or the result of practice. Caution during the approach to the turn has also not been reflected in a lower stroke rate in S11 swimmers. Stroke rate is the most common measure the swimmer and coach use to develop the desired race pattern, particularly as the swimmer can "feel" their arm rating and readily adjust this within their race. No significant differences in stroke rate were found between the Olympic or Paralympic swimmers, with stroke rate changes within 100 m only changing by ~7%. This sport science variable further highlights that Paralympic swimmers who reach the final have sufficient experience.

Technology and Paralympic swimming

Sport science has been the driver for technological developments within Paralympic and Olympic swimming. At the most recent 2008 Beijing Games,

Speedo™ launched their new LZR Racer Suit amid much debate about the performance-enhancement characteristics of these new suits. The suit's technology includes "polyurethane panels placed strategically around parts of the torso, abdomen, and lower back that experience high amounts of drag in the pool." A key feature of this suit that has caused speculation is the "corset-like structure" that may help to streamline the body, although this effect is yet to be confirmed in scientific literature. Advances in the manufacturing process, which employs "ultrasonic welding," have eliminated the need for seams, thus preventing absorption of water. At the 2008 Beijing Games, 94% of all swimming races were won by swimmers wearing the suit and, to date, 62 world records have been broken by swimmers in these suits.

Paralympic swimming generally follows the International Swimming Federation (FINA) rules, with some essential modifications, such as allowing one-handed touches for swimmers who can only extend one hand out in front. In some cases, the additional "technology" required is very simple. As shown in Figure 15.4, the swimmer has no arms and uses his teeth to hold onto the towel/rope to prepare them for the swimming start. As in Olympic swimming, athletes only wear a swimsuit, goggles, and cap, and Paralympic athletes are not permitted to use any prostheses or assistive devices while in the water. Currently, however, the most controversial issue in swimming is related to advances in the manufacture

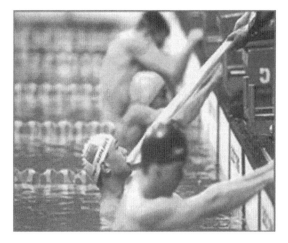

Figure 15.4 Image of a swimmer start with no hands.

of swimsuits, which can be considered to create an unfair advantage. The alleged buoyancy advantage provided by swimsuits, such as the Speedo™ LZR Racer and the Tyr™ Tracer Light, has provoked heated discussion on the technological ethics of the sport. Technological developments are fundamental to improving sporting performance and, although the first modern Olympic swimming races were held at the 1896 games, it was 80 years later in 1976 that swimming goggles were first allowed. Will the current swimsuit technology be considered "typical" in 80 years time? Perhaps the most important factor is equity of access to the new swimsuits, as they are very expensive and need frequent replacing.

Sport science technology developed for swimming

Sport science technology has been specifically developed to objectively measure aspects of the sport, such as the swimmer's start. To understand the relationships, it requires specific understanding of the forces generated on the starting block and the position, velocity, and acceleration of the human segments as they leave the block and enter the water. The development of synchronized above- and underwater cameras, the mounting of force plates onto swim starting blocks or the finishing pad on the wall have all enabled objective measures to be made in the swimming pool. This technology has enabled the kinematic analysis of segment movements such as rate of arm swing, path of the movement of the head, and the explosive power of the lower limbs to be quantified. Collectively, this movement pattern is then analyzed via the kinetic link chain to determine the relationships between variables such as the drive from the legs, arm movement, and head position. The influence of fine adjustments to the starting position has been quantified with swimming technology. For example, to determine the influence of the swimmer's upper-limb position on their center of gravity as they are poised on the starting block can be determined and used to guide the swimmer's starting position. Stability on the block is critical as any movement prior to the starter's gun will result in disqualification

under the one-start rule. Paralympic swimmers who have reduced balance control, such as lower-limb amputees or cerebral palsy, can find balancing on the starting block difficult.

The recent developments in microtechnology have enabled previously unknown swimming measures to be made, such as determining the swimmer's kick count and kick rate. The kick is typically hidden within the turbulent white water of the swimmer, and the kick rate is typically too fast to be measured by the human eye. Small inertial sensors, approximately 25-mm long and 8-mm thick, weighing less than 20 g, have been attached to the swimmer's leg to measure this new sport science variable. This knowledge can then be utilized by the swimming coach to effectively design the training program and to develop the appropriate swim race strategy.

Factors outside the pool that influence swimming performance

Equipment such as prostheses and wheelchairs are fundamental in allowing some people with disabilities to carry out the tasks of daily living. Lower-limb amputees rely on the technical attributes of their prosthetic limbs to ambulate and the specifications of these components have varied considerably in recent years. Of most importance are the not-so-obvious compensatory factors that can detrimentally influence the swimmer. At first glance, the impact of a lower-limb amputation seems to be confined to the lower limb. However, the skeletal image of an amputee identifies several compensatory factors, as shown in Figure 15.5. The amputation alters the orientation of the pelvis. As the pelvis is connected to the vertebral column, the change in pelvic angle causes a scoliosis of the spine. The altered orientation of the vertebral column in the cervical region then causes the shoulders to change alignment, as well as the orientation of the skull to be altered. Thus, the "compensatory" mechanisms resulting from the amputation can have far-reaching consequences on the functional ability of the swimmer. This phenomenon highlights the need to address the activities outside the pool to provide the most effective opportunities for the swimmer.

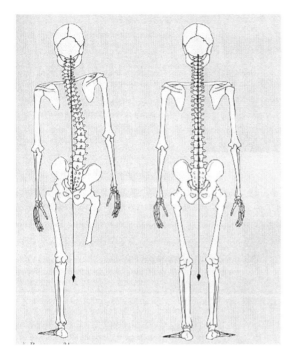

Figure 15.5 Image of an athlete with a lower-limb amputation and the compensatory influence.

Monitoring swimming technique—on the land

The coordination of the key body segments in swimming is of particular interest for the swimmer and coach, as understanding these body roll patterns can identify whether swimmer is maximizing the musculoskeletal leverage within the body, or potentially moving in an anatomically unsound path that could potentially cause injury. Studies of swimming have been investigated both in water and on dryland using equipment such as a swim bench to quantify the angle and timing of body roll. Debate exists around the timing of the body roll, i.e., the time point within the arm stroke when longitudinal rotation occurs, and the sequence in which the segments of head, chest/shoulders, and the hips move. This lack of data is most likely attributed to the difficulty in measuring human movement within the medium of water, with issues of parallax error for camera measurements and water turbulence hiding anatomical landmarks. For this reason, dryland simulators such as swim benches can enable three-dimensional movements to be quantified. Dryland

sport science research on the timing and sequence of body roll has found that for the breathing stroke, the head roll occurred at ~30% of the underwater propulsive phase, the chest at ~42%, and the hips at 47%. However, during the nonbreathing stroke, the timing and sequence changed, with maximum hip roll occurring early, at 20% of the propulsive phase, followed by the chest and hips at 34% of the propulsive phase. A reason for early hip roll may be to facilitate greater recruitment of the large torso muscles within the stroke or due to leg kick. The knowledge of timing and sequence has guided the coaching of swimmers and provided the coach with a greater understanding of swimming mechanics.

Putting Paralympic sport science knowledge into practice

There are several examples of putting this Paralympic sport science knowledge into practice; two examples are presented below. Firstly, the development and regular application of swimming test protocols is described. This is followed by the more individualized warm-down and recovery procedure, specific to the individual disability and athlete. The development of an individual management plan is fundamental for the effective performance of any elite athlete.

Swimming test protocols

To assist in understanding the current fitness status of the swimmer, and to enable the effectiveness of the progressive training program to be assessed, regular swimming test protocols have been developed. These measures enable the swimmer's ability to be quantified, and based on this knowledge, the training program can, if required, be modified. These protocols were first established for Olympic swimmers and will vary around the world, but in essence contain a step test and efficiency measures.

For Paralympic swimmers, the step tests contain six or seven 100-m repeat swims; Olympic swimmers tend to use seven 200-m swims (higher-level Paralympic swimmers could adopt this model if the coach desired). The step test is designed to train the swimmers to pace their main event as efficiently as possible and to determine the lactate threshold.

Using the swimmer's personal best 100-m time, plus 2 s as the target for their final swim, the six 100 s (or 200 s) are swam at a descending pace as listed below. The swimming variables of stroke rate, DPS, free swimming velocity, stroke count, turn time, lap time, total time, and lactates are recorded for each swim. All swims are conducted at the same time interval, so the intensity will progressively increase as with any test set. Starting at the personal best time plus 25 s, the swimmers are encouraged to evenly pace the 100-m or 200-m swim. The first four swims are to allow the athletes to pace themselves correctly at a slower velocity and to set themselves for an efficient fifth and sixth swim. The swimming zone and table for recording are listed below.

Swim 1—100 m at (+25 s) on 2:00 minute cycle

Swim 2—100 m at (+20 s) on 2:00 minute cycle

Swim 3—100 m at (+15 s) on 2:00 minute cycle

Swim 4—100 m at (+10 s) on 2:00 minutes 200 m swim down (easy swim)

Swim 5—100 m at (+5 s) on 2:00 minutes 200 m swim down, and dive the last

Swim 6—100 m at (+2 s) on 2:00 minute cycle

The step test data can then be plotted into a race analysis, as shown in Figure 15.6. The final swim can be videoed to provide feedback to the swimmer. Together, this information indicates the swimmers current race strategy. To improve their strategy, the aim is to reduce the drop in velocity (the dotted diamond line). This can be achieved by improving

the combination of their stroke rate (the dashed triangle line) and their DPS (the solid square line). Following this test, the swimmer completes their specific swim down and their blood lactate level is checked. Swimmers are encouraged to develop their individual recovery management plan. For example, a swimmer who is missing an arm and relies on the leg kick may recover better with recovery that consists of walking rather than the typical 1000 m of swimming.

A second measure is the stroke efficiency test protocol, which is designed to develop the swimmer's efficiency. The test involves swimming six 50-m swims at the swimmer's second 50-m of their 100-m pace. The swimmer counts the number of strokes they take to swim 50 m and the time for the swim is also recorded. These two values are added together (the stroke count and time) to produce a "golf" handicap score. The aim of the test is to reduce the swimmer's golf handicap by using either less strokes for the same time or a quicker time for the same number of strokes. Finally, variables such as the start and turn that are measured in the race analysis of the swimmer can also be tested on a regular basis within training. For example, to measure the swimmer's turn, the swimmer can be positioned at around 20 m out from the wall. This will enable the swimmer sufficient time to reach race velocity into the wall. To measure the "turn-in" part of the turn, the coach can measure the time the swimmer's head crosses the 5-m backstroke flag mark until the swimmer's feet touch the wall. The time from "feet on the wall" until the swimmer's head passes the 5-m window will determine the "turn-out" time. This simple sport science measure will enable the effectiveness of the turn to be quantified within the training session. A similar process can be applied for the swimmer's start, with timing measures made at the 5-, 10-, and 15-m intervals (or as required by the coach).

Individual recovery strategy

The appropriate recovery of an athlete is critical to the performance of the swimmer, particularly when the swimmer must recover from a morning heat session before the final that night. Furthermore, the 7- to 9-day demands of a World Championship or Paralympic Games will require the

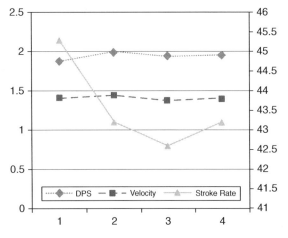

Figure 15.6 Typical output of swim race analysis.

athlete can suitably recover from an event early in the program and avoid any deterioration in performance as the competition goes on. Sport science has effectively guided the recovery strategies for Paralympic athletes, in particular, to address the unique physiological features each disability may possess.

Using the commonly accepted sport science measures of lactate production and RPE, an appropriate recovery strategy can be developed for each individual swimmer. Sport scientists have found that rather than employing the standard ~1000 m swimming warm-down for each swimmer, alternative modes of recovery are more effective. For example, the swimmer who has an arm disability (arm amputation or loss of function) relies predominately on the leg kick for swimming performance. Making this swimmer swim after a race has been found to in fact increase blood lactate levels, rather than reducing them. A more effective form of recovery includes a combination of swimming (~300 m) and walking to stimulate recovery.

A similar scenario has been found for the swimmer who utilizes a wheelchair. This swimmer is dependent on the shoulders for both swimming and daily mobility, only using swimming as the form of recovery has also elevated lactate levels. The alternative is a combination of swimming (~300 m) and pushing the wheelchair to stimulate recovery. From this new sport science knowledge, a better understanding of the appropriate recovery strategies has been established, and more importantly a specific regime can be developed for each individual swimmer.

Future directions

An understandable temptation for researchers is to research only "hot topics" that are more likely to be funded through research grants. As the majority of people with disabilities are aged, research and development has naturally focused on the older spectrum of the market. Paralympic athletes have created a new, albeit small market. Not only are these athletes significantly younger than the traditional aged person with a disability, they are also highly active and, as such, place far greater demands on the current established guidelines for swim coaching. The priority areas for future swimming knowledge are to better understand the adaptation process for people with a disability when in the aquatic environment, and to utilize this new knowledge to further enhance the Paralympic classification system.

References

Burkett, B. & Mellifont, R. (2008). Sport science and coaching in Paralympic swimming. *International Journal of Sports Science & Coaching*, **3(1)**, 105–112.

Daly, D., Djobova, S., Malone, L., Vanlandewijck, Y. & Steadward, R. (2003). Swimming speed patterns and stroking variables in the Paralympic 100-m freestyle. *Adapted Physical Activity Quarterly*, **20**, 260–278.

Fulton, S., Pyne, D., Hopkins, W. & Burkett, B. (2009). Variability and progression in competitive performance of Paralympic swimmers. *Journal of Sports Sciences*, **27(5)**, 535–539.

Index

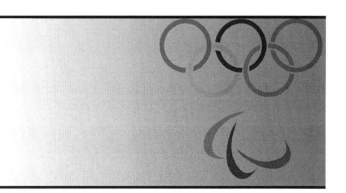

Printed in the USA/Agawam, MA
December 16, 2011